2013
YEAR BOOK OF
OPHTHALMOLOGY®

The 2013 Year Book Series

Year Book of Critical Care Medicine®: Drs Dries, Zanotti-Cavazzoni, Latenser, Martinez, Rincon, and Zwank

Year Book of Emergency Medicine®: Drs Hamilton, Bruno, Handly, Minczak, Quintana, and Ramoska

Year Book of Endocrinology®: Drs Schott, Apovian, Clarke, Eugster, Meikle, Oetgen, Ovalle, Schteingart, and Toth

Year Book of Hand and Upper Limb Surgery®: Drs Yao, Adams, Isaacs, and Rizzo

Year Book of Medicine®: Drs Barker, Garrick, Gersh, Khardori, LeRoith, Panush, Talley, and Thigpen

Year Book of Neonatal and Perinatal Medicine®: Drs Fanaroff, Benitz, Donn, Neu, Papile, and Van Marter

Year Book of Neurology and Neurosurgery®: Drs Klimo, Minagar, Gandhi, Liu, Panagariya, Rezania, Riel-Romero, Riesenburger, Robottom, Schwendimann, Shafazand, and Yang

Year Book of Obstetrics, Gynecology, and Women's Health®: Drs Dungan and Shulman

Year Book of Oncology®: Drs Arceci, Bauer, Chiorean, Gordon, Lawton, Murphy, Thigpen, and Tsao

Year Book of Ophthalmology®: Drs Rapuano, Flanders, Fudemberg, Gupta, Hammersmith, Milman, Myers, Nagra, Nelson, Penne, Pyfer, Sergott, Shields, Talekar, and Vander

Year Book of Orthopedics®: Drs Morrey, Huddleston, Rose, Swiontkowski, and Trigg

Year Book of Otolaryngology-Head and Neck Surgery®: Drs Sindwani, Balough, Franco, Gapany, and Mitchell

Year Book of Pathology and Laboratory Medicine®: Drs Raab and Bissell

Year Book of Pediatrics®: Dr Stockman

Year Book of Plastic and Aesthetic Surgery™: Drs Miller, Boehmler, Gosman, Gutowski, Ruberg, Salisbury, and Smith

Year Book of Psychiatry and Applied Mental Health®: Drs Talbott, Ballenger, Buckley, Frances, Krupnick, and Mack

Year Book of Pulmonary Disease®: Drs Barker, Jones, Maurer, Spradley, Tanoue, and Willsie

Year Book of Sports Medicine®: Drs Shephard, Cantu, Feldman, Galea, Jankowski, Janssen, Lebrun, and Nieman

Year Book of Surgery®: Drs Behrns, Daly, Fahey, Hines, Howe, Huber, Klodell, Mozingo, and Pruett

Year Book of Urology®: Drs Andriole and Coplen

Year Book of Vascular Surgery®: Drs Gillespie, Bush, Passman, Starnes, and Watkins

2013
The Year Book of OPHTHALMOLOGY®

Editor-in-Chief
Christopher J. Rapuano, MD
Professor of Ophthalmology, Jefferson Medical College of Thomas Jefferson University; Director, Cornea Service; Co-Director, Refractive Surgery Department, Attending Surgeon, Wills Eye Institute, Philadelphia, Pennsylvania

Wills Eye®

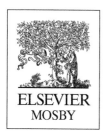

ELSEVIER
MOSBY

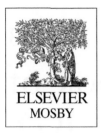

ELSEVIER
MOSBY

Senior Vice President, Content: Linda Belfus
Editor: Yonah Korngold
Production Supervisor, Electronic Year Books: Donna M. Skelton
Electronic Article Manager: Mike Rainey
Illustrations and Permissions Coordinator: Dawn Vohsen

2013 EDITION

Composition by TNQ Books and Journals Pvt Ltd, India

Editorial Office:
Elsevier
1600 John F. Kennedy Blvd.
Suite 1800
Philadelphia, PA 19103-2899

International Standard Serial Number: 0084-392X
International Standard Book Number: 978-1-4557-7284-1

Printed and bound by CPI Group (UK) Ltd, Croydon, CR0 4YY

Transferred to digital print 2012

Editorial Board

Table of Contents

Journals Represented

Journals represented in this YEAR BOOK are listed below.
Acta Ophthalmologica
American Journal of Ophthalmology
American Journal of Rhinology & Allergy
Annals of Neurology
Archives of Neurology
Archives of Ophthalmology
Archives of Pathology & Laboratory Medicine
British Journal of Ophthalmology
Cornea
Current Eye Research
Eye
Eye & Contact Lens
Investigative Ophthalmology and Visual Science
JAMA Ophthalmology
Journal of Cataract & Refractive Surgery
Journal of Clinical Endocrinology & Metabolism
Journal of Neuroinflammation
Journal of Neurological Sciences
Journal of Pediatric Ophthalmology and Strabismus
Journal of Refractive Surgery
Journal of Translational Medicine
Journal of the American Association for Pediatric Ophthalmology and Strabismus
Journal of the American Medical Association
Neurology
Ophthalmic Epidemiology
Ophthalmic Plastic and Reconstructive Surgery
Ophthalmic Surgery, Lasers & Imaging
Ophthalmology
Retina
Thyroid

STANDARD ABBREVIATIONS

The following terms are abbreviated in this edition: acquired immunodeficiency syndrome (AIDS), cardiopulmonary resuscitation (CPR), central nervous system (CNS), cerebrospinal fluid (CSF), computed tomography (CT), deoxyribonucleic acid (DNA), diopter (D), electrocardiography (ECG), health maintenance organization (HMO), human immunodeficiency virus (HIV), intensive care unit (ICU), intramuscular (IM), intravenous (IV), magnetic resonance (MR) imaging (MRI), ribonucleic acid (RNA), ultrasound (US), and ultraviolet (UV).

NOTE

The YEAR BOOK OF OPHTHALMOLOGY® is a literature survey service providing abstracts of articles published in the professional literature. Every effort is made to assure the accuracy of the information presented in these pages. Neither the editors nor the publisher of the YEAR BOOK OF OPHTHALMOLOGY® can be responsible for errors in the original materials. The editors' comments are their own opinions. Mention of specific products within this publication does not constitute endorsement.

To facilitate the use of the YEAR BOOK OF OPHTHALMOLOGY® as a reference tool, all illustrations and tables included in this publication are now identified as they appear in the original article. This change is meant to help the reader recognize that any illustration or table appearing in the YEAR BOOK OF OPHTHALMOLOGY® may be only one of many in the original article. For this reason, figure and table numbers will often appear to be out of sequence within the YEAR BOOK OF OPHTHALMOLOGY®.

1 Cataract Surgery

Argon Laser Iridoplasty to Improve Visual Function Following Multifocal Intraocular Lens Implantation
Solomon R, Barsam A, Voldman A, et al (Ophthalmic Consultants of Long Island, NY; et al)
J Refract Surg 28:281-283, 2012

Purpose.—To describe the use of argon laser iridoplasty following implantation of a multifocal intraocular lens (IOL) to improve visual function.

Methods.—Argon laser spots of 500-mW power, 500-μm spot diameter, and 500-ms duration were placed in the midperipheral iris in the area in which the iris was encroaching on the IOL.

Results.—Argon laser iridoplasty provided statistically significant improvement in visual function including corrected distance visual acuity (CDVA) and subjective quality of vision in 14 eyes from 11 patients. Mean CDVA improved from 0.24 (20/35 Snellen) to 0.10 (20/25 Snellen) logMAR ($P < .0001$), and mean subjective quality of vision improved from 2.9 to 7.5 ($P < .0001$).

Conclusions.—Argon laser iridoplasty should be considered in correcting visual problems associated with decentered multifocal IOLs.

▶ Finally, this work on argon laser pupilloplasty (ALP) for multifocal intraocular lens (MFIOL) patients was published. Discussed at many conferences anecdotally, now we can see the exact technique and review outcomes for a small cohort. This is useful information for surgeons trying to improve results of MFIOLs in less-than-happy patients using a noninvasive technique. IOL exchange may still be required in some patients ultimately, but there is little downside to trying ALP first. Furthermore, in some patients with small pupils who obtain inadequate near vision despite a well-centered MFIOL, symmetrical ALP may also be judiciously attempted, preferably after a successful trial of dilute topical phenylephrine, but this report does not address that application.

M. F. Pyfer, MD

Intracameral cefuroxime injection at the end of cataract surgery to reduce the incidence of endophthalmitis: French study

Barreau G, Mounier M, Marin B, et al (Faculté de Médecine, Limoges, France)

J Cataract Refract Surg 38:1370-1375, 2012

Purpose.—To determine whether an intracameral injection of cefuroxime at the end of cataract surgery decreases the incidence of postoperative endophthalmitis.

Setting.—Dupuytren Hospital, Ophthalmology Department, Limoges, France.

Design.—Clinical trials.

Methods.—Patients having cataract surgery between April 2003 and June 2008 were included in a survey of operative-site infection. Intracameral cefuroxime injections started in June 2006. Preoperative data (beta-lactam allergy, a history of endophthalmitis, age, sex), intraoperative data (use of trypan blue, use of capsular ring or iris retractors, surgical time, senior or junior surgeon, corticosteroid injection, iris retractors), and the incidence of postoperative infections at 8 days and 1 month were prospectively collected.

Results.—During the inclusion period, 5115 patients had cataract surgery; 2289 received cefuroxime and 2826 did not. The incidence of endophthalmitis was 35 (1.238%) of 2826 patients without intracameral cefuroxime and 1 (0.044%) of 2289 patients with intracameral cefuroxime; the difference was statistically significant ($P < .0001$). No intraoperative factor was significantly associated with postoperative infection. No allergic reaction was reported.

Conclusion.—Intracameral cefuroxime injection at the end of cataract surgery was safe and significantly decreased the incidence of endophthalmitis.

▶ This is a highly significant landmark study, providing convincing evidence in a large cohort, of a greatly reduced incidence of postoperative endophthalmitis using intracameral cefuroxime. However, it is not a randomized controlled trial, so that other changes that may have occurred in surgical technique around June 2006, such as the use of a smaller incision width, could influence the results. Taken along with several other large studies on the effectiveness of intracameral cefuroxime over the past few years, the evidence in favor of this method for cataract surgery postoperative endophthalmitis prophylaxis is hard to dispute.

M. F. Pyfer, MD

Comparison of Long-term Visual Outcome and IOL Position With a Single-optic Accommodating IOL After 5.5- or 6.0-mm Femtosecond Laser Capsulotomy

Szigeti A, Kránitz K, Takacs AI, et al (Semmelweis Univ Budapest, Hungary)
J Refract Surg 28:609-613, 2012

Purpose.—To evaluate the long-term visual outcome and intraocular (IOL) position parameters with a single-optic accommodating IOL after 5.5- or 6.0-mm femtosecond laser capsulotomy.

Methods.—This prospective, randomized, pilot study comprised 17 eyes from 11 patients (7 men) with a mean age of 65.82 ± 10.64 years (range: 51 to 79 years). All patients received a Crystalens AT-50AO (Bausch & Lomb) accommodating IOL after femtosecond laser refractive cataract surgery using either a 5.5-mm capsulotomy (5.5-mm group; 9 eyes) or 6.0-mm capsulotomy (6.0-mm group; 8 eyes). Near and distance visual acuities, manifest refraction spherical equivalent (MRSE), and IOL tilt and decentration were evaluated 1 year postoperatively.

Results.—No significant differences were noted between groups for postoperative uncorrected distance visual acuity, uncorrected near visual acuity, distance-corrected near visual acuity, and MRSE. Vertical and horizontal tilt were significantly higher in the 6.0-mm group than in the 5.5-mm group ($P = .014$ and $P = .015$, respectively). No significant difference was observed between groups regarding IOL decentration.

Conclusions.—A 5.5-mm capsulotomy created with a femtosecond laser is associated with less IOL tilt and therefore may be superior to a 6.0-mm capsulotomy when implanting a single-optic accommodating IOL.

▶ This is a small but well-controlled randomized study using validated measurement methods to quantify intraocular lens (IOL) tilt and centration after femtosecond laser-assisted cataract surgery. It is the first published study to take advantage of the precision and repeatability of the femtosecond laser capsulotomy to compare outcomes of different-sized capsulotomies using the same IOL. Hinged accommodating IOL designs are particularly dependent on anterior capsulotomy size, shape, and centration for optimal performance and to avoid known late complications such as the so-called Z syndrome (one hinge flexed forward while the other is flexed backward).

The study demonstrated a trend toward better uncorrected distance and near visual acuity with a 5.5-mm capsulotomy, but this did not reach statistical significance. Because the femtosecond laser excels at creating a near perfect anterior capsulotomy, we can expect more and larger studies on this topic in the near future.

M. F. Pyfer, MD

Risk of Age-related Macular Degeneration 3 Years after Cataract Surgery: Paired Eye Comparisons

Wang JJ, Fong CS-u, Rochtchina E, et al (Univ of Sydney, Australia; et al)
Ophthalmology 119:2298-2303, 2012

Objective.—To clarify possible associations between cataract surgery and progression of age-related macular degeneration (AMD).

Design.—Clinic-based cohort.

Participants.—We followed cataract surgical patients aged 65+ years in the Australian Cataract Surgery and Age-related Macular Degeneration (CSAMD) study. Patients who remained unilaterally phakic for at least 24 months after recruitment were included.

Methods.—We performed annual examinations with retinal photography. We assessed AMD using side-by-side grading of images from all visits. Paired comparisons between operated and nonoperated fellow eyes (defined as nonoperated or operated <12 months previously) were made using generalized estimating equation models.

Main Outcome Measures.—Incident early AMD was defined as the new appearance of soft indistinct/reticular drusen or coexisting retinal pigmentary abnormality and soft distinct drusen in eyes at risk of early AMD. Incident late AMD was defined as the new appearance of neovascular AMD or geographic atrophy (GA) in eyes at risk of late AMD.

Results.—Among 2029 recruited, eligible participants, 1851 had cataract surgery performed at Westmead Hospital, Sydney, and 1244 (70.7%) had 36-month postoperative visits. Of these participants, 1178 had gradable photographs at baseline and at least 1 follow-up visit. Of 308 unilaterally operated participants at risk of late AMD, this developed in 4 (1.3%) operated and 7 (2.3%) nonoperated fellow eyes (odds ratio [OR], 0.74; 95% confidence interval [CI], 0.23−2.36) after adjusting for the presence of early AMD at baseline. Of 217 unilaterally operated participants at risk of early AMD, this developed in 23 (10.6%) operated and 21 (9.7%) nonoperated fellow eyes (OR, 1.07; 95% CI, 0.74−1.65). Incident retinal pigment abnormalities were more frequent in operated than nonoperated fellow eyes (15.3% vs. 9.9%; OR, 1.64; 95% CI, 1.07−2.52). There was no difference in the 3-year incidence of large soft indistinct or reticular drusen between the 2 eyes (8.8% vs. 7.9%; OR, 1.12; 95% CI, 0.79−1.60).

Conclusions.—Prospective follow-up data and paired eye comparisons of this older surgical cohort showed no increased risk of developing late AMD, early AMD, or soft/reticular drusen over 3 years. There was a 60% increased detection of retinal pigmentary changes in surgical eyes.

▶ This is an interesting and well-done study. Its advantages are: (1) paired eye comparisons, which creates an internal control for systemic, environmental, or genetic risk factors for age-related macular degeneration (AMD), and (2) photographic documentation of examinations, which eliminates examiner bias. One disadvantage is that only 3-year follow-up was obtained.

A novel contribution here is the finding that early AMD is more common among cataract surgical candidates at baseline than in the general population. The presence of early AMD is established as the most significant risk factor for the development of late AMD. This apparent correlation of early AMD and need for cataract surgery may be caused by the combined effect of AMD and cataract on visual quality, which prompts patients to present with visual complaints earlier than their non-AMD, same-age healthy counterparts. The commentary by Klein et al[1] on this issue is also informative.

M. F. Pyfer, MD

Reference

1. Klein BE, Howard KP, Lee KE, Iyengar SK, Sivakumaran TA, Klein R. The relationship of cataract and cataract extraction to age-related macular degeneration: the Beaver Dam Eye Study. *Ophthalmology.* 2012;119:1628-1633.

Comparison of IOL Power Calculation and Refractive Outcome After Laser Refractive Cataract Surgery With a Femtosecond Laser Versus Conventional Phacoemulsification

Filkorn T, Kovács I, Takács A, et al (Semmelweis Univ Budapest, Hungary; et al)
J Refract Surg 28:540-544, 2012

Purpose.—To compare intraocular lens (IOL) power calculation and refractive outcome between patients who underwent laser refractive cataract surgery with a femtosecond laser and those with conventional cataract surgery.

Methods.—In this prospective study, 77 eyes from 77 patients underwent laser refractive cataract surgery (laser group; Alcon LenSx femtosecond laser), and conventional cataract surgery with phacoemulsification was performed in 57 eyes from 57 patients (conventional group). Biometry was done with optical low coherence reflectometry (Lenstar LS900, Haag-Streit AG), and IOL calculation was performed with third-generation IOL formulas (SRK/T, Hoffer Q, and Holladay). The refractive outcome was analyzed using the mean absolute error (MAE; difference between predicted and achieved postoperative spherical equivalent refraction), and multivariable regression analysis was performed to compare the two groups.

Results.—No significant differences were found between age, axial length, keratometry, and preoperative corrected visual acuity in the laser and conventional groups ($P > .05$; Mann-Whitney U test). At least 6 weeks after surgery, MAE was significantly lower in the laser group (0.38 ± 0.28 diopters [D]) than in the conventional group (0.50 ± 0.38 D) ($P = .04$). The difference was the greatest in short (axial length < 22.0 mm, 0.43 ± 0.41 vs 0.63 ± 0.48) and long (axial length > 26.0 mm, 0.33 ± 0.24 vs 0.63 ± 0.42) eyes.

Conclusions.—Laser refractive cataract surgery with a femtosecond laser resulted in a significantly better predictability of IOL power calculation than conventional phacoemulsification surgery. This difference is possibly due to a more precise capsulorrhexis, resulting in a more stable IOL position.

▶ This is one of the earliest studies to be published comparing outcomes of cataract surgery between conventional surgery and femtosecond laser-assisted cataract surgery. This study was not randomized, but subgroup analysis showed no significant effect for intraocular lens (IOL) type. However, there were more medium-long eyes in the manual surgery group compared with the laser-assisted group. If the IOL power calculation formulas used here are less accurate in this range of axial length, then this could bias the results in favor of laser-assisted surgery.

A good follow-up study would be to actually measure IOL position (depth), centration, and tilt for all eyes in this study to see if these parameters correlate with the reduced mean refractive error found in the laser-assisted surgical cohort.

M. F. Pyfer, MD

Biaxial microincision cataract surgery versus conventional coaxial cataract surgery: Metaanalysis of randomized controlled trials
Yu J-G, Zhao Y-E, Shi J-L, et al (Wenzhou Med College, Zhejiang Province, China)
J Cataract Refract Surg 38:894-901, 2012

A comprehensive literature search of Cochrane Library, PubMed, and Embase was performed to identify relevant prospective randomized controlled trials (RCTs) comparing biaxial microincision cataract surgery (MICS) and conventional coaxial phacoemulsification. A metaanalysis was performed on the following outcome measures: effective phacoemulsification time (EPT), phacoemulsification power (%), corrected distance visual acuity (CDVA), surgically induced astigmatism (SIA), laser flare photometry value, percentage of endothelial cell loss, change in central corneal thickness (CCT), and complications. Eleven RCTs describing a total of 1064 eyes were identified. There were no significant differences between the techniques in CDVA, mean percentage of endothelial cell loss, laser flare photometry value, CCT change, and intraoperative and postoperative complications. However, EPT was statistically significantly shorter and the mean phaco power was statistically significantly lower in the biaxial group than in the coaxial group, and biaxial MICS induced less SIA.

Financial Disclosure.—No author has a financial or proprietary interest in any material or method mentioned.

▶ If one accepts the principles of meta-analysis, then the conclusions of this study are stronger than those of any single study comparing coaxial and biaxial microincision cataract surgery (MICS). Still, the variation between the studies, including different phaco machines, incision sizes, and incision locations, limits the generalizability of these results for an individual surgeon trying to decide whether to adopt biaxial MICS.

Biaxial MICS represents a significant departure from the coaxial technique most cataract surgeons are so familiar with. It also requires an investment in new instruments and will undoubtedly increase total case duration at first, until the surgeon is comfortable with the new technique. This meta-analysis did not address the learning curve for biaxial surgery. Also, several articles over the past few years have found significant tearing or distortion of the biaxial incisions compared with coaxial, especially when the intraocular lens is implanted through one of the operative incisions.[1] This may influence sealing efficiency of the biaxial incisions and could increase the risk for postoperative endophthalmitis.

However, all of these technique-related issues aside, this meta-analysis provides compelling evidence that the results of the 2 techniques are comparable in experienced hands in all measures, except total ultrasound energy delivered into the eye during surgery, which was significantly lower using the biaxial approach. This should motivate cataract surgeons who are interested in rapid visual recovery for their patients to at least give biaxial MICS a try.

M. F. Pyfer, MD

Reference

1. Berdahl JP, DeStafeno JJ, Kim T. Corneal wound architecture and integrity after phacoemulsification evaluation of coaxial, microincision coaxial, and microincision bimanual techniques. *J Cataract Refract Surg.* 2007;33:510-515.

Postoperative increase in grey matter volume in visual cortex after unilateral cataract surgery
Lou AR, Madsen KH, Julian HO, et al (Copenhagen Univ Hosp Glostrup, Denmark; Copenhagen Univ Hosp Hvidovre, Denmark; et al)
Acta Ophthalmol 91:58-65, 2013

Purpose.—The developing visual cortex has a strong potential to undergo plastic changes. Little is known about the potential of the ageing visual cortex to express plasticity. A pertinent question is whether therapeutic interventions can trigger plastic changes in the ageing visual cortex by restoring vision.

Methods.—Twelve patients aged 50-85 years underwent structural high-resolution T1-weighted MRI of the whole brain 2 days and 6 weeks after unilateral cataract surgery. Voxel-based morphometry (VBM) based on T1-weighted magnetic resonance imaging (MRI) was employed to test whether cataract surgery induces a regional increase in grey matter in areas V1 and V2 of the visual cortex.

Results.—In all patients, cataract surgery immediately improved visual acuity, contrast sensitivity and mean sensitivity in the visual field of the operated eye. The improvement in vision was stable throughout the 6 weeks after operation. VBM revealed a regional expansion of grey matter volume in area V2 contralateral to the operated eye during the 6-week period after surgery. Individual increases in grey matter were predicted by the symmetry in visual acuity between the operated eye and nonoperated eye. The more symmetrical visual acuity became after unilateral cataract surgery, the more pronounced was the grey matter increase in visual cortex.

Conclusion.—The data suggest that cataract surgery triggered a use-dependent structural plasticity in V2 presumably through improved binocular integration of visual input from both eyes. We conclude that activity-dependent cortical plasticity is preserved in the ageing visual cortex and may be triggered by restoring impaired vision.

▶ This is a landmark study that demonstrates an increase in gray-matter brain volume in the visual cortex after unilateral cataract surgery. The increase occurred in the region known as V2, most associated with binocular or stereo visual processing. This finding received considerable attention in the lay press, and for good reason. It is significant because it is the first study to my knowledge of any kind to measure increased brain volume after cataract surgery, and because it may indicate unexpected plasticity in the adult brain. The phenomenon euphemistically termed "neuro-adaptation" by ophthalmologists describing the process of a patient learning to use multifocal intraocular lens (MFIOL) optics or monovision effectively now has a physical correlation that can be measured. I have had several patients who had cognitive limitations that were undetected before cataract surgery who showed no sign of "neuro-adaptation" to MFIOL implants even after an extended period. This article may offer a good explanation why, and confirms my personal conclusion to discourage use of MFIOLs in patients with cognitive disabilities. It would be intriguing to study patients with Alzheimer disease or other neurodegenerative conditions to see if the same increase in gray matter occurred after cataract surgery, and to determine if pharmacological or behavioral intervention could influence the effect. One significant limitation of this study is that there was no control group that did not have cataract surgery. We await with interest further brain imaging studies to corroborate and extend the results of this article.

M. F. Pyfer, MD

Short wavelength light filtering by the natural human lens and IOLs — implications for entrainment of circadian rhythm
Brøndsted AE, Lundeman JH, Kessel L (Univ of Copenhagen, Denmark)
Acta Ophthalmol 91:52-57, 2013

Purpose.—Photoentrainment of circadian rhythm begins with the stimulation of melanopsin containing retinal ganglion cells that respond directly to blue light. With age, the human lens becomes a strong colour filter attenuating transmission of short wavelengths. The purpose of the study was to examine the effect the ageing human lens may have for the photoentrainment of circadian rhythm and to compare with intraocular implant lenses (IOLs) designed to block UV radiation, violet or blue light.

Methods.—The potential for photoentrainment of circadian rhythm was computed for 29 human donor lenses (18−76 years) and five IOLs (one UV, two violet and two blue light blocking) based on the transmission properties of the lenses and the spectral characteristics of melanopsin activation and two of it's physiological outcomes; melanopsin-driven pupillary light reponse and light-induced melatonin suppression.

Results.—The potential for melanopsin stimulation and melatonin suppression was reduced by 0.6–0.7 percentage point per year of life because of yellowing of the natural lens. The computed effects were small for the IOLs and did not exceed that of a 22.2-year-old natural lens for the blue-blocking IOLs.

Conclusion.—The results show that photoentrainment of circadian rhythm may be significantly impaired in older subjects because of the colour filtering characteristics of the human lens, whereas the effects were small for all three types of IOLs studied. Consequently, the ageing process of the natural lens is expected to influence the photoentrainment of circadian rhythm, whereas IOLs are not expected to be detrimental to circadian rhythm.

▶ This is a theoretical laboratory-based study that provides convincing evidence that the blue-blocking intraocular lenses (IOLs) in common use today should not interfere with light-induced regulation of the circadian rhythm in patients with these implants. What was not discussed in this article is whether the blue light-activated melanopsin-containing photoreceptors, or their associated retinohypothalamic tract, degenerate with age. If they do, then more blue light could be necessary for regulation of circadian rhythm as patients age, regardless of the color of their crystalline lens or implant. However, at this time, based on the evidence in this study, surgeons should not hesitate to use blue-blocking IOLs out of concern for causing depression or seasonal affective disorder in their pseudophakic patients.

M. F. Pyfer, MD

Reverse Optic Capture of the Single-Piece Acrylic Intraocular Lens in Eyes With Posterior Capsule Rupture

Jones JJ, Oetting TA, Rogers GM, et al (Jones Eye Clinic and Surgery Ctr, Sioux City, IA; Univ of Iowa; et al)
Ophthalmic Surg Lasers Imaging 43:480-488, 2012

Background and Objective.—To evaluate the clinical results of reverse optic capture (ROC) with single-piece posterior chamber intraocular lenses (PC-IOLs) in cases of phacoemulsification cataract and IOL surgery with posterior capsular rupture.

Patients and Methods.—Preoperative diagnosis, intraoperative events, surgical parameters, intraoperative and postoperative complications, and preoperative and postoperative visual acuity and refraction of 16 eyes that underwent ROC were reviewed and analyzed. The fellow eye of 12 patients undergoing uneventful phacoemulsification without optic capture served as the control group.

Results.—Over a mean of 19 months' follow-up, 94% of eyes in the ROC group and 92% in the control group achieved a best-corrected visual acuity of 20/25 or better. Ninety-four percent of eyes in the ROC group and 100%

in the control group had postoperative spherical equivalent ± 1.00 D of the intended refraction. Refraction was stable between 1 month and final follow-up in both groups. In all eyes with ROC, the IOL remained well centered with a securely captured optic. There were no vision-threatening complications throughout the follow-up.

Conclusion.—The comparable outcomes in both groups suggests that optic capture of a single-piece acrylic IOL through an anterior capsulorhexis merits consideration for IOL placement in selected cases of insufficient posterior capsule support.

▶ This article describes a series of cases using the novel technique of reverse optic capture (haptics in the bag, optic in the sulcus) to assure long-term fixation and centration of a 1-piece intraocular lens (IOL) in the setting of an open posterior capsule. Visual outcomes were favorable, and no late complications were discovered. Reverse optic capture (ROC) is a useful technique, especially when the posterior capsule ruptures during or after IOL insertion. Removal of the 1-piece IOL from the capsular bag, a difficult task with an open posterior capsule, is avoided by using the ROC maneuver. Significantly, no cases of uveitis-glaucoma-hyphema syndrome or iris chafe occurred with ROC. These complications are very common if the haptics of a 1-piece IOL are placed in the sulcus, a situation to be avoided at all costs. A prerequisite to using the ROC maneuver is a well-centered continuous circular anterior capsulotomy about 1 mm smaller than the optic diameter.

M. F. Pyfer, MD

Fluctuations in corneal curvature limit predictability of intraocular lens power calculations

Norrby S, Hirnschall N, Nishi Y, et al (Leek, The Netherlands; Vienna Inst for Res in Ocular Surgery, Austria; Nishi Eye Hosp, Osaka, Japan)
J Cataract Refract Surg 39:174-179, 2013

Purpose.—To analyze fluctuations in corneal curvature over time.

Setting.—Moorfields Eye Hospital NHS Foundation Trust, London, United Kingdom.

Design.—Case series.

Methods.—A 3-piece IOL was implanted in 1 eye and a 1-piece IOL in the other eye through a 3.2 mm clear corneal temporal incision. Keratometry was performed preoperatively and at several points in time postoperatively. Differences between measurements were analyzed by power vectors. Statistical significance was assessed by monovariate, bivariate, and trivariate paired t tests. Acute angle shifts were determined as differences between meridians at 2 points in time.

Results.—Fifty patients were enrolled. From preoperatively to 1 year postoperatively, the changes in vector components (M, J0, J45) were, respectively, −0.02 diopter (D) ± 0.23 (SD) ($P=.38$), −0.07 ± 0.27 D ($P=.02$), and +0.04 ± 0.25 D ($P=.14$). Corresponding changes from 1 year to 2 years postoperatively were +0.01 ± 0.25 D ($P=.73$), +0.01 ± 0.23 D

TABLE 1.—Mean Changes in Vector Components and Monovariate *P* Values from Preoperatively to Several Postoperative Periods and from 1 Year to 2 Years Postoperatively. The Slight Differences in Values Between Text and Table for Preoperatively to 1 Year Postoperatively are Explained by the Different Numbers of Cases Included

Period	Cases (n)	M (D) Mean ± SD	P Value	J0 (D) Mean G SD	P Value	J45 (D) Mean G SD	P Value
Preop to 1 month	69	+0.11 ± 0.30	.00	−0.14 ± 0.31	.00	+0.07 ± 0.30	.05
Preop to 3 months	69	+0.11 ± 0.28	.00	−0.08 ± 0.56	.23	+0.02 ± 0.41	.67
Preop to 1 year	69	−0.02 ± 0.23	.58	−0.06 ± 0.25	.05	+0.05 ± 0.25	.10
Preop to 2 years	69	+0.01 ± 0.25	.79	−0.05 ± 0.30	.21	+0.06 ± 0.27	.06
1 year to 2 years	79	+0.01 ± 0.25	.73	+0.01 ± 0.23	.83	+0.01 ± 0.16	.40

($P =.83$), and +0.01 ± 0.16 D ($P =.40$). The meridian shift was −5 ± 32 degrees ($P =.13$) from preoperatively to postoperatively and +3 ± 22 degrees ($P =.23$) from 1 year to 2 years.

Conclusions.—Surgically induced astigmatism was composed of slight flattening in the horizontal meridian and slight steepening in the oblique meridian but was insignificant in relation to random fluctuations, which were almost equally large between postoperative measurements 1 year apart. The fluctuations were not due to imprecision in measurement (Table 1).

▶ This study is novel and quite significant, because it contradicts what might be called conventional wisdom among cataract surgeons, in that surgically induced astigmatism (SIA) from a temporal clear corneal incision of width 2.2 to 3.2 mm is about 0.25 D to 0.50 D. Prior studies have led to acceptance of this convention, but they rarely extended beyond 3 months postoperatively.[1,2]

This study followed patients out to 2 years and shows progressively decreasing SIA up to the 1-year point, where it is almost negligible (Table 1). Also, the authors demonstrate that the random fluctuation in astigmatism measurement over time is much greater than the SIA. This study also confirms that the small amount of flattening in the horizontal axis of the incision is balanced by steepening in the vertical axis, so there is no net power shift induced by the incision.

We know that incisional techniques to intentionally flatten the steep axis of the cornea, such as limbal relaxing incisions, diminish in effect over time, so it should not be surprising that the same is true for a beveled temporal clear corneal surgical incision.

One possible source of error here is that only the Zeiss IOL master was used to measure the corneal astigmatism, and the software version was not specified. However, this instrument has been verified against other accepted methods of keratometry, and many surgeons use only this device for all biometry prior to cataract surgery and achieve good outcomes.

Overall, if we are concerned with long-term refractive outcomes for 6 months and beyond in our cataract surgery patients, this study would indicate that it is best to ignore the effect of SIA as long as the incision is temporal and less than 3.2 mm wide.

M. F. Pyfer, MD

References

1. Visser N, Ruíz-Mesa R, Pastor F, Bauer NJ, Nuijts RM, Montés-Micó R. Cataract surgery with toric intraocular lens implantation in patients with high corneal astigmatism. *J Cataract Refract Surg.* 2011;37:1403-1410.
2. Hill W. Expected effects of surgically induced astigmatism on AcrySof toric intraocular lens results. *J Cataract Refract Surg.* 2008;34:364-367.

Initial Management of Acute Primary Angle Closure: A Randomized Trial Comparing Phacoemulsification with Laser Peripheral Iridotomy

Husain R, Gazzard G, Aung T, et al (Singapore Natl Eye Ctr and Singapore Eye Res Inst; et al)

Ophthalmology 119:2274-2281, 2012

Purpose.—To compare the 2-year efficacy of phacoemulsification and intraocular lens implant (phaco/IOL) with laser peripheral iridotomy (LPI) in the early management of acute primary angle closure (APAC) and coexisting cataract.

Design.—Randomized, controlled trial.

Participants.—We included 37 subjects presenting with APAC who had responded to medical treatment such that intraocular pressure (IOP) was ≤30 mmHg within 24 hours, and had cataract with visual acuity of ≤6/15.

Main Outcome Measures.—The primary outcome measure was failure of IOP control defined as IOP between 22 to 24 mmHg on 2 occasions (readings taken within 1 month of each other) or IOP ≥ 25 mmHg on 1 occasion, either occurring after week 3. Secondary outcome measures were complications, degree of angle opening, amount of peripheral anterior synechiae, visual acuity, and corneal endothelial cell count (CECC).

Methods.—Subjects were randomized to receive either LPI or phaco/IOL in the affected eye within 1 week of presentation and were examined at fixed intervals over 24 months. Patients underwent a standardized examination that included Goldmann applanation tonometry, gonioscopy, and CECC measurements. Logistic regression was used to estimate the effect of treatment on failure of IOP control. Time to failure was evaluated using the Kaplan—Meier technique and Cox regression was used to estimate the relative risk of failure.

Results.—There were 18 patients randomized to LPI and 19 to phaco/IOL. The average age of subjects was 66.0 ± 9.0 years and mean IOP after medical treatment was 14.5 ± 6.9 mmHg. The 2-year cumulative survival was 61.1% and 89.5% for the LPI and phaco/IOL groups, respectively ($P = 0.034$). There was no change in CECC for either group from baseline to month 6. There was 1 postoperative complication in the phaco/IOL group compared with 4 in the LPI group ($P = 0.180$).

TABLE 3.—Results of Primary Outcome (Failure)

	LPI (n = 18)	Phaco/IOL (n = 19)
Complete failure (loss of light perception attributable to glaucoma or the necessity for further glaucoma surgical intervention or recurrence of APAC)	7 (38.9)	0 (0)
Failure (IOP 22–24 mmHg on 2 occasions [readings taken within 1 month of each other] or IOP ≥25 mmHg on 1 occasion, either occurring after week 3)	0 (0)	2 (10.5)
Qualified success (IOP <22 mmHg at 2 years with the use of ocular hypotensive medications and failure not having occurred)	2 (11.1)	4 (21.1)
Complete success (IOP <22 mmHg at 2 years without the use of ocular hypotensive medications and failure not having occurred)	9 (50.0)*	13 (68.4)

APAC = acute primary angle closure; IOP = intraocular pressure (mmHg); LPI = laser peripheral iridotomy; Phaco/IOL = phacoemulsification and intraocular lens implantation.
P 0.020 (Fisher exact test).
Data shown as n (%).
*Of the 9 subjects who had LPI and who were regarded as complete successes at 2 years, 6 had subsequent cataract surgery, and this may have influenced IOP control.

Conclusions.—Performed within 1 week in patients with APAC and coexisting cataract, phaco/IOL resulted in lower rate of IOP failure at 2 years compared with LPI (Table 3).

▶ This is a landmark randomized, controlled trial that may change the management of acute angle closure glaucoma (ACG). The conclusion of this study, that urgent cataract surgery with intraocular lens implantation is more effective than laser peripheral iridotomy (LPI) for treatment of acute ACG, is surprising (Table 3). However, the result is similar to another study on treating uncontrolled chronic ACG using cataract surgery alone.[1]

It is increasingly obvious that ACG is precipitated by the crystalline lens and is best treated by lens extraction, whether or not it is indicated for visual improvement. However, in the case of acute ACG, why not perform LPI acutely after intraocular pressure is lowered medically enough to clear the cornea, as we do now, and then proceed to phacoemulsification cataract extraction in a timely manner? This method also alleviates any concerns that repeat angle closure could be precipitated by routine preoperative pupil dilation or by an unexpected delay in scheduling cataract surgery in eyes without a functioning peripheral iridotomy.

M. F. Pyfer, MD

Reference

1. Tham CC, Kwong YY, Baig N, Leung DY, Li FC, Lam DS. Phacoemulsification versus trabeculectomy in medically uncontrolled chronic angle-closure glaucoma without cataract. *Ophthalmology.* 2013;120:62-67.

Pseudo anterior capsule barrier for the management of posterior capsule rupture
Chee S-P (Natl Univ of Singapore)
J Cataract Refract Surg 38:1309-1315, 2012

A technique that uses an implanted intraocular lens (IOL) to create a barrier for the management of posterior capsule rupture is described. When a rupture occurs, surgery is halted and a dispersive ophthalmic visco-surgical device (OVD) injected into the anterior chamber to prevent vitreous prolapse. The remaining nucleus is maneuvered into the anterior chamber away from the pupillary space. The posterior capsule tear is converted into a continuous curvilinear capsulorhexis where possible. Dissociated anterior vitrectomy is performed as indicated, keeping the large nuclear fragments trapped in the OVD-filled anterior chamber. An IOL is implanted in the capsular bag or sulcus with optic capture through the anterior capsulorhexis. Using reduced parameters, phacoemulsification of the remaining fragments is completed over the IOL, which functions as a barrier to seal off the vitreous cavity. Residual nuclear fragments and vitreous are cleared from beneath the optic by placing the vitreous cutter under the optic, recapturing the optic before the instruments are removed from the eye (Figs 5B and 6B).

▶ This article presents a nice technique for handling an inadvertent open posterior capsule with residual lens fragments and vitreous prolapse during cataract surgery in the presence of adequate anterior capsule support for the intraocular lens (IOL) (Figs 5B and 6B). As usual, the anterior capsulotomy must be circular, continuous, and smaller than the IOL optic. One concern about this approach is the potential for corneal endothelial damage from anterior chamber sequestration and phacoemulsification of the residual nuclear fragments above the IOL. I would not advise using this technique in eyes with an anterior chamber depth less than 2.5 mm or in the presence of significant pre-existing corneal endothelial disease. The authors recommend cleaning up any residual vitreous and lens fragments beneath the IOL after the anterior chamber is clear by placing the vitreous cutter

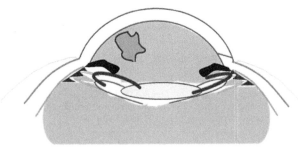

FIGURE 5.—B. Cross-section view of eye. *B*: A 3-piece IOL is implanted in the ciliary sulcus when there is adequate anterior but inadequate posterior capsule support. Posterior optic capture is done. (Reprinted from Journal of Cataract & Refractive Surgery. Chee S-P. Pseudo anterior capsule barrier for the management of posterior capsule rupture. *J Cataract Refract Surg.* 2012;38:1309-1315, Copyright 2012, with permission from ASCRS and ESCRS.)

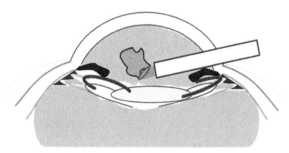

FIGURE 6.—B. Cross-section view of eye showing IOL in the sulcus with posterior optic capture (*B*). Phacoemulsification of the residual nuclear fragment is done over the pseudo anterior capsule barrier. (Reprinted from Journal of Cataract & Refractive Surgery. Chee S-P. Pseudo anterior capsule barrier for the management of posterior capsule rupture. *J Cataract Refract Surg.* 2012;38:1309-1315, Copyright 2012, with permission from ASCRS and ESCRS.)

beneath the IOL from an anterior approach. A preferred method for surgeons comfortable with the technique may be a dry pars plana approach to the residual prolapsed vitreous, with infusion from an anterior chamber maintainer. This would minimize the chance of damage to the anterior capsule rim and prevent further hydration and prolapse of vitreous around the IOL.

M. F. Pyfer, MD

Clinical Evaluation of Three Incision Size–Dependent Phacoemulsification Systems

Luo L, Lin H, He M, et al (Sun Yat-Sen Univ, Guangzhou, Guangdong, China)
Am J Ophthalmol 153:831-839.e2, 2012

Purpose.—To compare the outcomes of cataract surgery performed with 3 incision size–dependent phacoemulsification groups (1.8, 2.2, and 3.0 mm).

Design.—Prospective randomized comparative study.

Methods.—One hundred twenty eyes of 120 patients with age-related cataract (grades 2 to 4) were categorized according to the Lens Opacities Classification System III. Eligible subjects were randomly assigned to 3 surgical groups using coaxial phacoemulsification through 3 clear corneal incision sizes (1.8, 2.2, and 3.0 mm). Different intraoperative and postoperative outcome measures were obtained, with corneal incision size and surgically induced astigmatism as the main clinical outcomes.

Results.—There were no statistically significant differences in most of the intraoperative and postoperative outcome measures among the 3 groups. However, the mean cord length of the clear corneal incision was increased in each group after surgery. The mean maximal clear corneal incision thickness in the 1.8-mm group was significantly greater than for the other groups at 1 month. The mean surgically induced astigmatism in the 1.8- and 2.2-mm groups was significantly less than that in the 3.0-mm group after 1 month, without significant difference between the 1.8- and 2.2-mm groups.

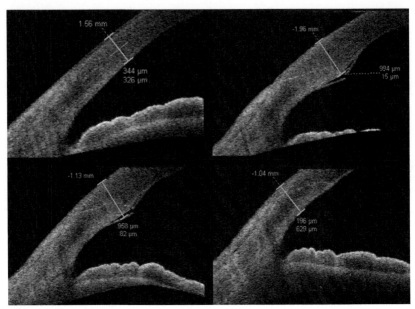

FIGURE 2.—Anterior segment optical coherence tomography images of changes in clear corneal incision thickness observed during the study. (Top left) Image showing preoperative corneal thickness. (Top right) Image showing corneal incision thickness with stromal swelling, endothelial wound gape, and Descemet membrane detachment at postoperative 1 day. (Bottom left) Image showing corneal incision thickness with stromal swelling, endothelial wound gape, and Descemet membrane detachment at postoperative 1 week. (Bottom right) Image showing corneal incision thickness without stromal swelling, endothelial wound gape, and Descemet membrane detachment at postoperative 1 month. (Reprinted from American Journal of Ophthalmology. Luo L, Lin H, He M, et al. Clinical evaluation of three incision size−dependent phacoemulsification systems. *Am J Ophthalmol.* 2012;153:831-839.e2, Copyright 2012, with permission from Elsevier.)

Conclusions.—With appropriate equipment, smaller incisions may result in less astigmatism, but the particular system used will influence incision stress and wound integrity, and may thus limit the reduction in incision size and astigmatism that is achievable (Figs 2 and 4).

▶ This is a well-documented, randomized study comparing outcomes with 3 different clear-corneal incision sizes in coaxial phacoemulsification cataract surgery. Using current terminology, the 1.8-mm and 2.2-mm incisions qualify as micro-incision cataract surgery (MICS), whereas 3.0 mm represents standard small-incision cataract surgery. Most US surgeons performing coaxial surgery use either a 2.4-mm or 2.75-mm incision size.

The results here showed some stretching of the smaller incisions after intraocular lens insertion, which is expected. Also, the 1.8-mm incision showed persistent thickening until 1 month after surgery relative to the larger incisions, but this resolved by 3 months (Fig 2). The rate of surgically induced astigmatism (SIA) was lower in the MICS groups at 1 month. Notably, the trend of the SIA curve indicates decreasing astigmatism with time that may continue beyond 1 month, but this was not reported (Fig 4).

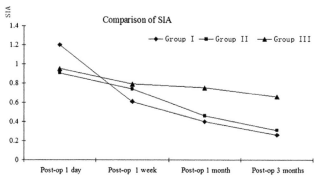

FIGURE 4.—Comparison of surgically induced astigmatism in the 1.8-, 2.2-, and 3.0-mm phacoemulsification groups at 1 day, 1 week, 1 month, and 3 months after surgery. At postoperative 1 day and 1 week, there was no significant difference in the mean induced astigmatism between the 3 groups. At 1 and 3 months after surgery, there were statistically significant differences in surgically induced astigmatism between Group I and Group III, and between Group II and Group III ($P = .001$ for both), but no statistically significant difference between Groups I and II ($P = .239$, $P = .154$ at 1 and 3 months respectively). SIA: surgically induced astigmatism; Group I: 1.8-mm incision; Group II: 2.2-mm incision; Group III: 3.0-mm incision. (Reprinted from American Journal of Ophthalmology. Luo L, Lin H, He M, et al. Clinical evaluation of three incision size—dependent phacoemulsification systems. *Am J Ophthalmol.* 2012;153:831-839.e2, Copyright 2012, with permission from Elsevier.)

All other measured outcome variables were similar between the 3 groups, including visual acuity and complication rate. There was a trend toward lower total ultrasound energy and less irrigation fluid use with the smaller incisions, but this did not reach statistical significance. Cataract surgeons who prefer the coaxial technique should consider migrating toward 2.2- to 2.4-mm MICS, but this move is not essential to obtaining good surgical results.

M. F. Pyfer, MD

The Relationship of Cataract and Cataract Extraction to Age-related Macular Degeneration: The Beaver Dam Eye Study

Klein BEK, Howard KP, Lee KE, et al (Univ of Wisconsin School of Medicine and Public Health, Madison; et al)
Ophthalmology 119:1628-1633, 2012

Objective.—To examine the associations of cataract and cataract surgery with early and late age-related macular degeneration (AMD) over a 20-year interval.

Design.—Longitudinal population-based study of age-related eye diseases.

Participants.—Beaver Dam Eye Study participants.

Methods.—Persons aged 43 to 86 years participated in the baseline examination in 1988−1990. Participants were followed up at 5-year intervals after the baseline examination. Examinations consisted of ocular examination with lens and fundus photography, medical history, measurements of blood pressure, height, and weight. Values of risk variables were updated, and incidences of early and late AMD were calculated for each 5-year interval. Odds ratios were computed using discrete linear logistic regression modeling with generalized estimating equation methods to account for correlation between the eyes and multiple intervals.

Main Outcome Measures.—Age-related macular degeneration.

Results.—After adjusting for age and sex, neither cataract nor cataract surgery was associated with increased odds for developing early AMD. Further adjusting for high-risk gene alleles (*CFH* and *ARMS2*) and other possible risk factors did not materially affect the odds ratio (OR). However, cataract surgery was associated with incidence of late AMD (OR 1.93; 95% confidence interval [CI], 1.28—2.90). This OR was not materially altered by further adjusting for high-risk alleles (*CFH Y402H, ARMS2*) or other risk factors. The OR for late AMD was higher for cataract surgery performed 5 or more years prior compared with less than 5 years prior.

Conclusions.—These data strongly support the past findings of an association of cataract surgery with late AMD independent of other risk factors, including high-risk genetic status, and suggest the importance of considering these findings when counseling patients regarding cataract surgery. These findings should provide further impetus for the search for measures to prevent or delay the development of age-related cataract.

▶ Population-based epidemiologic studies such as this one have to be interpreted very carefully. The only conclusion we can draw here is that in the study population, there is about a 2-fold higher incidence of late age-related macular degeneration (AMD) in patients who had cataract surgery 5 or more years prior to the examination than in those who had not yet had cataract surgery. No such association between early AMD and prior cataract surgery was found. The authors controlled for a known genetic risk factor for AMD and for other AMD risk factors, including age, sex, smoking history, and cardiovascular disease.

To conclude from this evidence that cataract surgery should be delayed in patients at risk for AMD is not justified. An epidemiologic association does not establish cause and effect. Cataract itself is not a disease; there is a significant element of patient choice and access to care involved, and surgical cataracts vary widely in density. For instance, a possible confounder is that patients who develop AMD experience diminished vision and become more symptomatic with early cataracts than those with a healthy macula, so they end up seeking treatment and having surgery sooner. This would mean that patients with undiagnosed AMD are more likely to choose to have cataract surgery, creating a bias in the data. Another problem with this study is that fundus photographs were used to make the diagnosis of AMD. The presence of a significant cataract hampers both fundus examination and photography. The addition of intravenous fluorescein angiography and ocular coherence tomography would increase the accuracy of diagnosis prior to cataract surgery.

A randomized, controlled trial is necessary to prove whether cataract surgery is an independent risk factor for development of AMD. Symptomatic patients with cataracts would have to be randomized to either observation or surgery, then monitored for at least 5 years without further intervention for development of AMD. This study is impractical and will likely never be done in a sufficient number of patients to answer this important question. However, several other well-controlled, nonrandomized studies over the past few years have found no increased risk for AMD after cataract surgery.[1-3]

M. F. Pyfer, MD

References

1. Wang JJ, Fong CS, Rochtchina E, et al. Risk of age-related macular degeneration 3 years after cataract surgery: paired eye comparisons. *Ophthalmology.* 2012;119: 2298-2303.
2. Xu L, You QS, Cui T, Jonas JB. Association between asymmetry in cataract and asymmetry in age-related macular degeneration. The Beijing Eye Study. *Graefes Arch Clin Exp Ophthalmol.* 2011;249:981-985.
3. Dong LM, Stark WJ, Jefferys JL, et al. Progression of age-related macular degeneration after cataract surgery. *Arch Ophthalmol.* 2009;127:1412-1419.

Glistenings on Intraocular Lenses in Healthy Eyes: Effects and Associations
Colin J, Orignac I (Centre Hospitalier et Universitaire de Bordeaux, France)
J Refract Surg 27:869-875, 2011

Purpose.—To assess glistenings in AcrySof (Alcon Laboratories Inc) intraocular lenses (IOLs), to quantify any effects of glistenings on the visual function of patients with healthy eyes, and to investigate whether glistenings were associated with demographic or lens characteristics.
Methods.—Case files from a consecutive series of healthy eyes were retrospectively analyzed. Subjective glistening grades were investigated for associations with the following parameters: contrast sensitivity, corrected distance visual acuity (CDVA), intraocular light scattering (measured by C-Quant [Oculus Optikgeräte GmbH]), posterior capsule opacification, demographic characteristics, lens power, and duration of pseudophakia.

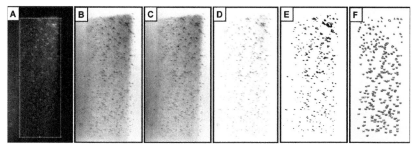

FIGURE 1.—Manipulation and analysis of images. A) Slit-lamp image of an intraocular lens with grade 2 glistenings, with the yellow rectangle showing the central 0.75×2-mm zone that was used for counting. B) Inversion of color. C) Conversion to 8-bit format. D) Subtraction of background and adjustment of contrast. E) Threshold set to recognize features of size up to 0.001 mm². F) Microvacuoles counted by the software are circled in red. The result (256 microvacuoles in this case) was divided by the area of the yellow analysis rectangle to yield the density of the microvacuoles. For interpretation of the references to color in this figure legend, the reader is referred to web version of this article. (Reprinted with permission from SLACK Incorporated. Colin J, Orignac I. Glistenings on intraocular lenses in healthy eyes: effects and associations. *J Refract Surg.* 2011;27:869-875.)

The subjective grading method was compared to objective software-based quantitation of glistenings.

Results.—The study cohort included 97 eyes from 65 patients with a mean age of 65 ± 11 years. Mean follow-up was 18 ± 17 months. Glistening grades did not vary by duration of pseudophakia ($P = .19$), although study design limited confidence in this result. Glistening grades had no associations with lens power ($P = .41$), intraocular light scattering ($P = .31$), logMAR CDVA ($P = .64$), contrast sensitivity at any spatial frequency (all $P \geq .22$), or with any other parameter under investigation. The software-based assessment confirmed the validity of the subjective grading method: glistening grades correlated with vacuoles/mm^2 ($P < .0001$) and mean values for vacuoles/mm^2 were statistically significant for each glistening grade (all $P \leq .004$).

Conclusions.—In healthy eyes, glistening grade was not associated with contrast sensitivity, CDVA, intraocular light scatter, or any lens or demographic characteristics that were investigated (Fig 1).

▶ The debate is over—glistenings do exist. These microscopic, bubblelike discontinuities in intraocular lenses (IOLs) can easily be seen on slit lamp examination. Glistenings have been documented in all common IOL materials: polymethylmethacrylate, silicone, and hydrophobic acrylic, but they are most commonly found in hydrophobic acrylic lenses. They have been found to be water-containing vacuoles within the substance of the lens. Glistenings may vary over time, with at least one study finding evidence of a decrease in glistening density over time in certain cases.

The unresolved questions are:

1. Do glistenings affect the light transmission quality and performance of the lens enough to impact vision?
2. Do they continue to increase in density over time?
3. Are any postimplantation environmental factors related to glistening formation?

Several studies, including this one, on visual performance of lenses with glistenings have found that they have minimal-to-no effect on visual acuity. This article is notable because it uses objective image analysis tools to verify the subjective slit lamp examination grading system (Fig 1). Also, glistening grade was found to be unrelated to time since implantation. However, this is not a longitudinal study of individuals, so it cannot determine if glistenings increase over time or assess risk factors for this increase.

M. F. Pyfer, MD

Capsular Adhesion to Intraocular Lens in Highly Myopic Eyes Evaluated in Vivo Using Ultralong-scan-depth Optical Coherence Tomography

Zhao Y, Li J, Lu W, et al (Wenzhou Med College, Zhejiang, China)
Am J Ophthalmol 155:484-491, 2013

Purpose.—To evaluate the in vivo capsular apposition to the intraocular lens (IOL) in subjects with high myopia by ultralong-scan-depth optical coherence tomography (OCT).

Design.—Prospective observational case series.

Methods.—Forty eyes from 40 cataract patients scheduled for phacoemulsification surgery at the Affiliated Eye Hospital, Wenzhou Medical College were studied, of which 20 eyes were highly myopic (axial length > 26 mm) and 20 eyes were emmetropic (22 mm < axial length < 24.5 mm). All eyes were examined with a custom-built ultralong-scan-depth OCT at 4 hours, 1 day, 7 days, 14 days, and 28 days after surgery.

Results.—Anterior capsule contact with the IOL was significantly delayed in highly myopic eyes. Complete apposition of the posterior capsule with the IOL was significantly less common among highly myopic eyes than in emmetropic eyes (4 vs 16 eyes; $P = .001$). Posterior capsule adhesion to the IOL was inversely correlated with axial length ($r = -0.494$, $P < .001$, nonparametric Spearman test). The 3 types of complete adhesive capsular bend configurations observed were classified as anterior adhesion, middle adhesion, and posterior adhesion. Incomplete adhesion patterns were classified as funnel adhesion, parallel adhesion, and furcate adhesion. Five highly myopic eyes had slight posterior capsule opacification (PCO) at the last follow-up, as did 1 emmetropic eye.

Conclusions.—Ultralong-scan-depth OCT revealed weak capsular adhesion and incompletely adhesive types of capsular bend in highly myopic eyes. These features presumably increase the likelihood of PCO during the early postoperative period (Fig 2).

▶ This is a very interesting and novel study that elucidates the behavior of the capsule around the intraocular lens (IOL) during early healing after routine phacoemulsification cataract extraction with implantation of a single-piece acrylic IOL. The images are of significantly higher quality and resolution than any prior human in vivo optical coherence tomography (OCT) studies of capsule—IOL interaction (Fig 2). The authors used a proprietary custom time-domain OCT mounted to a slit lamp with a 7.5-mm scan depth that is ideal for imaging the lens plane. The conclusion that highly myopic eyes have a delayed capsular adhesion to the IOL is the main point of the article; however, what I feel is more significant are the capsule morphology observations during the first 4 weeks postoperatively, especially the posterior capsule undulations imaged at day 7 in the myopic eye as in Fig 2. From my experience, these are quite common between 1 and 2 weeks after surgery and sometimes result in fixed posterior capsular folds or wrinkles that can be visually significant by causing a Maddox rod effect when they bisect the visual axis. Of course, the limitation on OCT imaging of the capsule periphery and IOL optic edge is that good pupil dilation is required. I look forward

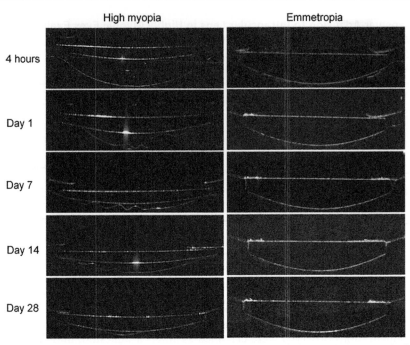

FIGURE 2.—Visualized adhesion of lens capsule to intraocular lenses by the ultralong-scan-depth optical coherence tomography in highly myopic and emmetropic eyes postoperatively. (Top row, left) In the highly myopic eye, a large shadow between the anteroposterior capsule and the intraocular lens (IOL) can be observed at 4 hours after the surgery. (Second row, left) The posterior capsule wrinkles 1 day after surgery, with the capsule clearly dissociated from the intraocular lens. The anterior and posterior capsule gradually appose to the IOL, while a shallow space remains between the capsule and the IOL in the highly myopic eye at days 7 (Third row, left) and 14 (Fourth row, left). (Bottom row, left) The anterior capsule and IOL are in complete apposition. A capsular bend has formed at 1 side of the IOL. A small space still exists at the center of the posterior capsule in a highly myopic eye. (Top row, right) In the emmetropic eye, the anterior capsule is in contact with the IOL at 4 hours after the surgery. The posterior capsule was completely adhered to the optic at days 1 (Second row, right) and 7 (Third row, right), while the capsular bend remains open. (Fourth row, right, and Bottom row, right) The capsule is completely wrapped around the IOL in an emmetropic eye. (Reprinted from American Journal of Ophthalmology. Zhao Y, Li J, Lu W, et al. Capsular adhesion to intraocular lens in highly myopic eyes evaluated in vivo using ultralong-scan-depth optical coherence tomography. Am J Ophthalmol. 2013;155:484-491, Copyright 2013, with permission from Elsevier.)

to the development of commercial OCT systems that are capable of this type of resolution in the lens plane.

M. F. Pyfer, MD

Accuracy of Intraocular Lens Calculation With Ray Tracing

Hoffmann P, Wahl J, Preußner P-R (Augen- und Laserklinik Castrop-Rauxel, Germany; Universitäts-Augenklinik Mainz, Germany)
J Refract Surg 28:650-655, 2012

Purpose.—To quantify the current accuracy limits of ray tracing for intraocular lens (IOL) calculations, compare results for spherical vs aspheric

IOLs, and determine the value of using crystalline lens thickness in IOL calculations.

Methods.—Of 591 eyes, 363 eyes were implanted with spherical IOLs (320 SA60AT [Alcon Laboratories Inc] and 43 Y-60H [Hoya Corp]) and 228 eyes had aspheric, aberration-correcting IOLs (57 SN60WF [Alcon Laboratories Inc], 112 Tecnis ZCB00 [Abbott Medical Optics], 21 CTAsphina404 [Carl Zeiss Meditec], and 38 iMics1 [Hoya Corp]), all calculated with OKULIX ray tracing (Tedics), based on Lenstar (Haag-Streit) measurements of axial length, corneal radii, and position and thickness of the crystalline lens. The measure of accuracy was the prediction error, ie, the difference between calculated refraction and manifest refraction (spherical equivalent) 1 month after surgery calculated as mean absolute error (MAE).

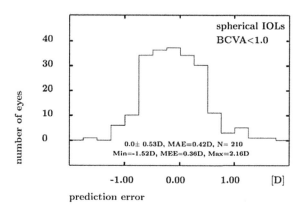

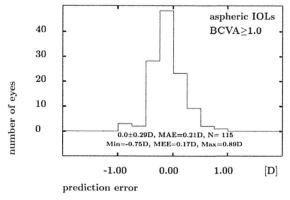

FIGURE 1.—Histograms of the distribution of the prediction errors are shown for the subgroups with the highest (top) and lowest (bottom) prediction errors. In the upper subgroup, 67% are within ± 0.50 D of the target refraction and 95% are within ± 1.00 D; in the lower subgroup, 91% are within ± 0.50 D and 100% are within ± 1.00 D. BCVA = best corrected visual acuity, MAE = mean absolute error, MEE = median absolute error. (Reprinted with permission from SLACK Incorporated. Hoffmann P, Wahl J, Preußner P-R. Accuracy of intraocular lens calculation with ray tracing. *J Refract Surg*. 2012;28:650-655.)

Results.—The prediction error with aspheric IOLs was lower than that with spherical IOLs (MAE 0.27 vs 0.36 D) and was lower for patients with corrected distance visual acuity (CDVA) ≥ 1.0 compared to CDVA <1.0 (MAE 0.26 vs 0.38 D). For aspheric IOLs and CDVA ≥ 1.0, MAE differed by a factor of two compared to spherical IOLs and CDVA <1.0 (MAE 0.21 vs 0.42 D). Taking the crystalline lens position and thickness into account improved the prediction error by $\sim 9\%$ overall (MAE 0.33 vs 0.36 D) and was most beneficial in patients with aspheric lenses and CDVA ≥ 1.0 (MAE improved from 0.26 to 0.21 D). All differences between the investigated subgroups were statistically significant ($P < .05$).

Conclusions.—Ray tracing for IOL calculation is particularly beneficial with aspheric IOLs and in eyes with good (20/20 or better) postoperative visual acuity (Fig 1).

▶ This study shows the accuracy of a ray-tracing method for performing intraocular lens (IOL) calculations based on reasonably precise biometry from a device currently available commercially (Lenstar by Haag-Streit). The prediction accuracy of the ray-tracing approach in the subset of 115 eyes implanted with aspheric IOLs and with postoperative best-corrected visual acuity of 20/20 or better is significantly better than the best published data for current third-generation biometry-based formulas. The authors achieved 91% within +0.5 diopters of emmetropia in these cases (Fig 1). This result was enhanced by estimating actual lens position from anterior chamber depth and lens thickness measurements. Corneal asphericity and posterior corneal measurements were not taken into account.

Soon, a significant leap forward in IOL calculations will occur by combining highly accurate anterior chamber measurements (most likely using ocular coherence tomography), including anterior and posterior corneal curvature, corneal thickness, and actual lens position, with currently accurate optical axial length measurements, and using a ray-tracing method as in this report for optical modeling. This will eliminate the need to use estimation for any parameter except for final IOL position, which cannot be truly measured until after surgery and healing takes place. However, intraoperative aberrometry may ultimately replace all of these preoperative calculations. Stay tuned for much more on this topic in the next few years.

M. F. Pyfer, MD

Association of biometric factors with anterior chamber angle widening and intraocular pressure reduction after uneventful phacoemulsification for cataract
Huang G, Gonzalez E, Lee R, et al (Univ of California, San Francisco; et al)
J Cataract Refract Surg 38:108-116, 2012

Purpose.—To evaluate anterior chamber biometric factors associated with the degree of angle widening and intraocular pressure (IOP) reduction after phacoemulsification.

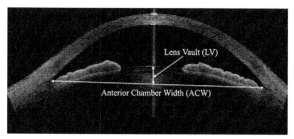

FIGURE 2.—The measurement of LV and ACW (AS-OCT). (Reprinted from Journal of Cataract & Refractive Surgery. Huang G, Gonzalez E, Lee R, et al. Association of biometric factors with anterior chamber angle widening and intraocular pressure reduction after uneventful phacoemulsification for cataract. *J Cataract Refract Surg*. 2012;38:108-116, Copyright 2012, with permission from ASCRS and ESCRS.)

Setting.—University of California, San Francisco, California, USA.

Design.—Case series.

Methods.—Anterior chamber parameters obtained by anterior segment coherence tomography were compared preoperatively and 3 months postoperatively. Measurements included the angle opening distance 500 μm anterior to the scleral spur (AOD500), trabecular—iris space area 500 μm from the scleral spur (TISA500), iris curvature (I-Curv), anterior chamber angle (ACA), trabecular-iris space area, anterior chamber volume, anterior chamber width, and lens vault (LV).

Results.—The study enrolled 73 eyes. The mean patient age was 77.45 years ± 7.84 (SD); 65.75% of patients were women. From preoperatively to 3 months postoperatively, the mean AOD500 increased significantly (0.254 ± 0.105 to 0.433 ± 0.108 mm) and the mean IOP decreased significantly (11.97 ± 3.35 to 12.62 ± 3.37 mm Hg) ($P < .001$). The reduction in IOP was correlated with the increase in AOD500 ($r = 0.240, P = .041$) and preoperative LV ($r = 0.235, P = .045$). After adjusting for related factors, AOD500 widening was positively correlated with LV ($\beta = 0.458, P = .044$) and I-Curv ($\beta = 0.235, P = .043$) and negatively correlated with preoperative TISA500 ($\beta = -0.269, P = .025$) and ACA ($\beta = -0.919, P = .027$).

Conclusions.—Surgically induced AOD widening was significantly correlated with anterior chamber biometric factors. Preoperative LV appears to be a significant factor in angle widening and IOP reduction after phacoemulsification (Fig 2).

▶ This study evaluates several anterior chamber (AC) measurements before cataract surgery and relates them to angle widening and reduction of intraocular pressure after surgery. Most significantly, a new parameter termed *lens vault* (LV) is discussed. LV (Fig 2) is easily obtained from anterior segment ocular coherence tomography and likely also from other noncontact optical imaging devices such as Scheimpflug-type scanning slit cameras like the Pentacam, although that was not evaluated in this study. Imaging of the posterior lens surface or behind the iris, which is not possible using optical imaging, is unnecessary for calculation of LV. The authors show with multivariate regression analysis that LV is the measurement most highly correlated with a postoperative increase in AC depth, angle opening distance, and reduction of intraocular pressure.

In light of this finding, simple software utilities for calculating lens vault should be added to all AC imaging devices. This report is one more bit of evidence that we are entering a new era of understanding via accurate noninvasive anterior segment imaging that will help predict (and eventually control) the anatomy of the pseudophakic eye, including actual lens position.

M. F. Pyfer, MD

2 Refractive Surgery

Early clinical outcomes, including efficacy and endothelial cell loss, of refractive lenticule extraction using a 500 khz femtosecond laser to correct myopia
Kamiya K, Igarashi A, Ishii R, et al (Univ of Kitasato School of Medicine, Kanagawa, Japan)
J Cataract Refract Surg 38:1996-2002, 2012

Purpose.—To assess the early clinical outcomes, including the efficacy and the endothelial cell loss, of femtosecond lenticule extraction using a 500 kHz femtosecond laser system to correct myopia.

Setting.—Department of Ophthalmology, Kitasato University, Kanagawa, Japan.

Design.—Case series.

Methods.—This study evaluated eyes with a spherical equivalent of −4.26 diopters (D) ± 1.39 (SD) that had femtosecond lenticule extraction for myopia. Before surgery and 1 week and 1, 3, and 6 months after surgery, the safety, efficacy, predictability, stability, and adverse events of the surgery were assessed.

Results.—The study enrolled 38 eyes of 20 patients. The uncorrected distance visual acuity and corrected distance visual acuity 6 months after surgery were −0.14 ± 0.10 logMAR and −0.21 ± 0.09 logMAR, respectively. The safety index was 0.96 ± 0.19 and the efficacy index, 0.82 ± 0.17. At 6 months, all eyes were within ±0.50 D of the targeted correction. The mean manifest refraction change from 1 week to 6 months was 0.02 ± 0.28 D. The endothelial cell density was 2814 ± 199 cells/mm^2 preoperatively and 2762 ± 213 cells/mm^2 postoperatively; the change was not significant ($P = .32$, Wilcoxon signed-rank test). No vision-threatening complications occurred during the observation period.

Conclusions.—Femtosecond lenticule extraction performed well in the correction of myopia. Neither significant endothelial cell loss nor serious complications occurred throughout the 6-month follow-up, suggesting femtosecond lenticule extraction is a viable surgical option to treat myopic eyes.

▶ Two of the most recent procedures in the field of corneal refractive surgery are performed completely with the femtosecond laser. One involves using the femtosecond laser to create a laser in situ keratomileusis flap and a refractive lenticule, after which the LASIK flap is lifted, the lenticule removed, and the LASIK flap replaced. Another version uses a femtosecond laser to perform essentially the same procedure, except only a small opening is made at the flap edge, and the lenticule is extracted through this small incision (small incision lenticule extraction). Neither of these procedures is currently approved by the US Food and Drug Administration.

The authors report good clinical results in this small study of 38 eyes of 20 patients followed for 6 months using the FLEX technique. They used a 120-μ flap thickness, 7.5-mm diameter flap, and 6.5-mm diameter lenticule. Minimal residual stromal bed thickness was at least 250 μ. The mean corneal endothelial cell count decreased from 2814 to 2762 cells/mm^2 (1.7%) from preoperatively to 6 months postoperatively. This rate of cell loss was not statistically significant, likely because of the small number of eyes and the large standard deviation. However, just because it was not statistically significant does not mean it was not clinically significant. The "normal" physiologic rate of endothelial cell loss is thought to be in the 0.6% per year range. The rate reported in this study is almost 3 times that. I await larger studies with longer follow-up to convince me that this procedure does not affect the health of the corneal endothelial cells.

C. J. Rapuano, MD

Small-incision lenticule extraction for moderate to high myopia: Predictability, safety, and patient satisfaction
Vestergaard A, Ivarsen AR, Asp S, et al (Aarhus Univ Hosp, Denmark)
J Cataract Refract Surg 38:2003-2010, 2012

Purpose.—To present initial clinical experience with small-incision lenticule extraction for the treatment of moderate to high myopia.

Setting.—Department of Ophthalmology, Aarhus University Hospital, Aarhus, Denmark.

Design.—Prospective clinical study.

Methods.—For small-incision lenticule extraction, an intrastromal lenticule was cut with a femtosecond laser and manually extracted without creation of a flap. Patients were treated and followed for 3 months. Only 1 randomly chosen eye of each patient was used in the statistical analyses.

Results.—The study enrolled 144 patients. The mean preoperative spherical equivalent was −7.18 diopters (D) ± 1.57 (SD). Of eyes with emmetropia as target refraction, 40% had an uncorrected distance visual acuity of 0.1 logMAR or less 1 day after surgery; this increased to 73% at 3 months. The mean corrected distance visual acuity (CDVA) improved significantly from −0.01 (logMAR) preoperatively to −0.03 3 months postoperatively. None of the 127 eyes lost 2 lines or more of CDVA and 6 eyes lost 1 line of CDVA after 3 months. In contrast, 1 eye gained 2 lines and 24 eyes gained 1 line of CDVA. The achieved refraction was a mean of −0.09 ± 0.45 D from the attempted refraction. Of the eyes, 77% were within ±0.50 D and 95% were within ± 1.00 D. Ninety-five percent of the patients would recommend the procedure to others.

Conclusions.—The refractive predictability, safety, and patient satisfaction 3 months after small-incision lenticule extraction were high and comparable to results in previous studies of femtosecond laser—assisted techniques.

▶ The small incision lenticule extraction version (SMILE) of the all- femtosecond laser corneal refractive surgery procedures has the advantage of a much smaller external incision compared with the hinged- laser in-situ keratomileusis (LASIK) flap of the femtosecond lenticule extraction (FLEX) technique. In this study, the "cap" diameter was 7.3 mm, the lenticule diameter was 6.0 to 6.5 mm, and the "cap" thickness was 110 to 120 μ. The external incision to remove the lenticule was made at the 12 o'clock position and was 40 to 60° in arc length. Residual stromal bed thickness was at least 250 μ. Ninety-four percent of eyes were treated for −4 to −10D of myopia (mean −7.2D); 88% of the 144 eyes had 3 months of follow-up.

The clinical results were very good for this level of myopia, although the follow-up was short, and the 3-month follow-up data were missing for 12% of eyes. Corneal endothelial cell counts were not reported. This report confirms the results of previous smaller studies, but with a larger number of eyes. As the authors stated, this procedure is still evolving and improving. I look forward to their 1-year results, although it is too bad they did not look at endothelial cell counts.

C. J. Rapuano, MD

Simultaneous corneal inlay implantation and laser in situ keratomileusis for presbyopia in patients with hyperopia, myopia, or emmetropia: Six-month results

Tomita M, Kanamori T, Waring GO IV, et al (Shinagawa LASIK Ctr, Tokyo, Japan; ReVision Advanced Laser Eye Ctr, Columbus, OH)
J Cataract Refract Surg 38:495-506, 2012

Purpose.—To evaluate the safety and efficacy of simultaneous Kamra corneal inlay implantation and laser in situ keratomileusis (LASIK) for the treatment of presbyopia in emmetropic, hyperopic, or myopic patients.

Setting.—Private center, Tokyo, Japan.

Design.—Cohort study.

Methods.—Patients had bilateral LASIK with simultaneous implantation of a corneal inlay in the nondominant eye to treat presbyopia and ametropia between September 2009 and April 2010. The efficacy and safety were determined by the spherical equivalent (SE) in the eye with the inlay.

Results.—The study enrolled 360 eyes of 180 patients with a mean age of 52.4 years ± 5.1 (SD) (range 41 to 65 years). Sixty-four patients were available for the 6-month postoperative examination. The mean logMAR uncorrected near visual acuity in the eye with the inlay improved 7 lines in hyperopic eyes, 6 lines in emmetropic eyes, and 2 lines in myopic eyes. The mean logMAR uncorrected distance visual acuity improved by 3 lines, 1 line, and 10 lines, respectively.

Conclusions.—Simultaneous intracorneal inlay implantation and LASIK to treat presbyopia with emmetropia, hyperopia, or myopia was clinically safe and effective, yielding improvement in distance and near visual acuity. Patients were satisfied with decreased dependence on reading glasses regardless of the preoperative SE range. However, postoperative symptoms, such as dry eyes, halo, glare, or night-vision disturbances, occurred occasionally.

▶ Most previous studies on the Kamra corneal inlay have been in emmetropic presbyopes. This study included primarily presbyopic myopes but also presbyopic emmetropes and presbyopic hyperopes. The 6-month results reported here include only 64 of the 180 patients enrolled in the study. Even so, the results are encouraging.

The authors implanted the Kamra inlay in the nondominant eye under a 200-micron Intralase LASIK flap. Minimal stromal bed depth was 260 microns. The target correction in the eye was "−0.75" diopters. Topical dexamethasone drops were prescribed every 1 h for 1 day, then 5 times a day for 2 weeks. It was then changed to fluorometholone 5 times a day tapering to once a day at 6 months and continuing for 12 months. Daily reading training without reading glasses was strongly encouraged to hasten neuroadaptation. Two eyes required surgical recentration of the Kamra inlay. Emmetropes, hyperopes, and myopes were all satisfied with their decreased dependence on reading glasses. As is not uncommon after LASIK, some patients complained of dry eye, glare, halos, and night vision disturbances. The authors note that implanting the inlay in a lamellar pocket might prevent some of these symptoms, but then myopic or hyperopic corrections could not be performed simultaneously. Hopefully, follow-up on the other two thirds of the patients in this study will reveal similarly good results.

C. J. Rapuano, MD

Reading Performance After Implantation of a Modified Corneal Inlay Design for the Surgical Correction of Presbyopia: 1-Year Follow-up
Dexl AK, Seyeddain O, Riha W, et al (Univ Eye Clinic, Salzburg, Austria)
Am J Ophthalmol 153:994-1001, 2012

Purpose.—To evaluate change in different reading performance parameters after monocular ACI7000PDT corneal inlay implantation for the improvement of near and intermediate vision.

Design.—Prospective, interventional case series.

Methods.—Twenty-four patients were scheduled for corneal inlay implantation in the nondominant eye in a university outpatient surgery center. Naturally emmetropic and presbyopic patients between 45 and 60 years of age, with uncorrected distance visual acuity of at least 20/20 in both eyes, without any additional ocular pathology were eligible for inclusion. Bilateral uncorrected reading acuity, mean and maximum reading speed, and smallest log-scaled print size were evaluated with the standardized Radner Reading Charts. Measurements of reading parameters and reading distance were performed with the Salzburg Reading Desk (SRD). Minimum postoperative follow-up was 12 months.

TABLE 2.—Reading Speed Measurements Over Time in Patients Implanted With the 3rd-Generation KAMRA Corneal Inlay (ACI7000PDT) for Improvement of Near and Intermediate Vision

	Mean ± SD	Mean Reading Speed (wpm) CI −95%	CI +95%	Min	Max
Preoperative	141 ± 20	133	150	112	180
1 month	150 ± 26	139	160	105	214
3 months	145 ± 22	135	154	96	211
6 months	150 ± 20	141	158	117	194
12 months	156 ± 26	145	167	104	222
	Mean ± SD	Maximum Reading Speed (wpm) CI −95%	CI +95%	Min	Max
Preoperative	171 ± 28	159	183	131	235
1 month	188 ± 35	173	203	135	268
3 months	177 ± 27	166	189	141	247
6 months	183 ± 23	174	193	141	242
12 months	196 ± 38	180	212	120	298

CI ± confidence interval; Min = minimum; Max = maximum; SD = standard deviation; wpm = words per minute.

Results.—The reading desk results showed significant changes in each parameter tested. After 12 months the mean reading distance changed from the preoperative value of 46.7 cm (95% CI: 44.1−49.3) to 42.8 cm (95% CI: 40.3−45.3, $P < .004$), and the mean reading acuity "at best distance" improved from 0.33 logRAD (95% CI: 0.27−0.39) to 0.24 logRAD (95% CI: 0.20−0.28, $P < .005$). Mean reading speed increased from 141 words per minute (wpm, 95% CI: 133−150) to 156 wpm (95% CI: 145−167, $P < .003$), maximum reading speed increased from 171 wpm (95% CI: 159−183) to 196 wpm (95% CI: 180−212, $P = .001$), and the smallest print size improved from 1.50 mm (95% CI: 1.32−1.67) to 1.12 mm (95% CI: 1.03−1.22, $P < .001$).

Conclusions.—After ACI7000PDT implantation, there were significant changes in all tested reading performance parameters in emmetropic presbyopic patients. These 1-year results indicate that the inlay seems to be an effective treatment for presbyopia (Table 2).

▶ Numerous studies have reported on the safety and efficacy of the KAMRA inlay to treat presbyopes. Tomita et al (see previous Year Book comment this chapter) demonstrated its effect while simultaneously treating myopia or hyperopia. This study continues the authors' work in evaluating the success of this device using the Salzburg Reading Desk. The benefit of the Salzburg Reading Desk is that it is a much more real-life test of reading vision than simply reading a near card. It tests uncorrected bilateral reading acuity, reading distance, and mean and maximum reading speed along with measuring the smallest print size patients could effectively read. This study was done only in ametropic patients. It used the newest KAMRA inlay that was implanted through a femtosecond laser-created pocket incision to minimize problems caused by a complete corneal flap.

The objective results were good with statistically significant improvement in all the measured parameters. However, mean reading speed improved only 11%, from 141 to 156 words per minute, and mean maximum reading speed improved only 15%, from 171 to 196 words per minutes, which doesn't seem that impressive to me. How was patient satisfaction? There was a statistically significant ($P < .001$) decrease in the need for patients to wear reading glasses, and 18 to 24 patients (75%) said they would undergo the procedure again. Time will tell whether this is good enough for this procedure to really catch on.

C. J. Rapuano, MD

Visual outcomes and corneal changes after intrastromal femtosecond laser correction of presbyopia
Menassa N, Fitting A, Auffarth GU, et al (Univ Hosp of Heidelberg, Germany)
J Cataract Refract Surg 38:765-773, 2012

Purpose.—To assess the effect of intrastromal femtosecond laser presbyopia treatment on uncorrected near visual acuity (UNVA) and corneal integrity over an 18-month period.

Setting.—Department of Ophthalmology, International Vision Correction Research Centre, University of Heidelberg, Heidelberg, Germany.

Design.—Clinical trial.

Methods.—The UNVA (at 40 cm), corneal pachymetry, and true net power were evaluated preoperatively and 1, 3, 6, 12, and 18 months after femtosecond intrastromal presbyopic treatment (Intracor). Endothelial cell density (ECD) was measured preoperatively and 3, 6, and 12 months postoperatively. Data were analyzed with the Wilcoxon test at a $P = .01$ level of significance.

Results.—The median UNVA improved significantly from 0.7 logMAR preoperatively to 0.4 logMAR, 0.2 logMAR, 0.2 logMAR, 0.3 logMAR, and 0.2 logMAR at 1, 3, 6, 12, and 18 months, respectively (all $P < .001$). The median corneal true net power increased significantly by 1.1 diopters (D) to 0.7 D, 0.8 D, 1.0 D, and 0.9 D, respectively (all $P < .001$); pachymetry showed no significant thinning postoperatively. There was no significant difference in ECD between preoperatively and postoperatively.

Conclusions.—Intrastromal femtosecond presbyopic treatment yielded a significant and stable gain of UNVA and corneal steepening without significant loss of endothelial cells or corneal thinning up to 18 months postoperatively. No significant regression of visual acuity or further corneal steepening occurred during the follow-up period (Fig 1, Table 3).

▶ The Intracor procedure uses the femtosecond laser to create 5 intrastromal ring ablations from an inner diameter of 1.8 mm to an outer diameter of 3.4 mm (Fig 1). These ablations steepen the very central cornea to create a multifocal cornea, theoretically achieving good reading vision while maintaining good uncorrected distance vision in presbyopic patients. Whenever I hear about a procedure that weakens the cornea to produce steepening, I am concerned about the induction

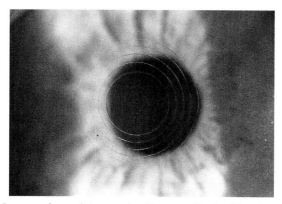

FIGURE 1.—Intrastromal corneal ring cuts placed in an eye. (Reprinted from Journal of Cataract & Refractive Surgery. Menassa N, Fitting A, Auffarth GU, et al. Visual outcomes and corneal changes after intrastromal femtosecond laser correction of presbyopia. *J Cataract Refract Surg.* 2012;38:765-773, Copyright 2012, with permission from ASCRS and ESCRS.)

TABLE 3.—Corneal Steepening (Difference of True Net Power) in the Treated Area in the Visual Axis After Treatment Compared with Preoperatively

Corneal Steepening (D)	1 Mo (n = 24)	3 Mo (n = 24)	6 Mo (n = 22)	12 Mo (n = 24)	18 Mo (n = 22)
Median	+1.05	+0.70	+0.80	+1.00	+0.90
Range	+0.1, +3.5	+0.1, +3.5	0.0, +3.6	0.0, +3.2	−0.8, +3.2
P value*	<.001	<.001	<.001	<.001	.001

*Compared with preoperative measurement (level of significance P =.01).

of corneal ectasia. Those of us who are older can remember the claims of "controlled ectasia" that was said to be created by automated lamellar keratoplasty to treat hyperopia. In these eyes deep (approximately 75% depth) cuts were made with a microkeratome to weaken the cornea. Admittedly, it worked well to weaken and steepen the cornea and improve hyperopia, but many of these eyes developed progressive myopia or excessive steepening, often leading to ectasia and occasionally requiring a corneal transplant.

The authors of this article looked at the results of Intracor in 25 eyes, all examined at 1 year, and 23 eyes, examined at 18 months. Inclusion criteria were presbyopia 2.00 D or more, hyperopia ranging from +0.50 to +1.25 D, and a corneal thickness of at least 500 μm. The most important results are those regarding safety and stability. No patient lost uncorrected near vision at any point. At 12 to 18 months, patients had gained between 1 and 9 lines of uncorrected near vision. At 12 to 18 months, 5 to 7 patients had lost 2 lines or more of uncorrected distance vision, and 5 to 6 patients had lost 2 or more lines of best-corrected distance vision. Some vision loss was said to be related to eye dryness and cataracts. Corneal pachymetry and endothelial cell counts were unchanged from preoperatively to 12 to 18 months postoperatively. Corneal steepening appeared fairly stable, with no trend toward progressive steepening from 1 to 18 months postoperatively (Table 3). Sixteen patients read newspaper print without glasses, while 9 used reading glasses. Intracor is minimally invasive and appears safe in the short term. I am hopeful the clinical results will improve with refinements of the technique and it remains safe and stable with longer-term follow-up.

C. J. Rapuano, MD

Mitomycin C: Biological effects and use in refractive surgery
Santhiago MR, Netto MV, Wilson SE (The Cleveland Clinic, OH)
Cornea 31:311-321, 2012

Purpose.—To provide an overview of the safety and efficacy of mitomycin C (MMC) as adjuvant therapy after refractive surgery procedures.
Methods.—Literature review.
Results.—Over the past 10 years, MMC has been used by refractive surgeons to prophylactically decrease haze after surface ablation procedures and therapeutically in the treatment of preexisting haze. Development of MMC treatments has had a significant role in the revival of surface ablation techniques. We reviewed the literature regarding mechanism of action of MMC, its role in modulating wound healing after refractive surgery, and its safety and efficacy as adjuvant therapy applied after primary photorefractive keratectomy surgery or after photorefractive keratectomy re-treatment after laser in situ keratomileusis and other corneal surgeries and disorders. The drug is a potent mitotic inhibitor that effectively blocks keratocyte activation, proliferation, and myofibroblast differentiation. Many studies have suggested that MMC is safe and effective in doses used by anterior surface surgeons, although there continue to be concerns regarding long-term safety. After initial depletion of anterior keratocytes, keratocyte density seems to return to normal 6 to 12 months after the use of MMC when corneas are examined with the confocal microscope. Most clinical studies found no difference between preoperative and postoperative corneal endothelial cell densities when MMC 0.02% was applied during refractive surgery, with exposure time of 2 minutes or less.
Conclusions.—After more than 10 years of use, MMC has been found to be effective when used for prevention and treatment of corneal haze. Questions remain regarding optimal treatment parameters and long-term safety.

▶ The authors reviewed the world literature on mitomycin-C (MMC) in the setting of refractive surgery. Although they conclude that the use of MMC is generally safe and effective, several questions remain. Most of the animal and human studies show little to no endothelial damage in the concentration and duration times generally used in refractive surgery, but not in all studies. MMC decreases the cellularity of the anterior stroma for at least 6 months, but the clinical significance of this finding is unknown. Fortunately, MMC does not appear to adversely affect re-epithelialization.

Other questions include the optimal concentration and application time. There seems to be a consensus that the best concentration is 0.02% (0.2 mg/mL), but there is no clear consensus on the application time. The authors use 30 seconds in primary cases of photorefractive keratectomy (PRK) and 1 minute in complicated cases, such as button-hole flaps after laser-assisted in-situ keratomileusis (LASIK), PRK after radial keratotomy, PRK after corneal transplantation, or PRK after LASIK. And lastly, should all primary cases of PRK get MMC or only higher risk eyes such as over −3 to −4 D or over 1 D of astigmatism, as many surgeons do? Having used MMC on most of my surface ablation and phototherapeutic keratectomy procedures for many years now, I am confident (and hopeful) that longer-term studies will continue to support the safety and efficacy of MMC.

C. J. Rapuano, MD

Vorinostat: A potent agent to prevent and treat laser-induced corneal haze
Tandon A, Tovey JC, Waggoner MR, et al (Harry S. Truman Memorial Veterans' Hosp, Columbia, MO)
J Refract Surg 28:285-290, 2012

Purpose.—This study investigated the efficacy and safety of vorinostat, a deacetylase (HDAC) inhibitor, in the treatment of laser-induced corneal haze following photorefractive keratectomy (PRK) in rabbits in vivo and transforming growth factor beta 1 (TGFβ1) -induced corneal fibrosis in vitro.

Methods.—Corneal haze in rabbits was produced with −9.00 diopters (D) PRK. Fibrosis in cultured human and rabbit corneal fibroblasts was activated with TGFβ1. Vorinostat (25 µm) was topically applied once for 5 minutes on rabbit cornea immediately after PRK for in vivo studies. Vorinostat (0 to 25 µm) was given to human/rabbit corneal fibroblasts for 5 minutes or 48 hours for in vitro studies. Slit-lamp microscopy, TUNEL assay, and trypan blue were used to determined vorinostat toxicity, whereas real-time polymerase chain reaction, immunocytochemistry, and immunoblotting were used to measure its efficacy.

Results.—Single 5-minute vorinostat (25 µm) topical application on the cornea following PRK significantly reduced corneal haze ($P < .008$) and fibrotic marker proteins (α-smooth muscle actin and f-actin; $P < .001$) without showing redness, swelling, or inflammation in rabbit eyes in vivo screened 4 weeks after PRK. Vorinostat reduced TGFβ1-induced fibrosis in human and rabbit corneas in vitro in a dose-dependent manner without altering cellular viability, phenotype, or proliferation.

Conclusions.—Vorinostat is non-cytotoxic and safe for the eye and has potential to prevent laser-induced corneal haze in patients undergoing PRK for high myopia.

▶ Several years ago I was involved in some studies at Wills Eye, Thomas Jefferson University, evaluating a transforming growth factor-β inhibitor to decrease corneal haze after photorefractive keratectomy (PRK) in rabbits.[1,2] I was the masked observer evaluating the rabbit eyes at a slit lamp for corneal health and corneal haze at various postoperative intervals. Although the compound was well tolerated and seemed to decrease haze, it never went anywhere. Currently, steroids and mitomycin-C are quite effective at minimizing corneal haze after surface ablation. However, they both have potential side effects and complications.

The authors performed in vitro and in vivo studies on 12 rabbits. They performed a -9.00 D PRK treatment in both eyes and applied vorinostat for 5 minutes in 1 eye, with the fellow eye acting as a control. They found no adverse effects and statistically significantly less corneal haze postoperatively in the vorinostat eyes over 4 weeks. Histochemical and histopathologic testing confirmed decreased fibrosis in the vorinostat-treated eyes.

Needless to say, this is a small animal study, but if future testing confirms its safety and efficacy, we may have an alternative to steroids and mitomycin-C to prevent and treat haze after surface ablation. Other uses of vorinostat could potentially include reduction of corneal scarring after corneal ulcers or corneal trauma.

C. J. Rapuano, MD

References

1. Myers JS, Gomes JA, Siepser SB, Rapuano CJ, Eagle RC Jr, Thom SB. Effect of transforming growth factor beta 1 on stromal haze following excimer laser photorefractive keratectomy in rabbits. *J Refract Surg.* 1997;13:356-361.
2. Thom SB, Myers JS, Rapuano CJ, Eagle RC Jr, Siepser SB, Gomes JA. Effect of topical anti-transforming growth factor-beta on corneal stromal haze after Photorefractive Keratectomy in rabbits. *J Cataract Refract Surg.* 1997;23:1324-1330.

Very late onset corneal scar triggered by trauma after photorefractive keratectomy
Gomes BAF, Smadja D, Espana EM, et al (Cleveland Clinic, OH)
J Cataract Refract Surg 38:1694-1697, 2012

A 54-year-old woman who had photorefractive keratectomy (PRK) more than 10 years earlier presented with a history of being hit in the eye by a tree branch and developing blurred vision a short time later. The corrected visual acuity was 20/100 with localized grade 3 stromal haze. The haze intensified despite initial response to corticosteroids and cyclosporine, and treatment with phototherapeutic keratectomy and 0.02% mitomycin-C (MMC) was effective in restoring corneal clarity and normal vision. Late-onset stromal scar can be triggered by trauma years after PRK. Phototherapeutic keratectomy with MMC can be an effective treatment for late-onset scar. Persistent haze or scar after trauma if PRK had not been performed previously is exceedingly rare.

▶ Excimer laser surface ablation (the term used to encompass a variety of techniques, including photorefractive keratectomy [PRK], LASEK [laser-assisted subepithelial keratomileusis], and epi-LASIK [laser-assisted in-situ keratomileusis) seems to have gained popularity over the past 5 years to avoid the complications of a LASIK flap. The downsides of surface ablation compared with LASIK are greater postoperative discomfort, slower visual recovery, and increased risk of haze. Mild haze within the first 3 to 6 months after surface ablation is common. Moderate haze can occur and often responds to topical steroids. Late haze is rare. The authors report a case of late onset corneal scarring 12 years after PRK without mitomycin-C for −4 D of myopia. The patient noted decreased vision and haze or scar soon after being hit in the eye with a tree branch. Haze is often associated with a myopic shift in the refraction, and in this case it was −1.75 D. Even late haze may respond to topical steroids, but it did not in this case. At this point the options include glasses, contact lenses, phototherapeutic keratectomy (PTK), or PRK with or without mitomycin-C. The authors performed PTK with mitomycin-C with an excellent result.

I saw a similar case recently in the resident Cornea Clinic at Wills Eye. Approximately 10 years after PRK, the patient developed significant corneal haze after trauma; he achieved 20/20 vision with −2.5 D sphere. The patient had been seen by several residents and attendings at Wills prior to seeing me. Most attendings wanted to perform a combination of PTK and PRK with mitomycin-C. Some wanted to treat the entire −2.5 D refraction, while others wanted to treat about half of that. I thought it was safest to just do PTK with mitomycin-C and then deal with any residual refractive error as needed at a later date, knowing that removing the haze often reduces the myopia. Six weeks after PTK with mitomycin-C, the patient achieved 20/20 uncorrected vision, which has been stable for 6 months. The take-home message is that post-surface ablation haze induces myopia, but simply treating the haze also treats some or all of the myopia.

C. J. Rapuano, MD

Outcomes of refractive surgery in patients with topographic superior corneal steepening
Kymionis GD, Kankariya VP, Grentzelos MA, et al (Univ of Crete, Greece)
J Refract Surg 28:462-467, 2012

Purpose.—To evaluate the outcomes of refractive surgery in patients with topographic superior corneal steepening.

Methods.—This retrospective, noncomparative, interventional, clinical study included 16 patients (29 eyes) with persistent superior corneal steepening as a variation of corneal curvature (inferior to superior topographic corneal difference of at least 1.00 diopter [D] at a 3-mm zone) not related to any underlying disease or condition who underwent corneal refractive surgery. Refractive, keratometric, and visual outcomes were evaluated preoperatively and at 1, 3, 6, 12, and 24 months postoperatively.

Results.—Twenty-two eyes underwent photorefractive keratectomy and 7 eyes underwent LASIK. Mean follow-up was 27.38 ± 2.37 months (range: 25 to 32 months). Mean preoperative inferior to superior keratometric difference was 1.61 ± 0.36 D (range: 1.20 to 2.63 D). Mean preoperative spherical equivalent refraction was -4.45 ± 1.66 D (range: -2.25 to -8.00 D), which decreased to -0.09 ± 0.61 D (range: +0.75 to -1.38 D) $(P < .05)$ at last follow-up. Mean preoperative topographic corneal astigmatism was

1.44 ± 0.79 D (range: 0.52 to 3.83 D), which decreased to 0.66 ± 0.39 D
($P < .05$) 3 months postoperatively and remained stable during follow-up
($P < .54$). Mean preoperative uncorrected distance visual acuity and corrected distance visual acuity in logMAR units were 1.57 ± 0.62 and
0.02 ± 0.06, respectively, which improved at last follow-up to 0.00 ± 0.05
and -0.02 ± 0.04, respectively. No intra- or postoperative complications
were noted; specifically, no patients developed postoperative ectasia.

Conclusions.—Corneal refractive surgery in patients with isolated topographic superior corneal steepening provided acceptable refractive and
visual outcomes without any intra- or postoperative complications. Dili-
gence is required to screen for the potential of ectatic corneal disorders
in this population. Photorefractive keratectomy may be a safer option
for these patients than LASIK.

▶ Inferior steepening is a red flag during a refractive surgery evaluation, and rightfully so, because it is associated with post-refractive surgery ectasia. But what
about isolated superior steepening? The authors report the 2-year results of photorefractive keratectomy (PRK) or laser in-situ keratomileusis (LASIK) in 29 eyes
of 16 patients with isolated superior steepening. They defined superior steepening
as a difference of > 1 D between the 90° and 270° meridians at the 3-mm zone. To
rule out contact lens warpage as a reason for the superior steepening, all contact
lens wearers were kept out of their contact lenses for 3 months and the topography repeated. Additionally, all patients were followed for 3 months before
surgery to confirm persistence of the superior steepening on topography.

Uncorrected vision improved from a mean of 20/751 to 20/20. Best-corrected
vision improved from a mean of 20/22 to 20/19 at 2 years. A total of 93% of eyes
did not gain or lose any lines of best-corrected vision, whereas 7% (2 eyes) lost
one line of best-corrected vision. The superior steepening persisted on topography in all eyes at 2 years. Although only 7 of the 29 eyes underwent LASIK,
the authors noted that there appeared to be "increased superior steepening over
time" in the LASIK eyes. Consequently, they concluded "PRK may be a safer
option for these patients than LASIK." I am extremely cautious about performing
any refractive surgery in any eye with inferior steepening. I am somewhat less concerned about other mild corneal asymmetries, including superior steepening, but I
agree with the authors that surface ablation is probably a safer option when
dealing with any slightly asymmetric corneal topographic pattern (assuming, of
course, that the rest of the exam is normal).

C. J. Rapuano, MD

Corneal wavefront-guided photorefractive keratectomy with mitomycin-C for hyperopia after radial keratotomy: Two-year follow-up

Ghanem RC, Ghanem VC, Ghanem EA, et al (Sadalla Amin Ghanem Eye Hosp, Joinville, Brazil)
J Cataract Refract Surg 38:595-606, 2012

Purpose.—To assess corneal wavefront-guided photorefractive keratectomy (PRK) to correct hyperopia after radial keratotomy (RK).

Setting.—Sadalla Amin Ghanem Eye Hospital, Joinville, Santa Catarina, Brazil.

Design.—Case series.

Methods.—Excimer laser corneal wavefront-guided PRK with intraoperative mitomycin-C (MMC) 0.02% was performed. Main outcome measures were uncorrected (UDVA) and corrected (CDVA) distance visual acuities, spherical equivalent (SE), corneal aberrations, and haze.

Results.—The mean time between RK and PRK in the 61 eyes (39 patients) was 18.8 years ± 3.8 (SD). Before PRK, the mean SE was +4.17 ± 1.97 diopters (D); the mean astigmatism, −1.39 ± 1.04 D; and the mean CDVA, 0.161 ± 0.137 logMAR. At 24 months, the mean values were 0.14 ± 0.99 D (*P* < .001), −1.19 ± 1.02 D (*P* = .627), and 0.072 ± 0.094 logMAR (*P* < .001), respectively; the mean UDVA was 0.265 ± 0.196 (*P* < .001). The UDVA was 20/25 or better in 37.7% of eyes and 20/40 or better in 68.9%. The CDVA improved by 1 or more lines in 62.3% of eyes. Two eyes (3.3%) lost 2 or more lines, 1 due to corneal ectasia. Thirty eyes (49.2%) were within ±0.50 D of intended SE and 45 (73.8%) were

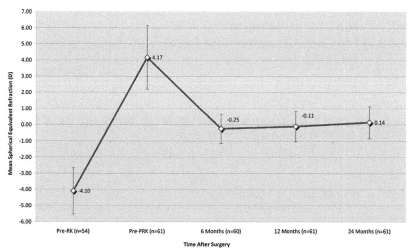

FIGURE 2.—Stability. Change in mean refractive SE over time. Error bars represent ± 1 standard deviation. (Reprinted from Journal of Cataract & Refractive Surgery. Ghanem RC, Ghanem VC, Ghanem EA, et al. Corneal wavefront-guided photorefractive keratectomy with mitomycin-C for hyperopia after radial keratotomy: two-year follow-up. *J Cataract Refract Surg.* 2012;38:595-606, Copyright 2012, with permission from ASCRS and ESCRS.)

within ± 1.00 D. From 6 to 24 months, the mean SE regression was +0.39 D ($P < .05$). A significant decrease in coma, trefoil, and spherical aberration occurred. Three eyes developed peripheral haze more than grade 1.

Conclusion.—Corneal wavefront-guided PRK with MMC for hyperopia after RK significantly improved UDVA, CDVA, and higher-order corneal aberrations with a low incidence of visually significant corneal haze (Fig 2).

▶ The hyperopic drift was one of the main factors that essentially ended the use of radial keratotomy (RK) about 15 years ago. However, we still see patients who are quite unhappy with their hyperopia, even years after RK. Although contact lenses work well in many patients, they aren't successful in everyone. Historically, we have not had a good surgical treatment for these patients.

This study is the largest with the longest follow-up I know of using custom photorefractive keratectomy (PRK) with mitomycin C to treat hyperopia after RK. Inclusion criteria were up to + 8.5 diopters (D) of hyperopia and up to −4.50 D of cylinder, with a central pachymetry of > 490 microns. Interestingly, the authors did not list refractive or topographic stability as a preoperative requirement. All patients were followed up for 2 years. The PRK treatment included mechanical epithelial debridement and mitomycin C for 20 to 40 seconds. (As an aside, you need to be very careful when removing the epithelium in these eyes, as you do not want to open up the old RK incisions.) A target refraction of −1.00 D was used to avoid undercorrection. The refractive and visual results were good to very good, certainly better than previous procedures, such as lasso suturing of the RK incisions and laser-assisted in-situ keratomileusis. The safety results were also quite good, although not perfect. Significant corneal haze did not develop, although one eye had widening of an inferior radial incision that required suturing and ended up with a good result. Although the refractions appeared relatively stable from 6 to 24 months (Fig 2), corneal topography showed a small but statistically significant regression over 1 to 2 years.

Even so, these results are encouraging enough for me to (cautiously) try PRK with mitomycin-C for hyperopia after RK.

C. J. Rapuano, MD

Visual stability of laser vision correction in an astronaut on a Soyuz mission to the International Space Station

Gibson CR, Mader TH, Schallhorn SC, et al (Coastal Eye Associates, Webster, TX; Alaska Native Med Ctr, Anchorage; Univ of California San Francisco, San Diego; et al)
J Cataract Refract Surg 38:1486-1491, 2012

This report documents the effects of photorefractive keratectomy (PRK) in an astronaut during a 12-day Russian Soyuz mission to the International Space Station in 2008. Changing environmental conditions of launch, microgravity exposure, and reentry create an extremely dynamic ocular environment. Although many normal eyes have repeatedly been subject to such stresses, the effect on an eye with a relatively thin cornea as a result of

PRK has not been reported. This report suggests that PRK is a safe, effective, and well-tolerated procedure in astronauts during space flight.

▶ Not that radial keratotomy is being performed much anymore, but fluctuating vision is widely known to be a significant side effect/complication. This was vividly illustrated in Jon Krakauer's superb book *Into Thin Air* about a doomed expedition to summit Mount Everest. Under normal conditions, photorefractive keratectomy (PRK) and laser-assisted in-situ keratomileusis (LASIK) do not experience this problem. PRK was demonstrated not to be susceptible to a refractive shift during 3 consecutive days at 14 000 feet at Pikes Peak, Colorado.[1] With the recent interest in commercial spaceflight, I thought this case report demonstrating stability of near and distance vision 14 years after bilateral PRK for −4D of myopia during a 12-day mission to the International Space Station was reassuring.

C. J. Rapuano, MD

Reference

1. Mader TH, Blanton CL, Gilbert BN, et al. Refractive changes during 72-hour exposure to high altitude after refractive surgery. *Ophthalmology.* 1996;103:1188-1195.

Custom vs Conventional PRK: A Prospective, Randomized, Contralateral Eye Comparison of Postoperative Visual Function

Mifflin MD, Hatch BB, Sikder S, et al (Univ of Utah, Salt Lake City; Univ of Utah School of Medicine, Salt Lake City; Wilmer Eye Inst, Baltimore, MD; et al)
J Refract Surg 28:127-132, 2012

Purpose.—To determine whether VISX S4 (VISX Inc) custom photorefractive keratectomy (PRK) results in better visual outcomes than VISX S4 conventional PRK.

Methods.—Photorefractive keratectomy was performed on 80 eyes from 40 patients in this randomized, prospective, contralateral eye study. Dominant eyes were randomized to one group with the fellow eye receiving the alternate treatment. Primary outcome measures included uncorrected distance visual acuity (UDVA), corrected distance visual acuity (CDVA), contrast sensitivity, and root-mean-square (RMS) higher order aberrations.

Results.—Mean UDVA was −0.023 ± 0.099 (20/19) in the custom group and −0.044 ± 0.080 (20/18) in the conventional group 6 months after surgery ($P = .293$). Mean CDVA was −0.073 ± 0.067 (20/17) in the custom group and −0.079 ± 0.071 (20/17) in the conventional group 6 months after surgery ($P = .659$). Total higher order aberration RMS and spherical aberration increased in both groups compared to preoperative values ($P < .05$). Coma increased in the conventional group ($P < .05$) whereas it was similar to preoperative values in the custom group. No significant differences were noted in induction of trefoil.

Conclusions.—Custom and conventional PRK were shown to be safe and effective with excellent visual acuity and contrast sensitivity performance at

6 and 12 months. Conventional PRK induced more coma than custom PRK; however, this did not seem to correlate with clinical outcomes.

▶ Most surgeons using the VISX excimer laser system believe that custom wavefront treatments are superior to conventional treatments. That would make sense. The preoperative wavefront analysis used for custom treatments has much more detail than the spherocylinder refractive correction used for conventional treatments. How can using all that additional information not give better results? But where is the proof?

This well-done prospective, randomized contralateral eye study looked at the results of 80 eyes of 40 patients undergoing photorefractive keratectomy (PRK). One eye had a custom wavefront treatment, and the fellow eye had a conventional treatment using the VISX laser. Uncorrected and best-corrected visual acuity, total higher order aberrations, and trefoil and spherical aberration were all essentially the same in the 2 groups (Tables 2 and 3 in the original article). Although total higher order aberration and trefoil and spherical aberration were the same in the 2 groups postoperatively, they were all greater than the preoperative values. Coma, on the other hand, was statistically significantly increased in the conventional group ($P < .05$) but was similar to preoperative values in the custom group.

So why do most surgeons feel custom treatments are better than conventional treatments? Perhaps the numbers in the study were too small to show a real difference. Perhaps the testing used just wasn't sensitive enough to show a real clinical difference. Or perhaps, many of us have just blindly accepted industry marketing regarding the superiority of custom treatments.

Larger studies, ideally with more sensitive visual function testing, should give us better answers in the future.

C. J. Rapuano, MD

Accelerated corneal crosslinking concurrent with laser in situ keratomileusis
Celik HU, Alagöz N, Yildirim Y, et al (Beyoglu Eye Training and Res Hosp, Istanbul, Turkey; et al)
J Cataract Refract Surg 38:1424-1431, 2012

Purpose.—To assess accelerated corneal collagen crosslinking (CXL) applied concurrently with laser in situ keratomileusis (LASIK) in a small group of patients.
Setting.—Beyoglu Eye Research and Training Hospital, Istanbul, Turkey.
Design.—Prospective pilot interventional case series.
Methods.—In May 2010, patients had LASIK with concurrent accelerated CXL in 1 eye and LASIK only in the fellow eye to treat myopia or myopic astigmatism. The follow-up was 12 months. The attempted correction (spherical equivalent) ranged from -5.00 to -8.50 diopters (D) in the LASIK–CXL group and from -3.00 to -7.25 D in the LASIK-only group. Main outcome measures were manifest refraction, uncorrected (UDVA) and corrected (CDVA) distance visual acuities, and the endothelial cell count.

Results.—Eight eyes of 3 women and 1 man (age 22 to 39 years old) were enrolled. At the 12-month follow-up, the LASIK–CXL group had a UDVA and manifest refraction equal to or better than those in the LASIK-only group. No eye lost 1 or more lines of CDVA at the final visit. The endothelial cell loss in the LASIK–CXL eye was not greater than in the fellow eye. No side effects were associated with either procedure.

Conclusions.—Laser in situ keratomileusis with accelerated CXL appears to be a promising modality for future applications to prevent corneal ectasia after LASIK treatment. The results in this pilot series suggest that evaluation of a larger study cohort is warranted.

▶ This is a small study: 8 eyes of 4 patients, where 1 eye received the collagen crosslinking, and the fellow eye did not. It was sponsored by Avedro, and 2 of the authors are paid consultants to Avedro. Having said that, this study brings up numerous interesting issues. Since the incidence of corneal ectasia after laser in situ keratomileusis (LASIK) is so low and often occurs many years postoperatively, how large and how long a study would be required to determine whether this treatment actually decreases the risk of ectasia? Although the authors stated that the purpose of the collagen crosslinking procedure was to avoid ectasia, another question is whether such a treatment decreases the incidence of regression of myopia after LASIK. That leads to the issue regarding which patients should receive this treatment—only those at higher risk for ectasia or everyone? Other questions are: Since the collagen crosslinking treatment often flattens keratoconic corneas, is a nomogram adjustment needed when used with LASIK? Are shorter treatment times using higher ultraviolet-A power (they used 30 mW/cm^2 for 3 minutes) better than the standard treatment (3 mW/cm^2 for 30 minutes)? What are the optimal power and exposure times? What should the additional cost to the patient be for this treatment? Only much larger studies with longer follow-up will begin to answer some of these questions.

C. J. Rapuano, MD

Elevated intraocular pressure-induced interlamellar stromal keratitis occurring 9 years after laser in situ keratomileusis
Lee V, Sulewski ME, Zaidi A, et al (Scheie Eye Inst, Philadelphia, PA)
Cornea 31:87-89, 2012

Elevated intraocular pressure-induced interlamellar stromal keratitis (PISK) is an entity of interface haze usually occurring weeks to months after laser in situ keratomileusis (LASIK) that is associated with elevated intraocular pressures and worsening with steroid treatment. There is evidence that this interface haze is the result of abnormal fluid dynamics that occur in the cornea after LASIK. We present a case of pressure-induced interlamellar stromal keratitis occurring 9 years after LASIK in the setting of anterior uveitis. This case emphasizes the importance of considering such diagnoses as pressure-induced interlamellar stromal keratitis in the differential diagnosis when presented with a patient with corneal haze and a history of LASIK.

▶ This case report brings up several important points:

1. Pressure-induced stromal keratitis (PISK) and diffuse lamellar keratitis (DLK), for that matter, can occur many years after laser in-situ keratomileusis (LASIK).

2. When asked about their ocular history, many patients will not state that they had LASIK, so technicians and physicians may have to ask patients specifically about this part of their ocular history.

3. PISK and DLK can look quite similar on slit-lamp examination. PISK can cause a fluid-filled cleft in the LASIK flap interface, which can give a falsely low intraocular pressure (IOP) measurement. This situation often reinforces the presumed diagnosis of DLK and steroids are increased, further raising the real IOP, causing more interface fluid and further lowering the IOP measurements. In these cases, the IOP should be measured peripherally to the LASIK flap. This is best done with a Tono-Pen and/or pneumotonometer. It is extremely important to get an accurate IOP measurement in the eyes with possible DLK or PISK.

4. PISK responds fairly rapidly when the IOP is normalized. You would think that 9 years after LASIK, the cornea would behave like a "virgin" cornea, but it just isn't so.

C. J. Rapuano, MD

Interface fluid syndrome in routine cataract surgery 10 years after laser in situ keratomileusis
Ortega-Usobiaga J, Martin-Reyes C, Llovet-Osuna F, et al (Instituto Oftalmológico Europeo, Madrid, Spain)
Cornea 31:706-707, 2012

Purpose.—Interface fluid syndrome is an unusual complication after laser in situ keratomileusis (LASIK). We present a case of interface fluid syndrome after cataract surgery in a patient who had previous LASIK surgery.

Methods.—A 62-year-old man underwent routine cataract surgery on the left eye 10 years after LASIK on both eyes. The day after surgery, the intraocular pressure (IOP) was 21 mm Hg and a pocket of fluid was present in the interface LASIK wound. The patient was treated with 0.50% timolol eye drops twice daily.

Results.—The problem resolved within 1.5 months. Two months later, the patient underwent routine cataract surgery of the right eye. The next day, the IOP was 11 mm Hg and LASIK interface fluid was present. The patient was treated with 0.5% timolol eye drops twice daily. Two months after the surgery, the problem had completely resolved.

Conclusions.—Ocular hypertension and traumatic endothelial cell damage could have been the causes of the syndrome. Although the IOP was not very high, previous LASIK could have led us to underestimate the IOP.

▶ The authors state that the "IOP [intraocular pressure] was not very high" but admit they measured the IOP with Goldmann applanation in the center portion of the cornea. Given the interface fluid they saw at the slit lamp, Goldmann applanation at the center of the cornea does NOT measure intraocular pressure but rather some sort of fluid cleft pressure. I suspect the real IOP was quite high, perhaps related to retained viscoelastic causing pressure-induced stromal keratitis. Even 10 years after laser in situ keratomileusis!

C. J. Rapuano, MD

IntraLase femtosecond laser vs mechanical microkeratomes in LASIK for myopia: A systematic review and meta-analysis
Chen S, Feng Y, Stojanovic A, et al (The Affiliated Eye Hosp, Zhejiang, China)
J Refract Surg 28:15-24, 2012

Purpose.—To evaluate the safety, efficacy, and predictability of Intra-Lase (Abbott Medical Optics) femtosecond laser-assisted compared to microkeratome-assisted myopic LASIK.
Methods.—A comprehensive literature search of Cochrane Library, PubMed, and EMBASE was conducted to identify relevant trials comparing LASIK with IntraLase femtosecond laser to LASIK with microkeratomes for the correction of myopia. Meta-analyses were performed on the primary outcomes (loss of ≥2 lines of corrected distance visual acuity [CDVA], uncorrected distance visual acuity [UDVA] 20/20 or better, manifest refraction spherical equivalent [MRSE] within ± 0.50 diopters [D], final refractive SE, and astigmatism), and secondary outcomes (flap thickness predictability, changes in higher order aberrations [HOAs], and complications).

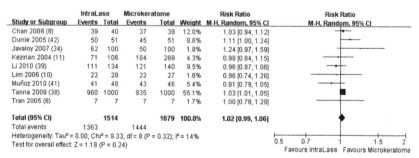

FIGURE 2.—Proportion of eyes with uncorrected distance visual acuity 20/20 or better after IntraLase femtosecond laser versus microkeratome LASIK. CI = confidence interval, df = degrees of freedom, I^2 = extent of inconsistency, Z = overall effect. (Reprinted with permission from SLACK Incorporated. Chen S, Feng Y, Stojanovic A, et al. IntraLase femtosecond laser vs mechanical microkeratomes in LASIK for myopia: a systematic review and meta-analysis. *J Refract Surg.* 2012;28:15-24, with permission from SLACK Incorporated.)

Study or Subgroup	IntraLase			Microkeratome			Weight	Mean Difference IV, Random, 95% CI	Mean Difference IV, Random, 95% CI
	Mean	SD	Total	Mean	SD	Total			
Alió 2008 (36)	0.041	0.17	20	0.032	0.19	40	2.0%	0.01 [-0.09, 0.10]	
Calvo 2010 (40)	-0.01	0.14	20	0.004	0.15	20	2.2%	-0.01 [-0.10, 0.08]	
Javaloy 2007 (34)	0.041	0.2	100	0.065	0.2	100	5.8%	-0.02 [-0.08, 0.03]	
Montés-Micó 2007 (9)	-0.04	0.09	100	-0.01	0.1	100	25.5%	-0.03 [-0.06, -0.00]	
Muñoz 2010 (41)	-0.02	0.06	48	-0.02	0.05	46	35.7%	0.00 [-0.02, 0.02]	
Patel 2007 (7)	0.01	0.11	21	-0.02	0.12	21	3.7%	0.03 [-0.04, 0.10]	
Rosa 2009 (37)	0.03	0.03	40	0.04	0.08	40	25.3%	-0.01 [-0.04, 0.02]	
Total (95% CI)			349			367	100.0%	-0.01 [-0.02, 0.00]	

Heterogeneity: Tau² = 0.00; Chi² = 4.65, df = 6 (P = 0.59); I² = 0%
Test for overall effect: Z = 1.56 (P = 0.12)

-0.2 -0.1 0 0.1 0.2
Favours IntraLase   Favours Microkeratome

FIGURE 3.—Mean uncorrected distance visual acuity (logMAR) after IntraLase femtosecond laser versus microkeratome LASIK. SD = standard deviation, CI = confidence interval, df = degrees of freedom, I² = extent of inconsistency, Z = overall effect. (Reprinted with permission from SLACK Incorporated. Chen S, Feng Y, Stojanovic A, et al. IntraLase femtosecond laser vs mechanical microkeratomes in LASIK for myopia: a systematic review and meta-analysis. *J Refract Surg.* 2012;28:15-24, with permission from SLACK Incorporated.)

Results.—Fifteen articles describing a total of 3679 eyes were identified. No significant differences were identified between the two groups in regards to a loss of ≥2 lines of CDVA ($P = .44$), patients achieving UDVA 20/20 or better ($P = .24$), final UDVA ($P = .12$), final mean refractive SE ($P = .74$), final astigmatism ($P = .27$), or changes in HOAs. The IntraLase group had more patients who were within ±0.50 D of target refraction ($P = .05$) compared to the microkeratome group, and flap thickness was more predictable in the IntraLase group ($P < .0001$). The microkeratome group had more epithelial defects ($P = .04$), whereas the IntraLase group had more cases of diffuse lamellar keratitis ($P = .01$).

Conclusions.—According to the available data, LASIK with the IntraLase femtosecond laser offers no significant benefits over LASIK with microkeratomes in regards to safety and efficacy, but has potential advantages in predictability (Figs 2 and 3).

▶ Meta-analyses combine data from multiple similar studies to increase the power of the findings. Although the 15 studies included in this meta-analysis are similar, they are not identical. The IntraLase was the only femtosecond laser used, but a variety of different modules, with different repetition rates, were employed. At least 5 different mechanical microkeratomes were used. Follow-up in these studies ranged from 3 to 48 months. Perhaps the biggest drawback of meta-analyses is that they are, by design, evaluating somewhat old data. Publication dates for studies included in this meta-analysis range from 2004 to 2010, meaning the actual surgeries were completed well before that. The fastest IntraLase in the studies included was 60 kHz. The current model is 150 kHz. Additionally, there are several other femtosecond laser flap makers available today. One of the most common mechanical microkeratomes used today, the Amadeus, was not included in any of the studies in this meta-analysis.

The results did not show any significant benefits of the femtosecond laser over the microkeratomes in either safety or efficacy (Figs 2 and 3). They did find more epithelial defects in the microkeratome eyes and more diffuse lamellar keratitis in the femtosecond laser eyes. Fortunately, both of these issues are less common today with newer technology. I believe the trend toward surgeons creating more femtosecond laser flaps and fewer microkeratome flaps will continue. The reasons include better predictability of flap size and thickness. Additionally, the size, thickness, shape, hinge location, and side-cut angle are infinitely more customizable with a femtosecond laser than a mechanical microkeratome. As technology continues to advance, femtosecond lasers may surpass the microkeratome in safety and efficacy at some point, but not quite yet according to this study.

C. J. Rapuano, MD

Clinical grading of post-LASIK ectasia related to visual limitation and predictive factors for vision loss
Brenner LF, Alió JL, Vega-Estrada A, et al (Vissum Instituto Oftalmologico de Alicante, Spain; et al)
J Cataract Refract Surg 38:1817-1826, 2012

Purpose.—To evaluate and characterize the main clinical features of post-laser in situ keratomileusis (LASIK) ectasia, propose a grading system based on visual limitation, and identify predictive factors related to the degree of visual loss.

Setting.—Vissum Corp., Alicante, Spain.

Design.—Retrospective case series.

Methods.—This study comprised consecutive eyes with corneal ectasia after LASIK from 1996 to 2010. Main outcomes were post-LASIK ectasia corrected distance visual acuity (CDVA), CDVA loss, spherical equivalent (SE), and the corneal bulge (delta K). These outcomes were correlated with the residual stromal bed, ablation depth, ablation ratio (ablation depth:pachymetry), corneal depth (flap + ablation depth), and corneal ratio (corneal depth:pachymetry) to characterize their role in the severity of the disease.

Results.—The mean post-LASIK ectasia CDVA, CDVA loss, SE, and delta K were 0.20 logMAR ± 0.18 (SD), −0.13 ± 0.15 logMAR, −3.80 ± 3.86 diopters (D), and 4.77 ± 4.23 D, respectively. The ablation ratio had the strongest correlation with post-LASIK ectasia CDVA ($\rho = 0.477$ and $P < .001$), whereas the corneal ratio had the strongest correlation with the post-LASIK ectasia SE and delta K ($\rho = -0.614$ and $\rho = 0.453$, respectively: $P < .001$). The ablation ratio was the main predictive factor for post-LASIK ectasia CDVA loss (relative risk, 2.04; $P = .049$).

Conclusions.—The grading system based on visual limitation was consistently represented by differences in CDVA loss, SE, and delta K. A high amount of tissue removed by the refractive procedure was associated with greater corneal biomechanical destabilization, increased corneal steepening, and a worse prognosis (Fig 1, Table 4).

► Because of the devastating visual consequences of post—laser-assisted in-situ keratomileusis (LASIK) ectasia, most published reports on this topic have, rightfully, focused on preoperative risk factors and ways to avoid performing LASIK in high-risk eyes. The authors of this article take a different but interesting approach. They studied all the eyes with post-LASIK ectasia in 2 large refractive surgery

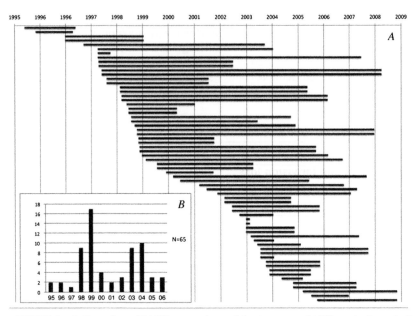

FIGURE 1.—*A*: Gantt chart of LASIK surgery date and the time to post-LASIK ectasia diagnosis. *B*: Bimodal distribution (1998 to 1999 and 2003 to 2004) of LASIK surgeries that resulted in post-LASIK ectasia. (Reprinted from Journal of Cataract & Refractive Surgery. Brenner LF, Alió JL, Vega-Estrada A, et al. Clinical grading of post-LASIK ectasia related to visual limitation and predictive factors for vision loss. *J Cataract Refract Surg.* 2012;38:1817-1826, Copyright 2012, with permission from ASCRS and ESCRS.)

centers. They included 96 eyes, but complete pre- and intraoperative data were not available for all eyes. Instead of looking at risk factors for the development of post-LASIK ectasia, they looked at the risk factors for severity of post-LASIK ectasia, primarily measured by visual loss.

They found an interesting bimodal distribution of when these eyes with ectasia were operated on, peaking in 1999 and again in 2004 (Fig 1), although they do not postulate a reason. Not surprisingly, 58 of the 77 eyes (75%) that had preoperative corneal topography available were considered keratoconus suspects. About half of the eyes had intraoperative pachymetry of the stromal bed performed and half did not. Mean residual stromal bed depth was 349 μm and 328 μm in the 2 groups, respectively. They looked at 2 specific ratios of the amount of tissue removed from individual corneas as possible predictors of the severity of post-LASIK ectasia. One was the ablation ratio, which is ablation depth/pachymetry. The other was the corneal ratio, which is corneal depth (flap thickness + ablation depth)/pachymetry.

The authors found that these 2 ratios had a stronger correlation with severity of ectasia than the residual stromal bed depth (Table 4). It makes sense to me that a theoretical safe residual stromal bed depth would be different for a cornea that started off at 500 μm thick than a cornea that started off at 600 μm thick. Although this is certainly interesting, the goal is to avoid post-LASIK ectasia. The next step is to compare these ratios with ratios in eyes that did not have post-LASIK ectasia and see if there is an ablation ratio or corneal ratio threshold that accurately

TABLE 4.—Intraoperative Data According to the Level of Visual Limitation

| | CDVA Ectasia Group (LogMAR) | | | | |
| | Group 1 | Group 2 | Group 3 | Group 4 | |
Parameter	CDVA ≤ 0.05	0.05 < CDVA ≤ 0.15	0.15 < CDVA ≤ 0.30	CDVA > 0.30	P Value*
CCT (μm)					
Mean ± SD	532.25 ± 19.98	527.05 ± 22.30	534.58 ± 23.52	538.31 ± 29.68	.850
Range	500 to 560	490 to 570	510 to 588	502 to 598	
AD (μm)					
Mean ± SD	88.20 ± 32.10	97.00 ± 42.62	107.66 ± 36.50	131.52 ± 36.65	.006†
Range	45 to 152	30 to 156	51 to 160	72 to 219	
AR (%)					
Mean ± SD	15.10 ± 5.44	17.92 ± 8.18	18.88 ± 6.93	23.25 ± 6.04	.014†
Range	8.49 to 27.14	6.12 to 29.43	10.00 to 30.53	13.16 to 34.21	
CD (μm)					
Mean ± SD	179.88 ± 37.81	197.94 ± 44.76	201.80 ± 38.70	233.73 + 36 46	005†
Range	103 to 262	121 to 257	131 to 256	175 to 298	
CR (%)					
Mean ± SD	33.81 ± 7.03	37.52 ± 8.13	37.40 ± 6.88	43.45 ± 7.38	.008‡
Range	19.00 to 46.79	22.32 to 48.30	25.69 to 47.23	31.99 to 55.19	
RSB (μm)					
Mean ± SD	352.37 ± 40.65	329.11 ± 44.52	337.20 ± 37.66	306.00 ± 49.37	.039†
Range	285 to 439	274 to 421	286 to 394	240 to 373	

AD = ablation depth; AR = ablation ratio; CCT = central corneal thickness; CD = corneal depth; CR = corneal ratio; RSB = residual stromal depth
*One-way analysis of variance except CCT (Kruskal-Wallis test)
†Statistical significance between Group 1 and Group 4 and between Group 2 and Group 4 (Student t test)
‡Statistical significance between all pairs of Groups, except between Group 2 and Group 3 (Student t test)

predicts post-LASIK ectasia. We could then apply these ratios preoperatively to decrease the risk of this complication.

C. J. Rapuano, MD

Prospective, Randomized Comparison of Self-reported Postoperative Dry Eye and Visual Fluctuation in LASIK and Photorefractive Keratectomy

Murakami Y, Manche EE (Stanford Univ School of Medicine, CA)
Ophthalmology 119:2220-2224, 2012

Purpose.—We sought to prospectively compare postoperative symptoms of dry eye, visual fluctuations, and foreign body sensation in patients undergoing LASIK and photorefractive keratectomy (PRK).

Design.—Randomized clinical trial.

Participants.—Sixty-eight eyes of 34 patients were treated with wavefront-guided LASIK and PRK.

Methods.—One eye was treated with LASIK and the fellow eye was treated with PRK. Eyes were randomized by ocular dominance. Patients completed a questionnaire preoperatively and at each postoperative visit evaluating symptoms of dry eye, dry eye severity, vision fluctuations, and foreign body sensation.

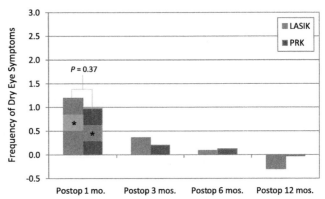

FIGURE 2.—Mean difference in frequency of dry eye symptom scores compared with the preoperative baseline evaluation (*P < 0.05). Postop = postoperative; PRK = photorefractive keratectomy. (Reprinted from Murakami Y, Manche EE. Prospective, randomized comparison of self-reported postoperative dry eye and visual fluctuation in LASIK and photorefractive keratectomy. *Ophthalmology.* 2012;119:2220-2224, with permission from the American Academy of Ophthalmology.)

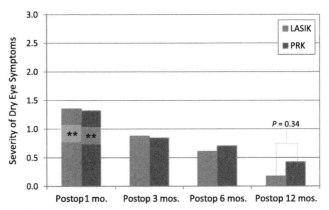

FIGURE 3.—Mean difference in severity of dry eye symptom scores compared with the preoperative baseline evaluation (**P < 0.01). Postop = postoperative; PRK = photorefractive keratectomy. (Reprinted from Murakami Y, Manche EE. Prospective, randomized comparison of self-reported postoperative dry eye and visual fluctuation in LASIK and photorefractive keratectomy. *Ophthalmology.* 2012;119:2220-2224, with permission from the American Academy of Ophthalmology.)

Main Outcome Measures.—Change in self-reported dry eye with secondary outcome measure of visual fluctuations and foreign body sensation scores after LASIK and PRK.

Results.—Both groups of eyes experienced significant increases in symptoms of dry eye, vision fluctuation, and foreign body sensation after LASIK and PRK at postoperative months 1, 3, and 6. However, by the 12-month postoperative visit, there was no increase in dry eye symptoms over the preoperative baseline levels in either group. Patients undergoing PRK experienced significantly higher levels of vision fluctuation at postoperative month 1 than those undergoing LASIK.

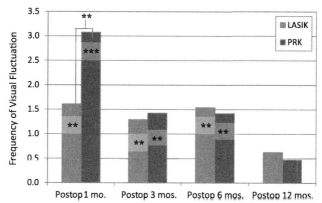

FIGURE 4.—Mean difference in frequency of visual fluctuation scores compared with the preoperative baseline evaluation (**$P < 0.01$; ***$P < 0.001$). Postop = postoperative; PRK = photorefractive keratectomy. (Reprinted from Ophthalmology. Murakami Y, Manche EE. Prospective, randomized comparison of self-reported postoperative dry eye and visual fluctuation in LASIK and photorefractive keratectomy. *Ophthalmology*. 2012;119:2220-2224, Copyright 2012, with permission from the American Academy of Ophthalmology.)

Conclusions.—Both LASIK and PRK caused an increase in dry eye symptoms and severity, vision fluctuations, and foreign body sensation over baseline in the early postoperative period. At postoperative month 1, PRK caused greater vision fluctuations than LASIK. By 1 year postoperatively, all symptoms of dry eye, vision fluctuations, and foreign body sensation returned to their baseline, preoperative levels (Figs 2-4).

▶ This well-done study looked at an important clinical question—does laser assisted in-situ keratomileusis (LASIK) cause more or worse dry eye than photorefractive keratectomy (PRK)? The LASIK technique in this study involved a 9.2-mm diameter, superior-hinged, 100-μm thick, femtosecond laser flap. The PRK technique was not specified (for some reason). They excluded patients with greater than 6 diopters (D) of spherical myopia and with greater than 3 D of astigmatism. They also, understandably, excluded patients with severe dry eyes or severe blepharitis.

They found increased visual fluctuations compared with preoperative levels in both the LASIK and PRK eyes at 1, 3, and 6 months but not at 12 months (Fig 4). The frequency and severity of dry eye symptoms increased significantly at 1 month but was back to baseline by 3 months, in both the LASIK and PRK eyes (Figs 2 and 3). Also of interest, they found no effects of patient age or central corneal ablation depth on any reported symptoms.

My main issue with this study is that they did not evaluate slit lamp findings, including vital dye staining, punctate epithelial erosions, or Schirmer's testing. They relied solely on answers to preoperative and postoperative questions. Although patients' symptoms are extremely important, objective data from the corneal surface would have been very nice to see.

C. J. Rapuano, MD

Precision of a Commercial Hartmann-Shack Aberrometer: Limits of Total Wavefront Laser Vision Correction

López-Miguel A, Maldonado MJ, Belzunce A, et al (Univ of Valladolid, Spain; Clínica Universidad de Navarra, Pamplona, Spain; et al)

Am J Ophthalmol 154:799-807.e5, 2012

Purpose.—To assess the intrasession and intersession precision of higher-order aberrations (HOAs) measured using a commercial Hartmann-Shack wavefront sensor (Zywave; Bausch & Lomb) in refractive surgery candidates.

Design.—Prospective, experimental study of a device.

Methods.—To analyze intrasession repeatability, 1 experienced examiner measured 30 healthy eyes 5 times successively. To study intersession reproducibility, the same clinician obtained measurements from another 30 eyes in 2 consecutive sessions at the same time of day 1 week apart.

Results.—For intrasession repeatability, excellent intraclass correlation coefficients (ICCs) were obtained for total ocular aberrations, total HOAs, and second-order terms (ICC, > 0.94). The ICCs for third-order terms also were high (ICCs, > 0.87); however, fourth-order ICCs varied from 0.71 to 0.90 ($Z_4^0 = 0.90$); and fifth-order ICCs were less than 0.85. For intersession reproducibility, only total ocular aberrations, total ocular HOAs, second-order terms, Z_4^0, Z_3^1, and Z_3^3 had ICCs of 0.90 or more. Bland-Altman analysis showed that the limits of agreement (were clinically too wide for most higher-order Zernike terms, especially for the third-order terms (>0.21 µm).

Conclusions.—Total ocular aberrations, total HOAs, and second-order terms can be measured reliably by Zywave aberrometry without anatomic recognition. Third-order terms and Z_4^0 are repeatable, but not as reproducible between visits. Fourth-order terms, except for Z_4^0, and fifth-order terms are not sufficiently reliable for clinical decision making or treatment. Because the variability of Zywave can be a major limitation of a truly successful wavefront-guided excimer laser procedure, surgeons should consider treating HOA magnitudes that are more than the intrasession repeatability values ($2.77 \times S_w$) as those presented in this study.

▶ The promise of wavefront-guided treatments was super visual acuity in addition to super quality of vision in most, if not all, patients. Why has this not occurred? There are certainly a large number of reasons, but these authors highlight one reason for this particular aberrometer. It could not reproduce third-order aberrations between visits and most fourth-order and all fifth-order aberrations on multiple measurements on the same visit. You have to be able to accurately measure something if you want to reliably get rid of it. Other aberrometers, especially those with some type of anatomic recognition such as iris registration or tracking, may be better, but then again, they may not.

C. J. Rapuano, MD

Intraoperative cyclorotation and pupil centroid shift during LASIK and PRK

Narváez J, Brucks M, Zimmerman G, et al (Loma Linda Univ, CA)
J Refract Surg 28:353-357, 2012

Purpose.—To determine the degree of cyclorotation and centroid shift in the x and y axis that occurs intraoperatively during LASIK and photorefractive keratectomy (PRK).

Methods.—Intraoperative cyclorotation and centroid shift were measured in 63 eyes from 34 patients with a mean age of 34 years (range: 20 to 56 years) undergoing either LASIK or PRK. Preoperatively, an iris image of each eye was obtained with the VISX WaveScan Wavefront System (Abbott Medical Optics Inc) with iris registration. A VISX Star S4 (Abbott Medical Optics Inc) laser was later used to measure cyclotorsion and pupil centroid shift at the beginning of the refractive procedure and after flap creation or epithelial removal.

Results.—The mean change in intraoperative cyclorotation was $1.48 \pm 1.11°$ in LASIK eyes and $2.02 \pm 2.63°$ in PRK eyes. Cyclorotation direction changed by $>2°$ in 21% of eyes after flap creation in LASIK and in 32% of eyes after epithelial removal in PRK. The respective mean intraoperative shift in the x axis and y axis was 0.13 ± 0.15 mm and 0.17 ± 0.14 mm, respectively, in LASIK eyes, and 0.09 ± 0.07 mm and 0.10 ± 0.13 mm, respectively, in PRK eyes. Intraoperative centroid shifts >100 μm in either the x axis or y axis occurred in 71% of LASIK eyes and 55% of PRK eyes.

Conclusions.—Significant changes in cyclotorsion and centroid shifts were noted prior to surgery as well as intraoperatively with both LASIK and PRK. It may be advantageous to engage iris registration immediately prior to ablation to provide a reference point representative of eye position at the initiation of laser delivery.

▶ The importance of accurate alignment of the axis of astigmatism for refractive surgery (or for glasses, for that matter) should be a no-brainer to anyone performing refractive surgery. Correction for the centroid shift is not as intuitive. Because laser treatments are generally centered on the middle of the entrance pupil, and it is well-known that the middle of the pupil typically shifts slightly nasally as the pupil shrinks (such as under the bright light of the laser), the laser will treat slightly different areas of the cornea depending on the pupil size. Laser system software can correct for this centroid shift. There is some evidence that $> 2°$ of cyclorotation or > 100 micron pupil centroid shift can adversely affect the clinical results of laser refractive surgery.

It is old news that cyclotorsion and centroid shift can change substantially from the seated WaveScan measurement to the supine position under the laser. What this article demonstrates is that both of these parameters can change from before laser in-situ keratomileusis (LASIK) flap creation or epithelial removal in photorefractive keratectomy (PRK) to after LASIK flap creation or epithelial removal. A total of 21% and 32% of eyes during LASIK and PRK, respectively, had a greater than $2°$ of cyclorotation during surgery. A total of 71% and 55% of eyes during

LASIK and PRK, respectively, had a centroid shift > 100 microns intraoperatively. The authors conclude that it may be better to engage iris registration just prior to the laser ablation rather than before LASIK flap creation or epithelial removal during PRK, to achieve the best results.

They also acknowledge that cyclorotation and centroid shift likely change during the actual ablation that is not compensated for in static systems such as the VISX laser. Presumably these changes are small. Then the authors go on to recommend that preoperative limbal marks should be considered. It is inexplicable to me how limbal marks are at all useful when iris registration is captured preoperatively and intraoperatively. The surgeon certainly cannot move the eye or head with any accuracy during the laser treatment to compensate for slight cyclotorsion or centroid shift during the laser ablation. The time when limbal marks are useful is when iris registration cannot be captured preoperatively or intraoperatively. Interestingly, in this study, iris registration could be captured in 100% of eyes before LASIK flap creation or epithelial removal for PRK, but only 93% to 94% after LASIK flap lift or epithelial removal. Limbal marks may be beneficial in these 6% to 7% of eyes. The problem is, you can't necessarily predict preoperatively which eyes will or won't be captured with iris registration intraoperatively, and therefore limbal marks may be useful in everyone, especially if they have a high degree of astigmatism.

C. J. Rapuano, MD

Initial surface temperature of PMMA plates used for daily laser calibration affects the predictability of corneal refractive surgery
Wernli J, Schumacher S, Wuellner C, et al (IROC Science to Innovation AG, Zurich, Switzerland)
J Refract Surg 28:639-644, 2012

Purpose.—To investigate the relevance of initial temperature of the polymethylmethacrylate (PMMA) plates used as a target for photoablation during calibration of excimer lasers performed in daily clinical routine.

Methods.—An experimental argon fluoride excimer laser with a repetition rate of 1050 Hz, a radiant exposure of 500 mJ/cm^2, and single pulse energy of 2.1 mJ was used for photoablation of PMMA plates. The initial plate temperature varied from 10.1°C to 75.7°C. The initial temperature was measured with an infrared camera and the central ablation depth of a myopic ablation of −9.00 diopters (D) with an optical zone of 6.5 mm was measured by means of a surface profiling system.

Results.—The ablation depth increased linearly from 73.9 to 96.3 μm within a temperature increase from 10.1°C to 75.7°C (increase rate of 0.3192 μm/K). The linear correlation was found to be significant ($P < .05$) with a coefficient of determination of $R^2 = 0.95$. Based on these results and assuming a standard room temperature of 20°C, optimal plate temperature was calculated to be 15°C to 25°C to maintain an ablation within 0.25 D.

Conclusions.—The temperature of PMMA plates for clinical laser calibration should be controlled ideally within a range of approximately

± 5°C, to avoid visually significant refractive error due to calibration error. Further experimental investigations are required to determine the influence of different initial corneal temperatures on the refractive outcome.

▶ It is well known that environmental conditions in the laser room, especially ambient temperature and humidity, can affect the accuracy of the excimer laser ablation. For example, high humidity can lead to undercorrection, most likely because of a combination of (1) the humid air blocking some of the intensity of the excimer laser beam and (2) the humid air decreasing evaporation of water from the corneal surface so more water and less tissue is ablated per laser pulse. Some of this variability is compensated for by the calibration of the plastic plate performed just prior to surgery.

Most other lasers that are used in ophthalmology (eg, the argon or Nd:YAG) can be adjusted intraoperatively if the initial power seems too strong or too week. However, it is impossible to determine whether too much or too little power is being emitted from the excimer laser during a treatment. Therefore, we rely on how the laser ablates a polymethylmethacrylate test plate prior to treating a patient. The test plate is ablated, the plate is measured to see exactly how much was ablated, and the laser is adjusted accordingly. Each laser has its own specific recommendation as to how to measure and adjust the power emitted from the laser prior to treating a patient.

The authors investigate the interesting question of whether the temperature of the test plate affects its ablatability. As it turns out, it does. Warmer test plates ablate more easily. Having said that, they tested plates ranging from 10.1°C (50°F) to 75.7°C (168°F), which is quite a large range. But given the fact that there are no regulations or even recommendations on the storage of the plates, one could imagine plates being kept in a box in a vehicle parked in freezing cold or extremely hot temperature or being stored indoors next to a heating vent or in direct sunlight. Fig 4 in the original article illustrates the "allowed range" of temperatures that would result in less than 0.25 D error for treatments from low to high myopia, assuming a room temperature of 68°F. The authors conclude that test plates should be kept between 64°F and 72°F to maintain excellent refractive accuracy. Test plate temperature is another variable to keep in mind when trying to obtain the best possible clinical laser vision correction outcomes.

C. J. Rapuano, MD

3 Glaucoma

A Comparison of Active Ingredients and Preservatives Between Brand Name and Generic Topical Glaucoma Medications Using Liquid Chromatography-Tandem Mass Spectrometry

Kahook MY, Fechtner RD, Katz LJ, et al (Univ of Colorado Hosp Eye Ctr, Aurora; UMDNJ-New Jersey Med School, Newark; Thomas Jefferson Univ, Philadelphia, PA; et al)

Curr Eye Res 37:101-108, 2012

Background.—This work compares the concentration of active ingredients and preservatives in commonly used brand name versus generic glaucoma medications.

Materials and Methods.—Active ingredient and benzalkonium chloride (BAK) concentrations in brand name latanoprost and dorzolamide-timolol were each compared to two generic counterparts using liquid chromatography—mass spectrometry at baseline and after exposure to 25°C and 50°C for 30 days. Micro flow imaging was used to quantify particulate material greater than one micron in diameter.

Results.—Brand name formulations contained active ingredients and BAK in concentrations that were generally in agreement with their package inserts at baseline. The two generic formulations of latanoprost contained baseline levels of active ingredients that were 10% greater than their labeled value. Generic latanoprost formulations had significant loss of active ingredient concentration after exposure to 25°C and 50°C for 30 days. Both generic and brand name dorzolamide-timolol appeared relatively resistant to degradation. BAK concentrations remained stable at 25°C but decreased in some bottles at 50°C. Bottles of both generic medications had higher levels of particulate matter compared to brand name versions.

Conclusions.—Exposure to temperatures at the high end of the labeled value may lead to a significant decrease in concentration of active ingredients in generic formulations that could influence clinical efficacy. Re-evaluation of intraocular pressure lowering efficacy may be indicated in glaucoma patients switching from brand name to generic formulations.

▶ Patients and physicians often wonder if generic medications are truly the same as innovator products. Historically, this is a valid question because regulations of the US Food and Drug Administration (FDA) have changed over the years, and products introduced prior to certain dates are not the same. In 1984, Congress passed the Hatch-Waxman Act (Drug Price Competition and Patent Term Restoration Act) to facilitate approval of lower cost generic alternatives to innovator drugs through abbreviated applications. Prior to 1992, the FDA required generic products to have the same active ingredients, but not the same inactive ingredients. However, it is now widely known that using different inactive ingredients results in different efficacy and tolerability profiles. Further, similar but different innovator products may be mistaken for generic equivalents of each other. Prior to 1962, companies submitted products with the same active ingredients for approval that were never intended to be the same products—prednisolone acetate and prednisolone phosphate are a good example.[1] After 1992, FDA requirements for generics stipulate that all components, active and inactive, must be present in the same concentration as the innovator drug.

Despite improved regulation of the composition of generic products, there is still concern in the ophthalmic community that generics and innovator products are not equivalent. This study indicates that generic products behave differently in certain, albeit extreme, circumstances. In general, generic products work well for most patients and are significantly less expensive.

J. S. Myers, MD

Reference

1. Chambers WA. Ophthalmic generics—are they really the same? *Ophthalmology.* 2012;119:1095-1096.

Macular assessment using optical coherence tomography for glaucoma diagnosis

Sung KR, Wollstein G, Kim NR, et al (Univ of Ulsan, Seoul, Korea; Univ of Pittsburgh School of Medicine, PA; Inha Univ School of Medicine, Incheon, Korea; et al)
Br J Ophthalmol 96:1452-1455, 2012

Optical coherence tomography (OCT) is an interferometry-based imaging modality that generates high-resolution cross-sectional images of the retina. Circumpapillary retinal nerve fibre layer (cpRNFL) and optic disc assessments are the mainstay of glaucomatous structural measurements. However, because these measurements are not always available or precise, it would be useful to have another reliable indicator. The macula has been suggested as an alternative scanning location for glaucoma diagnosis. Using time-domain (TD) OCT, macular measurements have been shown to provide good glaucoma diagnostic capabilities. Performance of cpRNFL measurement was generally superior to macular assessment. However, macular measurement showed better glaucoma diagnostic performance and progression detection capability in some specific cases, which suggests that these two measurements may be combined to produce a better diagnostic strategy. With the adoption of spectral-domain OCT, which allows a higher image resolution than TD-OCT, segmentation of inner macular layers becomes possible. The role of macular measurements for detection of glaucoma progression is still under investigation. Improvement of image quality would allow better visualisation, development of various scanning modes would optimise macular measurements, and further refining of the analytical algorithm would provide more accurate segmentation. With these achievements, macular measurement can be an important surrogate for glaucomatous structural assessment.

▶ According to our current understanding of glaucoma, in which structural changes precede changes in function, devices that reveal glaucomatous damage earlier in the disease course may help prevent functional vision loss from glaucoma. Further, by identifying damage earlier in the disease course, we might be able to better separate glaucoma suspects that will progress from those that will never need treatment. Optical coherence tomography (OCT) is a particularly appealing technology because current machines collect massive amounts of data about tissues that succumb to glaucoma damage. However, the technology evolved rapidly in the recent past, so it has been difficult to produce a long-term prospective study that provides good information on OCT changes that are predictors of glaucoma progression. We are left using OCT to monitor for change and trying to separate sensitivity for glaucoma damage from hypersensitivity.

Harnessing data about the macula for use in glaucoma has captured much interest in the literature because of the macula's unique anatomic characteristics. Glaucoma damages retinal ganglion cells (RGCs), and the greatest density of RGCs is in the macula (50% of all RGCs). Peripheral RGC layers are 1 cell thick, but in the macula there are up to 7 layers of RGC bodies. Therefore, any glaucomatous loss should be easiest to detect in the macular region. However, peripapillary measurements with OCT have, thus far, proven superior to macular measurements. Perhaps this is because the tissues of primary interest in glaucoma comprise only one-third of the total macular thickness. The other two-thirds might introduce confounding effects from nonglaucomatous pathology.[1] Also, circumpapillary retinal nerve fiber layer measurement may be advantageous because it captures all retinal axons as they head to the optic disc as opposed to measuring only those found in the macula.

Given the interest level in evaluation of the macula with OCT for glaucoma, it seems likely that algorithms will be developed to help tap the potential in this important tissue to guide glaucoma diagnosis and management.

S. Fudemberg, MD, FACS

Reference

1. Kotowski J, Folio LS, Wollstein G, et al. Glaucoma discrimination of segmented cirrus spectral domain optical coherence tomography (SD-OCT) macular scans. *Br J Ophthalmol.* 2012;96:1420-1425.

Prevalence, Progression, and Impact of Glaucoma on Vision After Boston Type 1 Keratoprosthesis Surgery

Talajic JC, Agoumi Y, Gagné S, et al (Université de Montréal, Quebec, Canada; et al)
Am J Ophthalmol 153:267-274, 2012

Purpose.—To report glaucoma outcomes after Boston type 1 kerato-prosthesis (KPro) surgery, in particular, glaucoma prevalence, progression, and treatment.

Design.—Consecutive, retrospective, interventional case series.

Methods.—*Setting:* Tertiary care institution.

Study Population: Thirty-eight eyes in 38 patients.

Intervention: KPro surgery.

Main Outcome Measures: Visual acuity (VA), intraocular pressure, visual fields, optic nerve status, and glaucoma treatment.

Results.—Glaucoma diagnosis was known before surgery in 29 patients (76%; 14 had undergone previous surgery) and was diagnosed after surgery in 34 patients (89%) after a mean ± standard deviation of 16.5 ± 4.7 months of follow-up. The number of patients taking intraocular pressure-lowering medications increased from 19 (50%) before surgery to 28 (76%) after surgery ($P = .017$). Twenty-four patients (63%) were taking at least 1 additional glaucoma medication at their most recent postoperative visit. Eight patients (21%) had glaucoma progression (visual field progression, need for surgery, or both). Fifteen patients (40%) had a cup-to-disc ratio of 0.85 or more. Five patients required glaucoma surgery. VA was limited by glaucoma in 14 patients (37%), 11 of whom had a VA of 20/200 or worse. Five such patients (13%) had a dramatic improvement in VA, then progressed to end-stage glaucoma with fixation loss. Visual fields were limited by glaucoma in 25 patients (66%; mean Swedish Interactive Threshold Algorithm Fast mean defect, -20.3 ± 8.8 decibels; $n = 18$).

Conclusions.—Most KPro candidates have glaucoma, which may deteriorate in a subset of patients after surgery. Dramatic VA improvement after KPro surgery does not preclude the need for rigorous monitoring for glaucoma progression. A low threshold should be used to treat suspicion of even slightly elevated intraocular pressure.

▶ The Boston keratoprosthesis (KPRO) revolutionized corneal transplant surgery by providing an option for patients with a history of failed full-thickness transplants and/or high risk of transplant failure. The refractory nature of the problems for which KPRO is a treatment means that these eyes commonly have multiple ophthalmic diseases processes, including glaucoma. Additionally, those patients without preoperative glaucoma are likely to develop glaucoma following KPRO implantation. As modifications to the device improve its retention rates, glaucoma is becoming the biggest postoperative threat to vision. Outcomes with the KPRO may be life-changing for patients, so refining glaucoma management to maintain visual improvement offered by the KPRO is critical.

The etiology of glaucoma after KPRO is incompletely understood. It is likely that progressive angle closure is a major contributing factor. However, Netland and associates reported a series with total iridectomy during KPRO implantation to prevent secondary angle closure, but the prevalence of postoperative glaucoma was still 58%.[1] Inflammation, bleeding, and vitreous debris are also possible causes of intraocular pressure (IOP) elevation following KPRO. Further, glaucoma is a significant complication of traditional full-thickness transplant that affects up to one third of patients.

Unfortunately, glaucoma management following KPRO is difficult. The IOP cannot be measured by preferred methods, so we must rely on digital palpation. Laser trabeculoplasty is impossible after KPRO placement and trabeculectomy is, at best, not a good option. Obstruction of the tube lumen is a problem when tube shunts are placed in the anterior chamber before, during, or after KPRO implantation. Pars plana tube shunts are a good option, relatively, but corneal opacity preoperative typically prevents vitrectomy for pars plana placement of the tube. After KPRO implantation, the view for vitrectomy is much improved, but it may still be limited in the far periphery; close shaving of the vitreous peripherally (especially in the quadrant where the tube is placed) helps prevent occlusion of the tube with vitreous.

It is particularly disappointing to see patients experience tremendous visual recovery after KPRO placement only to ultimately lose vision from glaucoma. Although glaucoma management is difficult in the context of a KPRO, aggressive management is justified.

J. S. Myers, MD

Reference

1. Netland PA, Terada H, Dohlman CH. Glaucoma associated with keratoprosthesis. *Ophthalmology.* 1998;105:751-757.

Glaucoma Filtration Surgery Following Sustained Elevation of Intraocular Pressure Secondary to Intravitreal Anti-VEGF Injections
Skalicky SE, Ho I, Agar A, et al (Univ of Sydney, New South Wales, Australia; Prince of Wales Hosp, New South Wales, Australia)
Ophthalmic Surg Lasers Imaging 43:328-334, 2012

■ *Background and Objective.*—To document cases of sustained elevation of intraocular pressure (IOP) while receiving intravitreal anti-vascular endothelial growth factor (VEGF) agents and subsequent management.

■ *Patients and Methods.*—A retrospective series of all cases managed by the authors and colleagues was performed.

■ *Results.*—Six patients developed sustained elevated IOP; five received ranibizumab and one bevacizumab. Four received unilateral and two received bilateral injections. Two had preexisting primary open-angle glaucoma and one had pseudoexfoliative glaucoma, all with stable IOP prior to anti-VEGF treatment. Angles were open in all cases. Peak IOP averaged

43 mm Hg (range: 34 to 60 mm Hg). The mean number of injections preceding the IOP increase was 10 (range: 1 to 20). Four patients required trabeculectomy, one selective laser trabeculoplasty, and one multiple topical medications.

■ *Conclusion.*—A sustained increase in IOP requiring glaucoma filtering surgery is a rare but important treatment complication for patients receiving intravitreal anti-VEGF therapy, especially those with preexisting glaucoma or glaucoma risk factors.

▶ Anti-vascular endothelial growth factor (VEGF) therapy for retinal disease has already saved a significant number of people from profound vision loss and serious disability. In a very small percentage of cases, it seems that intravitreal anti-VEGF injections cause a sustained increase in intraocular pressure (IOP). IOP elevation immediately following intravitreal injections is well documented and short lived. In contrast, sustained IOP elevation may require IOP lowering therapy including surgical filtration. An increasing number of reports provide variable information regarding the incidence of this problem, but rates are typically in the single digits. It is likely that multiple factors contribute to the rate at which sustained IOP elevation occurs. Intuitively, processes that challenge the outflow apparatus should also increase the likelihood of poor IOP control in patients receiving intravitreal anti-VEGF therapy. Pre-existing glaucoma has been linked to increased risk of sustained IOP elevation. Neovascularization in the anterior segment may certainly cause glaucoma and some patients now receive anti-VEGF injections for vein occlusions and diabetic retinopathy. Perhaps these patients are more likely to have a sustained IOP elevation. Patients chronically treated with anti-VEGF agents may undergo an impressive number of injections, which one might also expect to increase the rate of persistent IOP spike, but this problem has been reported even after a single injection.

The etiology has not been completely elucidated. Damage to the trabecular meshwork was shown in vitro, but at a concentration 4 times that of the clinical dose of bevacizumab.[1] Ranibizumab was not toxic even at the elevated concentration.[1] Contaminants may be present in injections, and these contaminants could affect aqueous outflow. Research has shown a wide range of particle levels in solutions from different compounding pharmacies.[2] There are other issues related to mishandling of the syringes that could yield higher levels of microdroplets and subsequently greater risk of IOP spike. Also, patients receiving injections at regular and relatively frequent intervals are having their IOP measured frequently, so glaucoma may be identified in this population as a result of selection bias.

Sustained IOP elevation in patients treated with anti-VEGF agents is a phenomenon that bears consideration, but it also affects a small portion of the patients treated with these revolutionary agents.

S. Fudemberg, MD, FACS

References

1. Kahook MY, Ammar DA. In vitro effects of antivascular endothelial growth factors on cultured human trabecular meshwork cells. *J Glaucoma*. 2010;19:437-441.

2. Liu L, Ammar DA, Ross LA, Mandava N, Kahook MY, Carpenter JF. Silicone oil microdroplets and protein aggregates in repackaged bevacizumab and ranibizumab: effects of long-term storage and product mishandling. *Invest Ophthalmol Vis Sci.* 2011;52:1023-1034.

Subspecialization in Glaucoma Surgery

Campbell RJ, Bell CM, Gill SS, et al (Queen's Univ, Kingston, Canada; Inst for Clinical Evaluative Sciences, Ontario, Canada; et al)
Ophthalmology 119:2270-2273, 2012

Purpose.—To evaluate trends in glaucoma surgery subspecialization.

Design.—Population-based analysis of incisional glaucoma surgery and laser trabeculoplasty practice patterns among all ophthalmologists in Ontario, Canada, from 1995 through 2010.

Participants.—All ophthalmologists in Ontario, Canada, providing universal health care for the provincial population of approximately 12 million.

Methods.—The province of Ontario provides government-funded universal health care insurance to all citizens through the Ontario Health Insurance Plan (OHIP). Anonymized physician services data were obtained from the OHIP database, which has excellent accuracy for procedure performance.

Main Outcome Measures.—Proportion of ophthalmologists providing incisional glaucoma surgery and laser trabeculoplasty and the distribution of these surgical and laser procedures among ophthalmologists.

Results.—Between 1995 and 2010, the median number of ophthalmologists in Ontario was 427 (35.1 per 1 million population), ranging from 417 to 453 (32.9—40.3 per 1 million population). The percentage of ophthalmologists providing incisional glaucoma surgery dropped from 35% in 1995 to 19% in 2010, a 47% decline. Over the same period, the mean number of incisional glaucoma surgeries performed per surgeon doubled, and the percentage of incisional glaucoma operations provided by high-volume surgeons rose from 23% to 59%. The percentage of ophthalmologists performing laser trabeculoplasty was relatively stable (48% in 1995 to 50% in 2010).

Conclusions.—Over the past 16 years, the proportion of ophthalmologists providing incisional glaucoma surgery has declined significantly. At the same time, the proportion of incisional glaucoma surgery provided by high-volume glaucoma surgeons has more than doubled. These trends will have important implications for stakeholders from policy makers and hospitals to academic departments and residency education programs.

▶ This article supports a commonly held belief that glaucoma surgery is increasingly being performed by specialists. Analyzing the use of services in Canada is appealing because the universal health insurance program there provides access to data on a large population. As the authors point out, understanding trends in delivery of surgical glaucoma care may be important for thoughtful physician human resource planning, certification rules, and quality improvement.

This study provides dramatic evidence that incisional glaucoma surgery is being concentrated among a smaller group of surgeons. During the 15-year study period, the percentage of ophthalmologists providing incisional glaucoma surgery was roughly cut in half. Correspondingly, the number of procedures performed per surgeon roughly doubled. High-volume glaucoma surgeons were considered those performing 100 or more procedures annually, and by 2010 the percentage of cases they performed increased 2.5 times to almost 60%. Both early- and late-career ophthalmologists were progressively less likely to perform any glaucoma surgery. The percentage of surgeons performing 5 or fewer cases per year declined as well. Meanwhile, the percentage of ophthalmologists performing laser trabeculoplasty was roughly stable, but the number of procedures per year increased significantly.

This article notes many factors that probably push glaucoma surgery toward specialists today. Surgical glaucoma training is increasingly reserved for fellowship programs. Although practice patterns in Ontario, Canada, may not mimic those in the United States, American residency programs are 1 year shorter than those in Canada and may put even more stress on US graduates to limit the scope of their practice. As fellowship opportunities grow, access to specialists and referrals for glaucoma care increase. Finally, higher surgeon volumes have been associated with better outcomes for many therapies.

Nonetheless, new glaucoma surgical procedures are often marketed to cataract surgeons. The volume of cataract surgery dwarfs that of glaucoma surgery, so companies are financially incentivized to attach glaucoma and cataract surgery. The ultimate goal in surgical glaucoma management is to create a simple, quick, low-risk, and highly effective procedure. Such a procedure would be an excellent adjunct to cataract extraction. However, during the process of developing new procedures, the comprehensive ophthalmologist may be increasingly exposed to the challenges associated with managing glaucoma patients.

S. Fudemberg, MD, FACS

3-T Diffusion tensor imaging of the optic nerve in subjects with glaucoma: correlation with GDx-VCC, HRT-III and Stratus optical coherence tomography findings
Nucci C, Mancino R, Martucci A, et al (Univ of Rome Tor Vergata, Italy; et al)
Br J Ophthalmol 96:976-980, 2012

Objectives.—To correlate diffusion-tensor imaging (DTI) of the optic nerve with morphological indices obtained by scanning laser polarimetry (GDx-VCC); confocal scanning laser ophthalmoscopy (Heidelberg III retinal tomograph; HRT-III) and optical coherence tomography (Stratus OCT).

Methods.—Thirty-six subjects (12 with no eye disease and 24 with perimetrically diagnosed glaucoma) were examined. One eye for each participant was studied with 3-Tesla DTI (with automatic generation of mean diffusivity (MD) and fractional anisotropy (FA) values); GDx-VCC,

HRT-III and OCT. Single and multiple regression analyses of all variables studied were performed.

Results.—MD displayed the strongest correlation with linear cup/disc ratio (LCDR) from HTR-III (r = 0.662), retinal nerve fibre layer (RNFL) thickness (avThickn) from OCT (r = −0.644), and nerve fibre index (NFI) from GDx (r = 0.642); FA was strongly correlated with the LCDR (r = −0.499). In multiple regression analyses, MD correlated with LCDR (*p* = 0.02) when all variables were considered; with avThickn (*p* < 0.01) (analysis of all RNFL parameters); with NFI (*p* < 0.01) (analysis of all GDx parameters); with avThickn (*p* < 0.01) (analysis of OCT parameters); with LCDR (*p* = 0.01) (analysis of HRT-III morphometric parameters) and with linear discriminant function (RB) (*p* = 0.02) (analysis of HRT-III indices). As for FA, it correlated with avThickn (*p* = 0.02) when we analysed the OCT parameters and with RB (*p* = 0.01) (analysis of HRT-III indices).

Conclusions.—DTI parameters of the axonal architecture of the optic nerve show good correlation with morphological features of the optic nerve head and RNFL documented with GDx-VCC, HRT-III and OCT.

▶ This article is a pioneering look at the application of evolving magnetic resonance imaging (MRI) techniques to the optic nerve in glaucoma. It compares them with current clinical tools for following morphologic changes in the retinal nerve fiber layer (RNFL) and optic nerve. A background on MRI is essential to interpret the results of this study.

Over the past 20 years, the field of neuroscience experienced significant growth in the use of neuroimaging to determine function and anatomy. In general, functional MRI measures hemodynamic changes in the gray matter as a response to physical, cognitive, or emotional tasks. Diffusion tensor imaging (DTI) complements functional MRI by mapping white matter tracts essential for flow of information to and between sites of activity.

Functional MRI works on the principle that neural activity in a gray matter region causes increased blood consumption in that region. Deoxyhemoglobin is paramagnetic, and as the ratio of deoxyhemoglobin to oxyhemoglobin increases with activity, this may be registered by signal changes in the MRI. This signal is considered blood oxygenation level dependent (BOLD), and it is assumed that changes in BOLD signals reflect changes in neural activity, but this relationship is incompletely understood.[1]

DTI is based on principles of water molecule diffusion. According to the rules of diffusion, the less spatial constraints to which a molecule is subject, the larger the diffusion. For example, ventricles in the brain are large spaces, and molecules inside them will diffuse in all directions randomly, which is called isotropic diffusion. In contrast, molecules in tubular structures, such as axons, will experience limited motion and diffuse mainly in a directional pattern, called anisotropic diffusion.[1] The strength of local diffusion directionality may be quantified by the fractional anisotropy (FA), which will be high in axons. Additionally, the mean diffusivity (MD), which is a measure of the total diffusion, will be low in axons.

Interestingly, advancing glaucoma was associated with changes in the optic nerve using DTI. MD significantly increased and FA progressively decreased.

This supports the belief that ultrastructural damage to the optic nerve from glaucoma correlates with functional changes. Additionally, this study identified links between the DTI and certain parameters of optic nerve and RNFL analyzers used in clinical practice.

Although we are a long way from regularly ordering MRI studies on glaucoma patients, this article is an important step toward the use of biomarkers to help identify changes in the function of neural tissues like the optic nerve and retina in response to glaucoma.

S. Fudemberg, MD, FACS

Reference

1. Bick AS, Mayer A, Levin N. From research to clinical practice: implementation of functional magnetic imaging and white matter tractography in the clinical environment. *J Neurol Sci.* 2012;312:158-165.

Effects of caffeinated coffee consumption on intraocular pressure, ocular perfusion pressure, and ocular pulse amplitude: a randomized controlled trial
Jiwani AZ, Rhee DJ, Brauner SC, et al (Harvard Med School, Boston, MA; et al)
Eye 26:1122-1130, 2012

Purpose.—To examine the effects of caffeinated coffee consumption on intraocular pressure (IOP), ocular perfusion pressure (OPP), and ocular pulse amplitude (OPA) in those with or at risk for primary open-angle glaucoma (POAG).

Methods.—We conducted a prospective, double-masked, crossover, randomized controlled trial with 106 subjects: 22 with high tension POAG, 18 with normal tension POAG, 20 with ocular hypertension, 21 POAG suspects, and 25 healthy participants. Subjects ingested either 237 ml of caffeinated (182 mg caffeine) or decaffeinated (4 mg caffeine) coffee for the first visit and the alternate beverage for the second visit. Blood pressure (BP) and pascal dynamic contour tonometer measurements of IOP, OPA, and heart rate were measured before and at 60 and 90 min after coffee ingestion per visit. OPP was calculated from BP and IOP measurements. Results were analysed using paired t-tests. Multivariable models assessed determinants of IOP, OPP, and OPA changes.

Results.—There were no significant differences in baseline IOP, OPP, and OPA between the caffeinated and decaffeinated visits. After caffeinated as compared with decaffeinated coffee ingestion, mean mm Hg changes ($\pm$ SD) in IOP, OPP, and OPA were as follows: 0.99 ($\pm$ 1.52, $P < 0.0001$), 1.57 ($\pm$ 6.40, $P = 0.0129$), and 0.23 ($\pm$ 0.52, $P < 0.0001$) at 60 min, respectively; and 1.06 ($\pm$ 1.67, $P < 0.0001$), 1.26 ($\pm$ 6.23, $P = 0.0398$), and 0.18 ($\pm$ 0.52, $P = 0.0006$) at 90 min, respectively. Regression analyses revealed sporadic and inconsistent associations with IOP, OPP, and OPA changes.

Conclusion.—Consuming one cup of caffeinated coffee (182 mg caffeine) statistically increases, but likely does not clinically impact, IOP and OPP in those with or at risk for POAG.

▶ There is a significant focus in popular media on the potential effects of what we eat. Recommendations for healthy living continue to evolve and change. Perhaps concern about the epidemic of obesity accelerates the drive to develop new diet strategies including movements toward organic food. Understandably, glaucoma patients are anxious to find inexpensive and easy ways to treat their disease. Some patients find the possibility of medicine side effects and drug interactions daunting and out of sync with their desire for an organic lifestyle. Therefore, today's glaucoma patient is particularly interested in lifestyle modifications and their effect on glaucoma management.

Generally, lifestyle changes have not proven effective for long-term glaucoma treatment. Nonetheless, we know that some of the things we do and ingest may affect intraocular pressure (IOP). Marijuana is in the spotlight with the adoption of medical marijuana laws in some states. The American Glaucoma Society produced a position paper explaining why marijuana (although it lowers IOP) is not a treatment for glaucoma.[1] Alcohol may also lower IOP, but drinking it would not be a treatment for glaucoma. Transient increases in IOP after caffeine consumption have been reported. Caffeinated coffee is the primary source of dietary caffeine and is reported among the most common beverages in the world.

This well-designed and relatively large prospective study confirms that consuming a cup of coffee causes an increase in IOP that is statistically, but not clinically, significant. However, it is still possible that extreme caffeine consumption might have a greater impact on IOP and glaucoma or that consistent intake over a period of many years might be more deleterious. In a perfect world, we need a large, long-term, prospective study that could evaluate the link between caffeine consumption and glaucoma progression as opposed to IOP elevation. Practically, this study is a great step toward answering a common question for patients using evidence-based medicine.

If you ask, you might be surprised how many cups of coffee some patients drink in a day. Currently, there is not enough evidence to recommend that patients with glaucoma withhold caffeine intake, but using it in moderation seems reasonable.

S. Fudemberg, MD, FACS

Reference

1. Jampel H. American glaucoma society position statement: marijuana and the treatment of glaucoma. *J Glaucoma.* 2010;19:75-76.

Cataract surgery with trabecular micro-bypass stent implantation in patients with mild-to-moderate open-angle glaucoma and cataract: Two-year follow-up

Craven ER, for the iStent Study Group (Wills Eye Inst, Philadelphia, PA; et al)
J Cataract Refract Surg 38:1339-1345, 2012

Purpose.—To assess the long-term safety and efficacy of a single trabecular micro-bypass stent with concomitant cataract surgery versus cataract surgery alone for mild to moderate open-angle glaucoma.

Setting.—Twenty-nine investigational sites, United States.

Design.—Prospective randomized controlled multicenter clinical trial.

Methods.—Eyes with mild to moderate glaucoma with an unmedicated intraocular pressure (IOP) of 22 mm Hg or higher and 36 mm Hg or lower were randomly assigned to have cataract surgery with iStent trabecular micro-bypass stent implantation (stent group) or cataract surgery alone (control group). Patients were followed for 24 months postoperatively.

Results.—The incidence of adverse events was low in both groups through 24 months of follow-up. At 24 months, the proportion of patients with an IOP of 21 mm Hg or lower without ocular hypotensive medications was significantly higher in the stent group than in the control group ($P = .036$). Overall, the mean IOP was stable between 12 months and 24 months (17.0 mm Hg ± 2.8 [SD] and 17.1 ± 2.9 mm Hg, respectively) in the stent group but increased (17.0 ± 3.1 mm Hg to 17.8 ± 3.3 mm Hg, respectively) in the control group. Ocular hypotensive medication was statistically significantly lower in the stent group at 12 months; it was also lower at 24 months, although the difference was no longer statistically significant.

Conclusions.—Patients with combined single trabecular micro-bypass stent and cataract surgery had significantly better IOP control on no medication through 24 months than patients having cataract surgery alone. Both groups had a similar favorable long-term safety profile.

▶ Minimally invasive glaucoma surgery is an important topic. Transscleral filtration of aqueous humor has long been the gold standard for surgical treatment of glaucoma. Unfortunately, transscleral filtration is inherently imprecise because we are unable to finely modulate the eye's healing response in the subconjunctival space. This results in a Catch-22 between aggressive use of antiscarring agents that increase the risk of avascular conjunctiva and infection or sparing use that risks failure. Ab-interno approaches extricate us from the problems of transscleral filtration, but so far they don't work as well. Historically, the original intention of trabeculectomy was removal of the trabeculum to free the flow of aqueous into Schlemm's canal. However, trabeculectomy worked well only in the context of transscleral filtration.[1] In recent years, attention has refocused on developing techniques that might effectively lower intraocular pressure (IOP) by bypassing the trabecular apparatus.

The iStent was approved by the US Food and Drug Administration for use with cataract surgery in 2012. The device is L-shaped, with a snorkel that resides in the anterior chamber and a foot that resides in Schlemm's canal. This article reveals the 2-year data on iStent success for patients with mild-to-moderate open-angle glaucoma. The success of cataract surgery alone for IOP lowering in this patient population is impressive. Patients treated with the iStent were more likely to have an IOP less than 21 on no glaucoma medicines. These patients were treated with one iStent device, but it may be possible to achieve better results implanting multiple devices. Also, it is likely that trabecular bypass devices will undergo further refinement that may yield better IOP control, but at this point it does not achieve the low pressures needed to treat significant glaucoma. An additional benefit of iStent is that the conjunctiva remains untouched if future filtration surgery is indicated.

S. Fudemberg, MD, FACS

Reference

1. Razeghinejad MR, Fudemberg SJ, Spaeth GL. The changing conceptual basis of trabeculectomy: a review of past and current surgical techniques. *Surv Ophthalmol.* 2012;57:1-25.

Continuous 24-Hour Monitoring of Intraocular Pressure Patterns With a Contact Lens Sensor: Safety, Tolerability, and Reproducibility in Patients With Glaucoma
Mansouri K, Medeiros FA, Tafreshi A, et al (Univ of California at San Diego)
Arch Ophthalmol 130:1534-1539, 2012

Objective.—To examine the safety, tolerability, and reproducibility of intraocular pressure (IOP) patterns during repeated continuous 24-hour IOP monitoring with. contact lens sensor.

Methods.—Forty patients suspected of having glaucoma (n = 21) or with established glaucoma (n = 19) were studied. Patients participated in two 24-hour IOP monitoring sessions (S1 and S2) at. 1-week interval (SENSIMED Triggerfish CLS; Sensimed AG). Patients pursued daily activities, and sleep behavior was not controlled. Incidence of adverse events and tolerability (visual analog scale score) were assessed. Reproducibility of signal patterns was assessed using Pearson correlations.

Results.—The mean (SD) age of the patients was 55.5 (15.7) years, and 60% were male. Main adverse events were blurred vision (82%), conjunctival hyperemia (80%), and superficial punctate keratitis (15%). The mean (SD) visual analog scale score was 27.2 (18.5) mm in S1 and 23.8 (18.7) mm in S2 ($P =.22$). Overall correlation between the. sessions was 0.59 (0.51 for no glaucoma medication and 0.63 for glaucoma medication) ($P =.12$). Mean (SD) positive linear slopes of the sensor signal from wake to. hours into sleep were detected in both sessions for the no glaucoma medication group (S1: 0.40 [0.34], $P < .001$; S2: 0.33 [0.30], $P < .01$) but not for the glaucoma medication group (S1: 0.24 [0.60], $P =.06$; S2: 0.40 [0.40], $P < .001$).

Conclusions.—Repeated use of the contact lens sensor demonstrated good safety and tolerability. The recorded IOP patterns showed fair to good reproducibility, suggesting that data from continuous 24-hour IOP monitoring may be useful in the management of patients with glaucoma. *Trial Registration.*—clinicaltrials.gov Identifier: NCT01319617.

▶ Evidence from sleep laboratories shows that intraocular pressure (IOP) may be highest during the nocturnal/sleep period with the patient supine. Measurement of IOP during sleep and the effect of therapies on nocturnal IOP have been receiving greater attention. Further, we manage glaucoma by making treatment decisions with very little IOP data. An average patient may be followed up with 3 to 4 times per year with changes in therapy based, in part, on the IOP level at those visits. Unlike blood pressure, which may be measured by sticking one's arm in an automated machine at the nearest pharmacy, efforts to develop and adopt a home monitoring device for IOP have been unsuccessful. As technology advances, continuous home monitoring of IOP is becoming a more realistic possibility.

The Triggerfish (Sensimed AG) is a single-use contact lens made of silicone with a passive and active strain gauge embedded in the silicone that monitors changes in the diameter of the corneoscleral junction. Changes in the corneal curvature and circumference are assumed to correspond to changes in IOP. The output of the sensor is expressed in arbitrary units, not millimeters of mercury. A disposable adhesive antenna is worn periorbitally and connects via a cable to a portable recorder that is worn around the patient's waist. The external system sends energy to the contact lens sensor and receives measurement data. The contact lens sensor is available in 3 different base curves (flat, medium, steep). It collects data for 30 seconds every 5 minutes.

This is a very well-designed study to determine the tolerability and reproducibility of the Triggerfish, which are fundamentally important for its clinical application. Although most patients experienced an adverse event, these events were mild and short lived. When asked to rate the tolerability of the device, only about 10% of patients considered it poor. Statistical tools indicated fair-to-good agreement between the two 24-hour sessions monitored.

The Triggerfish is not yet approved for sale in the United States. It may ultimately be limited by its novel strategy to monitor IOP. The relationship between the data obtained and the magnitude of IOP in millimeters of mercury requires further study. In addition, data on the variability of IOP must be correlated with risk of glaucoma progression.

S. Fudemberg, MD, FACS

4 Cornea

Risk of Corneal Transplant Rejection Significantly Reduced with Descemet's Membrane Endothelial Keratoplasty
Anshu A, Price MO, Price FW Jr (Cornea Res Foundation of America, Indianapolis, IN; Price Vision Group, Indianapolis, IN)
Ophthalmology 119:536-540, 2012

Purpose.—To evaluate the relative risk of immunologic rejection episode in patients who underwent Descemet's membrane endothelial keratoplasty (DMEK), Descemet's stripping endothelial keratoplasty (DSEK), and penetrating keratoplasty (PK).

Design.—Comparative case series.

Participants.—One hundred forty-one eyes treated with DMEK at Price Vision Group, Indianapolis, Indiana.

Methods.—The patients in the DMEK group were compared retrospectively with cohorts of DSEK (n = 598) and PK (n = 30) patients treated at the same center, with similar demographics, follow-up duration, and indications for surgery. The postoperative steroid regimen and rejection criteria were identical in the 3 groups. Kaplan—Meier survival analysis, which takes varying length of follow-up into consideration, was performed to determine the cumulative probability of a rejection episode 1 and 2 years after surgery. Proportional hazards analysis was used to determine the relative risk of rejection episodes between the 3 groups. $P < 0.05$ was considered significant and calculated using the log-rank test.

Main Outcome Measures.—Rejection-free survival and cumulative probability of a rejection episode.

Results.—The mean recipient age was 66 years (56% females and 94% Caucasian) and median follow-up duration was 13 months (range, 3—40) in the DMEK group. Fuchs' dystrophy was the most common indication for surgery (n = 127; 90%) followed by pseudophakic bullous keratopathy (n = 4; 4%) and regrafts (n = 9; 6.4%). Only 1 patient (0.7%) had a documented rejection episode in the DMEK group compared with 54 (9%) in the DSEK and 5 (17%) in the PK group. The Kaplan—Meier cumulative probability of a rejection episode at 1 and 2 years was 1% and 1%, respectively, for DMEK; 8% and 12%, respectively, for DSEK; and 14% and 18%, respectively, for PK. This was a highly significant difference ($P = 0.004$). The DMEK eyes had a 15 times lesser risk of experiencing a rejection episode than DSEK eyes (95% confidence limit [CL], 2.0—111; $P = 0.008$) and 20 times lower risk than PK eyes (95% CL, 2.4—166; $P = 0.006$).

Conclusions.—Patients undergoing DMEK had a significantly reduced risk of experiencing a rejection episode within 2 years after surgery compared with DSEK and PK performed for similar indications using the same corticosteroid regimen.

▶ Descemet's membrane endothelial keratectomy (DMEK) has well-known advantages, such as improved visual acuity and faster visual rehabilitation, compared with Descemet's stripping endothelial keratoplasty (DSEK) and penetrating keratoplasty (PK) as well as known disadvantages, namely intraoperative difficulties with graft management and high risk of graft dislocation and need for rebubbling. This article evaluates the risk of rejection, comparing DMEK with DSEK and PK.

The authors retrospectively compared 141 DMEK eyes with 598 DSEK eyes and 30 PK eyes. The DMEK group, with a median follow-up of 13 months, only had 1 eye (0.7%) develop rejection compared with 9% of the DSEK eyes (median follow-up of 11 months) and 17% of the PK eyes (median follow-up 17 months). DMEK eyes were noted to have a significantly decreased risk of rejection, whereas the rejection rates in DSEK were not significantly lower than PK. All 3 groups were treated with the same steroid regimen.

The marked difference in rejection rates between DMEK and DSEK/PK suggest the importance of the stroma in the development of rejection, in addition to other previously recognized factors, such as sutures and neovascularization. Given the decreased rejection rate in DMEK eyes, the authors consider the future possibility of reduction in steroid dosage for these patients, potentially decreasing risk of steroid-induced glaucoma as well as health care costs of both medications and glaucoma management.

There are several limitations to this study, including its retrospective comparison, the small number of PK eyes, and the relatively short follow-up period. However, this study has greatly enhanced our understanding of rejection, while introducing many questions, such as: Why is DMEK superior regarding rejection? Is the stromal pro-antigenic? How do endothelial cells compare? How can we use this information to benefit our patients? What is the ideal steroid regimen? We look forward to more studies further assessing these issues.

P. K. Nagra, MD

Rotational Autokeratoplasty in Pediatric Patients for Nonprogressive Paracentral Corneal Scars
Ramappa M, Pehere NK, Murthy SI, et al (L.V. Prasad Eye Inst, Hyderabad, India)
Ophthalmology 119:2458-2462, 2012

Objective.—To report the outcomes of ipsilateral rotational autokeratoplasty (RAK) for nonprogressive paracentral corneal opacities in children <16 years of age.

Design.—Retrospective, consecutive, interventional case series.

Participants.—Thirty-three eyes of 33 children aged <16 years undergoing RAK for nonprogressive paracentral scars.

Methods.—Medical records were retrospectively reviewed for the primary etiology of corneal opacity, time of onset, duration of opacity, preoperative visual acuity, formula used for calculation of trephine size, size of the trephine used, and duration of follow-up. Any intraoperative and early and late postoperative complications were noted for all patients. Postoperative visual acuity and astigmatism were noted. Visual acuity was converted to logarithm of the minimum angle of resolution units for analysis.

Main Outcome Measures.—Primary outcome was postoperative visual acuity. Graft clarity and complications were analyzed as secondary outcomes.

Results.—The mean age at surgery was 7.2 ± 3.9 months. The mean follow-up duration was 27 ± 37 months. The commonest etiology of corneal opacity was trauma (62.5%), followed by resolved microbial keratitis (21.9%). Postoperative visual acuity (1.25 ± 0.84) was significantly better ($P < 0.001$) than preoperative visual acuity (2.05 ± 0.96). The mean astigmatism at last visit was 4.04 ± 2.21 diopters. Postoperative visual acuity was better in older children ($\beta = -0.01$; $P = 0.03$) and had a shorter delay in presentation ($\beta = 0.02$; $P = 0.05$). At the last follow-up, the graft was clear in 27 cases (81.25%). The cumulative probability of graft survival was 85% at 2 years and 65% at 5 years. Complications included wound leak in 4 eyes, secondary glaucoma in 2 eyes, graft infiltrate and traumatic dehiscence in 1 eye each.

Conclusions.—Rotational is a autokeratoplasty viable alternative surgical option to allogenic keratoplasty. Graft survival at 2 years seems to be better than allogenic keratoplasty. Younger age and delay in presentation contribute to poorer visual outcomes after surgery.

▶ Given the availability of corneal tissue in this country, rotational autokeratoplasty is an uncommon option for patients with corneal scars. However, as these authors suggest, in developing countries in which corneal tissue may be scarce, this is a reasonable option for patients, especially those in the amblyopic age group for whom waiting for corneal tissue may not be a good option. The authors note significant improvement in postoperative visual acuity as well as favorable graft survival. Interestingly, the most common postoperative complication was wound leak noted in 4 patients, all of whom were treated with resuturing on postoperative day 1. As they hypothesize, the mismatch between central and peripheral corneal thickness may have led to difficulty with wound closure, potentially compounded by the same-size graft wound.

Unfortunately, the authors did not have data on amblyopia treatment and outcomes after this procedure. The real benefit in this procedure for these children is visual rehabilitation, while still in the amblyopic age range, to allow for additional visual development.

While these results are encouraging, fortunately, the availability of corneal tissue may preclude the necessity of rotational autokeratoplasty in this country. However, as these authors demonstrate, it is a reasonable option with good success, especially when delay caused by lack of availability of graft tissue may lead to development or progression of amblyopia.

P. K. Nagra, MD

The Mycotic Ulcer Treatment Trial: A Randomized Trial Comparing Natamycin vs Voriconazole

Prajna NV, for the Mycotic Ulcer Treatment Trial Group
Arch Ophthalmol 1-8, 2012

Objective.—To compare topical natamycin vs voriconazole in the treatment of filamentous fungal keratitis.

Methods.—This phase 3, double-masked, multicenter trial was designed to randomize 368 patients to voriconazole (1%) or natamycin (5%), applied topically every hour while awake until reepithelialization, then 4 times daily for at least 3 weeks. Eligibility included smear-positive filamentous fungal ulcer and visual acuity of 20/40 to 20/400.

Main Outcome Measures.—The primary outcome was best spectacle-corrected visual acuity at 3 months; secondary outcomes included corneal perforation and/or therapeutic penetrating keratoplasty.

Results.—A total of 940 patients were screened and 323 were enrolled. Causative organisms included Fusarium (128 patients [40%]), Aspergillus (54 patients [17%]), and other filamentous fungi (141 patients [43%]). Natamycin-treated cases had significantly better 3-month best spectacle-corrected visual acuity than voriconazole-treated cases (regression coefficient = -0.18 logMAR; 95% CI, -0.30 to -0.05; $P=.006$). Natamycin-treated cases were less likely to have perforation or require therapeutic penetrating keratoplasty (odds ratio = 0.42; 95% CI, 0.22 to 0.80; $P=.009$). Fusarium cases fared better with natamycin than with voriconazole (regression coefficient = -0.41 logMAR; 95% CI, -0.61 to -0.20; $P<.001$; odds ratio for perforation = 0.06; 95% CI, 0.01 to 0.28; $P<.001$), while non- Fusarium cases fared similarly (regression coefficient = -0.02 logMAR; 95% CI, -0.17 to 0.13; $P=.81$; odds ratio for perforation = 1.08; 95% CI, 0.48 to 2.43; $P=.86$).

Conclusions.—Natamycin treatment was associated with significantly better clinical and microbiological outcomes than voriconazole treatment for smear-positive filamentous fungal keratitis, with much of the difference attributable to improved results in Fusarium cases.

Application to Clinical Practice.—Voriconazole should not be used as monotherapy in filamentous keratitis.

Trial Registration.—clinicaltrials.gov Identifier: NCT00996736.

▶ Unlike bacterial ulcers, for which we have a number of available topical medication options, there are fewer antifungal choices. Natamycin is the only topical antifungal approved by the US Food and Drug Administration; other available options include compounded medications such as amphotericin B and, more recently, topical voriconazole.

This prospective, randomized multicenter trial compared topical natamycin with topical voriconazole as monotherapy in the treatment of fungal keratitis. All 368 patients enrolled in the study had smear-positive filamentous fungal ulcers in one of 3 centers in India. The authors found natamycin was superior to voriconazole in the treatment of *Fusarium* ulcers and similar for *Aspergillus* and other fungal infections. Visual acuity results at 3 months were better with natamycin, and faster healing with smaller scar formation was noted with natamycin in Fusarium ulcers. Recruitment in the study was stopped early after review of the data, which showed more corneal perforations and therapeutic penetrating keratoplasties were associated with topical voriconazole use. At that time, all patients enrolled in the study were started on natamycin.

Although there are a few limitations of this study (all patients were from South India and from an agrarian background), this is a well-designed, large study that should impact our practice of clinical medicine and understanding of fungal keratitis. Natamycin should be considered the treatment of choice for filamentous fungal keratitis, and especially Fusarium. In addition, topical voriconazole should not be used as monotherapy in filamentous fungal keratitis. Further, we should understand in vivo response to antimicrobial treatment may be different from that of in vitro response. The authors point out that voriconazole was more effective against *Fusarium* in vitro compared with natamycin based on susceptibility studies. In vivo, however, this study showed the opposite to be true, underscoring the importance of other factors in antimicrobial efficacy, such as absorption and drug pharmacodynamics.

We laud the efforts of these investigators and look forward to additional reports, such as the results of MUTT II, evaluating the use of oral voriconazole in severe fungal ulcers.

P. K. Nagra, MD

Relationship of Fuchs Endothelial Corneal Dystrophy Severity to Central Corneal Thickness
Kopplin LJ, for the Fuchs' Endothelial Corneal Dystrophy Genetics Multi-Center Study Group (Case Western Reserve Univ, Cleveland, OH; et al)
Arch Ophthalmol 130:433-439, 2012

Objective.—To define the relationship between Fuchs endothelial corneal dystrophy (FECD) severity and central corneal thickness (CCT).

Methods.—We examined 1610 eyes from a subset of index cases, family members, and unrelated control subjects with normal corneas from the FECD Genetics Multi-Center Study. To estimate the association between FECD severity grade (7-point severity scale based on guttae confluence) and CCT measured by ultrasonographic pachymetry, a multivariable model was used that adjusted for eye, age, race, sex, history of glaucoma or ocular hypertension, diabetes mellitus, contact lens wear, intraocular pressure, and familial relationship to the index case. An interaction between FECD severity grade and edema (stromal or epithelial) on slitlamp examination findings was used to investigate whether the effect of FECD severity grade on CCT differed between those with and without edema.

Results.—Average CCT was thicker in index cases for all FECD grades compared with unaffected controls ($P \le .003$) and in affected family members with an FECD grade of 4 or greater compared with unaffected family members ($P \le .04$). Similar results were observed for subjects without edema. Average CCT of index cases was greater than that of affected family members with grades 4, 5, and 6 FECD ($P \leq .02$). Intraocular pressure was also associated with CCT ($P = .01$).

Conclusions.—An increase in CCT occurs with increasing severity of FECD, including at lower FECD grades in which clinically observable edema is not present. Monitoring CCT changes serially could be a more sensitive measure of disease progression with surgical therapeutic implications.

▶ With recent advances in the surgical management of Fuchs endothelial corneal dystrophy (FECD), specifically the continued evolution of endothelial keratoplasty, our understanding of this condition is also continuing to evolve. This article, focusing on the relationship between the severity of Fuchs and central corneal thickness (CCT), involved a large study with 1610 eyes of 969 patients and employed ultrasound pachymetry to measure CCT. The authors found that CCT gradually increased as FECD severity increased. Interestingly, even patients with early stages of FECD had significantly different CCT compared with normal corneas, although clinically these patients may be asymptomatic and have few clinical signs on examination. The results suggest the importance of routine CCT measurements in our FECD patients as a means of assessing severity and following progression.

Although this was a well-designed study, it does have limitations related to its cross-sectional design. Truly assessing the relationship between severity of disease and CCT as a measure of the severity would be best evaluated by measuring the cohort over time. As the authors acknowledged, some patients have below average CCT at baseline. Their progression in CCT is more important than the absolute CCT, considering that some of these patients may be quite symptomatic with CCT only mildly above average if their baseline was below 500. This would best be demonstrated through a longitudinal study.

Nonetheless, this is an important study suggesting the importance of CCT in evaluating severity of FECD. Although absolute CCT may be helpful, change in CCT over time may be a better marker of the progression and severity of FECD and, in conjunction with clinical exam, may be useful in determining the timing of surgical intervention.

P. K. Nagra, MD

Combined Transepithelial Phototherapeutic Keratectomy and Corneal Collagen Cross-Linking for Progressive Keratoconus
Kymionis GD, Grentzelos MA, Kounis GA, et al (Univ of Crete, Heraklion, Greece)
Ophthalmology 119:1777-1784, 2012

Purpose.—To compare the outcomes of corneal collagen cross-linking (CXL) for the treatment of progressive keratoconus using 2 different techniques for epithelial removal: transepithelial phototherapeutic keratectomy (t-PTK) versus mechanical epithelial debridement.

Design.—Prospective, comparative, interventional case series.

Participants.—Thirty-four patients (38 eyes) with progressive keratoconus were enrolled.

Methods.—All patients underwent uneventful CXL treatment. Sixteen patients (19 eyes) underwent epithelial removal using t-PTK (group 1) and 18 patients (19 eyes) underwent mechanical epithelial debridement using a rotating brush (group 2) during CXL treatment. Visual and refractive outcomes were evaluated along with corneal confocal microscopy findings preoperatively and at 1, 3, 6, and 12 months postoperatively.

Main Outcome Measures.—Uncorrected distance visual acuity (UDVA), corrected distance visual acuity (CDVA), manifest refraction, and keratometry readings.

Results.—No intraoperative or postoperative complications were observed in any of the patients. In group 1, logarithm of the minimum angle of resolution mean UDVA and mean CDVA improved from 0.99 ± 0.71 and 0.30 ± 0.26 preoperatively to 0.63 ± 0.42 $(P = 0.02)$ and 0.19 ± 0.18 $(P = 0.008)$ at 12 months postoperatively, respectively. In group 2, neither mean UDVA nor mean CDVA demonstrated a significant improvement at 12 months postoperatively $(P > 0.05)$. In group 1, mean corneal astigmatism improved from -5.84 ± 3.80 diopters (D) preoperatively to -4.31 ± 2.90 D $(P = 0.015)$ at the last follow-up, whereas in group 2 there was no significant difference at the same postoperative interval $(P > 0.05)$. No endothelial cell density alterations were observed throughout the follow-up period for both groups $(P > 0.05)$.

Conclusions.—Epithelial removal using t-PTK during CXL results in better visual and refractive outcomes in comparison with mechanical epithelial debridement.

▶ While debates continue regarding epithelial-off versus transepithelial collagen cross-linking, this article attempts to evaluate another question: What is the best procedure for epithelial debridement prior to cross-linking?

This prospective study involving 38 eyes of evenly divided participants into transepithelial phototherapeutic keratectomy (t-PTK) versus mechanical epithelial debridement with a rotating brush prior to collagen cross-linking. They found the t-PTK eyes had a statistically significant improvement in uncorrected visual acuity and best corrected visual acuity as well as corneal astigmatism at 1 year. The patients who underwent mechanical debridement did not demonstrate a statistically significant improvement in vision or astigmatism.

In the t-PTK group, an ablation depth of 50 microns was used. In these patients, the central corneas are typically thinner as well as potentially more irregular. The authors hypothesize that the transepithelial approach allowed the patient's epithelium to serve as a masking agent, potentially decreasing surface irregularities. In addition, the 50-micron depth may have led to ablation of anterior stroma at the apex, or other areas where the epithelium may be thinner than 50 microns, leading to a smoother, more regular corneal surface, and therefore a better visual result.

Although this is a very interesting study, longer follow-up is necessary to evaluate the long-term effect of t-PTK treatment, and whether some patients may respond better to this approach than others. One specific concern is the long-term stability of these eyes, particularly those in which more anterior stromal tissue was ablated, given concern regarding further weakening of the stroma and possible progression. Further, follow-up with the mechanical debridement eyes would also be helpful to better understand why those patients did not experience significant improvement following treatment. Nevertheless, as we aim to improve techniques and maximize results with our procedures, this is a noteworthy study that impacts the evolution of collagen cross-linking.

P. K. Nagra, MD

Riboflavin-UVA-induced corneal collagen cross-linking in pediatric patients
Caporossi A, Mazzotta C, Baiocchi S, et al (Siena Univ, Italy)
Cornea 31:227-231, 2012

Purpose.—Evaluation of stability and functional response after riboflavin-UVA—induced cross-linking in a population of patients younger than 18 years with progressive keratoconus after 36 months of follow-up.

Methods.—Prospective nonrandomized phase II open trial conducted at the Department of Ophthalmology, Siena University, Italy. The "Siena CXL Pediatrics" trial involved 152 patients aged 18 years or younger (10—18 years) with clinical and instrumental evidence of keratoconus progression. The population was divided into 2 groups according to corneal thickness (>450 and <450 μm) at the time of enrollment. The riboflavin-UVA—induced corneal cross-linking was performed in all patients according to the standard epi-off protocol. Parameters recorded preoperatively and postoperatively were as follows: uncorrected visual acuity, best spectacle—corrected visual acuity, corneal topography and surface aberrometry (CSO Eye Top topographer; Florence, Italy), optical pachometry (Visante OCT; Zeiss Meditec, Jena, Germany), and HRT II confocal microscopy (Rostock Cornea Module, Heidelberg, Germany).

Results.—Functional data at 36 months showed an increase of +0.18 and +0.16 Snellen lines for uncorrected visual acuity and best spectacle-corrected visual acuity, respectively, in the thicker group (corneal thickness >450 μm) and +0.14 and +0.15 Snellen lines, respectively, in the thinner group (corneal thickness <450 μm). Patients in the latter group already showed a better and faster functional recovery than the thicker group at 3-month follow-up. Topographic results showed statistically significant improvement in K readings and asymmetry index values. Coma reduction was also statistically significant.

Conclusions.—The study demonstrated significant and rapid functional improvement in pediatric patients younger than 18 years with progressive keratoconus, undergoing riboflavin-UVA—induced cross-linking. In pediatric age, a good functional response and keratoconus stability was obtained after corneal cross-linking in a 36-month follow-up.

▶ Keratoconus is a progressive, bilateral cornea condition that often presents in young patients. These patients, in their teenage years or even younger, tend to have rapid disease progression and often develop more advanced disease than those patients who present at a later age. These are the patients who may most benefit from a procedure such as collagen cross-linking; if performed at the earliest sign of progression, these patients may retain good visual function with glasses or contact lenses, minimizing the need for corneal transplantation.

This study was a prospective, nonrandomized trial involving 152 children ages 10 to 18 years with documented progression over a 3-month interval. The patients were divided into 2 groups based on their corneal thickness (> 450 μm or < 450 μm), and all patients received treatment. The authors found improvement in uncorrected visual acuity and best-corrected visual acuity, keratometry readings, and coma reduction over a 3-year period. In spite of their young age, all patients tolerated the procedure, and no adjunctive sedation was required. Further, the authors state no adverse events were recorded, although they note 55% of patients had transient corneal edema with glare disability" in the first 4 to 6 weeks, which responded to topical steroids without adversely affecting visual acuity.

Interestingly, they found that patients with thinner corneas had faster functional improvement at 3 months compared with patients with thicker corneas, as noted in Fig 2 of the original article. Thicker corneas were slower to respond, but by 36 months, there was no difference between the 2 groups. The authors explained this early difference by noting that thinner corneas may have a higher percentage of newly cross-linked tissue compared with thicker corneas, leading to the early improvement. Because thinning corneas may be associated with more advanced keratoconus, the patients with thinner corneas ended up with poorer final visual acuities overall.

This study, as well as another similar study published this year by Vinciguerra et al,[1] evaluated progression over a 3-month interval. Vinciguerra and his group followed these young keratoconus patients every 3 months to identify early progression before cross-linking. Before the availability of cross-linking in this country we would not routinely follow up with these patients as frequently; now that we are able to intervene at the earliest sign of progression, more frequent assessments are warranted.

This is an important study, which adds to the growing literature suggesting the safety and efficiency of corneal cross-linking in children, a patient population very vulnerable to rapid progression of keratoconus. Given these findings, this procedure should be considered in all young keratoconus patients with progression.

P. K. Nagra, MD

Reference

1. Vinciguerra P, Albé E, Freuh BE, Trazza S, Epstein D. Two-year corneal cross-linking results in patients younger than 18 years with documented progressive keratoconus. *Am J Ophthalmol.* 2012;154:520-526.

Trends in the Indications for Corneal Graft Surgery in the United Kingdom: 1999 Through 2009

Keenan TDL, for the National Health Service Blood and Transplant Ocular Tissue Advisory Group and Contributing Ophthalmologists (Ocular Tissue Advisory Group Audit Study 8) (Univ of Manchester, England; et al)

Arch Ophthalmol 130:621-628, 2012

Objective.—To examine trends in the indications for corneal graft surgery in the United Kingdom.

Methods.—National Health Service Blood and Transplant data were analyzed for keratoplasty operations performed in the United Kingdom between April 1, 1999, and March 31, 2009, distinguishing the type of graft and the surgical indication.

Results.—The total number of annual keratoplasty operations increased from 2090 in 1999-2000 to 2511 in 2008-2009. Among these, the annual number of grafts performed for endothelial failure increased from 743 (35.6%) in 1999-2000 to 939 (37.4%) in 2008-2009. The performance of penetrating keratoplasty (PK) for endothelial failure decreased from 98.3% of all grafts in 1999-2000 to 46.6% of all grafts in 2008-2009, while the performance of endothelial keratoplasty increased from 0.3% of all grafts in 1999-2000 to 51.2% of all grafts in 2008-2009. The annual number of grafts performed for keratoconus increased from 514 (24.6%) in 1999 to 564 (22.5%) in 2008-2009. The performance of PK for keratoconus decreased from 88.4% of all grafts in 1999-2000 to 57.1% of all grafts in 2008-2009, while the performance of deep anterior lamellar keratoplasty increased from 8.8% of all grafts in 1999-2000 to 40.1% of all grafts in 2008-2009. The number of annual regraft operations increased from 249 (11.9%) in 1999-2000 to 401 (16.0%) in 2008-2009, most commonly for endothelial failure. In 2008-2009, PK regrafts (78.1%) far outnumbered endothelial keratoplasty regrafts (17.0%).

Conclusions.—Endothelial failure is the most common indication for keratoplasty in the United Kingdom, and endothelial keratoplasty is performed more commonly than PK for this indication. The number of grafts performed for pseudophakic bullous keratopathy has remained stable, while the number of grafts performed for Fuchs endothelial dystrophy is likely to continue increasing. Keratoconus is the second most common indication for keratoplasty, and deep anterior lamellar keratoplasty numbers are approaching those for PK. Regraft surgery is the third most common indication for keratoplasty, required in most cases because of endothelial failure.

▶ Corneal transplantation has evolved significantly over the last decade, with the introduction of endothelial keratoplasty and growing popularity of lamellar keratoplasty. This study evaluated the trends in keratoplasty over a 10-year span in the United Kingdom, highlighting the evolution of cornea transplantation during this period.

The authors evaluated the National Health Service Blood and Transplant data between 1999 and 2009, assessing the number, type, and indication for corneal transplantation performed. Over this 10-year period, they documented an increase in the number of transplants performed, from 2090 to 2511 between the first and final years of the study. The most common indication over this period was endothelial failure. During this period, techniques for endothelial transplantation evolved, and the authors noted a definite change starting 2005 to 2006, with a decrease in penetrating keratoplasty (PK) and increase in endothelial keratoplasty (EK). By the final year of the study, EK was performed more commonly than PK for endothelial dysfunction (Fig 5 in the original article).

A similar transition in surgical management was noted for keratoconus, which was the indication for a mean of 24% of cornea transplants performed. Over the 10-year span, a slow increase in the percentage of deep anterior lamellar keratoplasty (DALK) was noted, and by 2008 to 2009, 40% of transplants for keratoconus were DALK procedures.

The authors also noted a downward trend for PK because of viral infections, which they attributed to improved antiviral agents. On the other hand, an increase in PK for bacterial keratitis was noted, which they associated with increased contact lens—associated infections.

Overall, this is an interesting study, assessing corneal transplantation trends over one decade in the United Kingdom. As corneal transplantation for endothelial failure continues to develop, especially with the advent of Descemet membrane endothelial keratoplasty and Descemet membrane automated endothelial keratoplasty, as well as the addition of collagen crosslinking for keratoconus, I suspect the next 10 years will show new or different trends in the surgical management of these conditions.

P. K. Nagra, MD

Comparison of Penetrating Keratoplasty and Deep Lamellar Keratoplasty for Macular Corneal Dystrophy and Risk Factors of Recurrence

Cheng J, Qi X, Zhao J, et al (Qingdao Univ Med College, China; Qingdao Eye Hosp, China)
Ophthalmology 120:34-39, 2013

Purpose.—To compare the therapeutic effects of penetrating keratoplasty (PK) and deep anterior lamellar keratoplasty (DALK) on patients with macular corneal dystrophy (MCD) and to analyze the risk factors of postoperative recurrence.

Design.—Retrospective, interventional, comparative case series.

Participants.—Fifty-one patients (78 eyes) with MCD treated by PK or DALK at Shandong Eye Institute between January 1992 and December 2010.

Methods.—The medical records of the patients were reviewed retrospectively.

Main Outcome Measures.—Best-corrected visual acuity, corneal endothelial density, complications, recurrence, graft survival, and risk factors for recurrence.

Results.—Penetrating keratoplasty was performed in 57 eyes, and DALK was performed in 21 eyes. The mean follow-up time was 5.1 ± 4.1 years (range, 1.0–18.0 years). The best-corrected visual acuity of the PK group was much better than that of the DALK group at 1, 2, 3, and 5 years. The corneal endothelial density was reduced to 1000 cells/mm^2 or less within 5 years in 21.6% (11/51) of eyes treated by PK and in none of the eyes treated by DALK. The 1-year incidence rate of complications was 21.1% in the PK group, higher than the 4.8% rate in the DALK group. At the last visit, the rate of graft clarity was 87.7% and 85.7% in the 2 groups, respectively. Ten eyes (17.5%) treated by PK had recurrent MCD, with a rate of 0.8%, 7.7%, and 40% at 1, 5, and 10 years, respectively, whereas 9 eyes (42.9%) treated by DALK demonstrated recurrence, with a rate of 14.3% and 49.5% at 1 and 5 years, respectively. The recurrence risk was higher in patients whose age was 18 years or younger at onset or younger than 30 years at surgery. The recurrence risk after DALK was 5.066 times higher than that after PK.

Conclusions.—Penetrating keratoplasty more often immediately improves the visual acuity of patients with MCD, but many complications seem to be inevitable, especially continuous loss of corneal endothelium. Despite poor visual acuity and recurrence after surgery, DALK may produce fewer complications overall and more durable stability of the ocular surface compared with PK. The selection of PK or DALK for MCD should depend on the actual need and situation of certain patients (Fig 1).

▶ Patients with macular corneal dystrophy, a rare autosomal recessive condition, may develop significant visual loss because of their corneal changes, necessitating corneal transplant for visual rehabilitation. Deep anterior lamellar keratoplasty (DALK) may be considered a preferred procedure over penetrating keratoplasty for many conditions, such as keratoconus, corneal scars, and other stromal pathology. This study evaluated DALK compared with penetrating keratoplasty (PK) for patients with macular dystrophy.

Seventy-eight eyes were included in this study; PK was performed in 57 eyes compared with DALK in 21 eyes. Visual acuity was significantly better in the PK

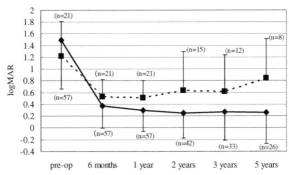

FIGURE 1.—Graph showing change in best-corrected visual acuity after deep anterior lamellar keratoplasty (DALK) and penetrating keratoplasty (PK). logMAR = logarithm of the minimum angle of resolution. -◆- = PK; -■- = DALK. (Reprinted from Cheng J, Qi X, Zhao J, et al. Comparison of penetrating keratoplasty and deep lamellar keratoplasty for macular corneal dystrophy and risk factors of recurrence. Ophthalmology. 2013;120:34-39, Copyright 2013, with permission from the American Academy of Ophthalmology.)

group compared with the DALK eyes (Fig 1). As expected, the PK eyes had decreased endothelial cell counts compared with DALK eyes. In addition, PK eyes were noted to have increased postoperative complications, such as rejection, endothelial decompensation, elevated intraocular pressure, cataract, and corneal wound dehiscence. DALK eyes had fewer complications, including rejection and cataract.

Recurrent disease was more common in DALK eyes (42.9%) compared with PK eyes (17.5%). At 5 years, graft survival in the PK eyes was 87.2% (failures caused by endothelial decompensation or recurrence) compared with 72.7% in the DALK eyes (failures caused by recurrence); the survival rate between the 2 groups was not significantly different. The authors were able to identify risk factors for disease recurrence, including age less than 18 years at time of diagnosis and less than 30 years at time of surgery and treatment with DALK.

Recurrent disease in PK eyes was noted to start at the graft margin and sutures and then gradually progress centrally. In DALK eyes, recurrence manifested as opacification in the interface followed by progression to the graft. The authors hypothesize the retention of "more genetically defective tissue" in DALK compared with PK led to the earlier onset and faster rate of recurrences. The decreased visual acuity results in DALK compared with PK were most likely related to the central location as well as earlier onset of recurrence.

As the authors discuss, we can use this information to help in the management of our patients with macular dystrophy requiring corneal transplantation. While there are benefits as well as risks associated with both PK and DALK for this condition, younger patients with more severe disease may be better served with a PK, given the improved vision and associated lower and slower risk of recurrent disease. Older patients, however, may be better candidates for DALK given the fewer postoperative complications.

P. K. Nagra, MD

Long term visual outcomes, graft survival and complications of deep anterior lamellar keratoplasty in patients with herpes simplex related corneal scarring

Lyall DAM, Tarafdar S, Gilhooley MJ, et al (Gartnavel General Hosp, Glasgow UK; Southern General Hosp, Glasgow, UK; et al)
Br J Ophthalmol 96:1200-1203, 2012

Aims.—To report long term visual outcomes, complications and graft survival of patients undergoing deep anterior lamellar keratoplasty (DALK) to treat corneal scarring secondary to herpes simplex virus (HSV) keratitis.

Methods.—Retrospective, non-comparative case series. 18 patients who underwent DALK for HSV keratitis related corneal scarring between January 2004 and February 2007 were included. DALK was performed by Anwar's big bubble technique. Data collected for analysis included preoperative characteristics, intraoperative complications and postoperative acuity, complications and subsequent operations.

Results.—Mean best corrected distance visual acuity (LogMAR) improved from 1.51 ± 0.90 preoperatively to 0.82 ± 0.85 at the last follow-up

($p = 0.05$). 27% of patients with more than 4 years follow-up had a best corrected distance visual acuity of 6/12 or better and 64% were 6/24 or better. Six patients (33%) experienced a recurrence of HSV keratitis and 9 (50%) experienced an episode of graft rejection. There were five cases (28%) of graft failure, four of whom had had a previous episode of graft rejection. Logistic regression did not find an association with graft rejection, HSV recurrence, any other observed postoperative host corneal vascularisation and any postoperative complication. The majority of patients underwent a second operation with 50% requiring cataract surgery.

Conclusions.—DALK for the treatment of HSV related corneal scarring is associated with a high percentage of postoperative complications. DALK in this context is also associated with a large percentage of secondary operations. Patients should be aware of this when giving informed consent for DALK to treat HSV related corneal scars (Fig 1).

▶ Over the last decade, an increase in lamellar keratoplasty and, specifically, deep anterior lamellar keratoplasty (DALK) has occurred, especially in the management of keratoconus. DALK also is indicated in the treatment of other anterior corneal pathology, such as corneal scars from bacterial or viral infections like herpes simplex virus (HSV) keratitis. Given the chronic nature of HSV keratitis, these patients may be prone to reactivation of the virus or other inflammatory postoperative complications after penetrating keratoplasty, although little data are available on the success of DALK for this indication.

This article focuses on the results of DALK in patients with HSV-related corneal scars. The authors present a retrospective case series of 18 eyes that underwent DALK with a mean follow-up period of 56 months. Mean postoperative best-corrected distance visual acuity was significantly improved from preoperative levels as noted in Fig 1. HSV keratitis recurrence was noted in 6 cases, and rejection

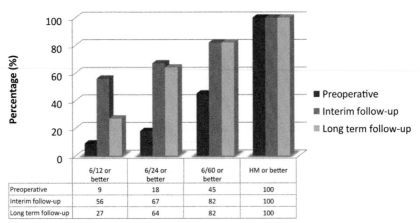

	6/12 or better	6/24 or better	6/60 or better	HM or better
Preoperative	9	18	45	100
Interim follow-up	56	67	82	100
Long term follow-up	27	64	82	100

FIGURE 1.—Cumulative best-corrected distance visual acuity (BDVA) of patients with >4 years follow-up. Preoperative BDVA is compared with BDVA at the last follow-up. HM, Hand movements. (Reprinted from Lyall DAM, Tarafdar S, Gilhooley MJ, et al. Long term visual outcomes, graft survival and complications of deep anterior lamellar keratoplasty in patients with herpes simplex related corneal scarring. *Br J Ophthalmol.* 2012;96:1200-1203, with permission from the BMJ Publishing Group Ltd.)

was diagnosed in 9 eyes (50%). Graft failure was found in 5 eyes (28%), including 2 eyes that had reactivation of HSV keratitis. Most patients required additional procedures, including 50% who underwent cataract extraction and intraocular lens implantation; other procedures included repeat transplantation, astigmatic incisions, trabeculectomy, and conjunctival flaps.

Graft survival after DALK for HSV keratitis was 72%. The authors found active inflammation preoperatively was a significant risk factor for graft failure. Interestingly, corneal neovascularization (both superficial and deep) was not found to be significantly associated with HSV reactivation, graft rejection, or graft failure. All patients were placed on prophylactic acyclovir postoperatively for 1 year.

These findings underscore the importance of treating active HSV keratitis medically and waiting for a period of inactive disease before performing keratoplasty. We typically wait for at least 6 months of quiescence before proceeding with surgery, and similar to the study, all of our patients are maintained on oral antiviral perioperatively and postoperatively.

While this is a small, retrospective study, the authors do suggest DALK is a reasonable option for visual rehabilitation for patients with HSV keratitis. However, both physician and patients should be aware of the higher risk of rejection and HSV reactivation as well as the high likelihood of requiring additional surgical procedures.

P. K. Nagra, MD

Diagnosis and treatment of ocular chronic graft-versus-host disease: report from the German-Austrian-Swiss Consensus Conference on Clinical Practice in chronic GVHD
Dietrich-Ntoukas T, Cursiefen C, Westekemper H. et al (Univ Med Ctr, Regensburg, Germany)
Cornea 31:299-310, 2012

Purpose.—Ocular chronic graft-versus-host disease (cGVHD) is one of the most frequent long-term complications after hematopoietic stem cell transplantation and is often associated with significant morbidity and reduced quality of life.

Methods.—The German/Austrian/Swiss Consensus Conference on Clinical Practice in cGVHD aimed to summarize the currently available evidence for diagnosis and (topical) treatment and to summarize different treatment modalities of ocular cGVHD. The presented consensus was based on a review of published evidence and a survey on the current clinical practice including transplant centers from Germany, Austria, and Switzerland.

Results.—Ocular cGVHD often affects the lacrimal glands, the conjunctiva, the lids (including meibomian glands), and the cornea but can also involve other parts of the eye such as the sclera. Up to now, there have been no pathognomonic diagnostic features identified. The main therapeutic aim in the management of ocular cGVHD is the treatment of inflammation and dryness to relieve patients' symptoms and to maintain ocular integrity and function. Therapy should be chosen in the context of the patient's overall condition, systemic immunosuppressive therapy, symptoms, ocular surface integrity, and inflammatory activity. The consensus conference proposed new grading criteria and diagnostic recommendations for general monitoring of patients with graft-versus-host-disease for use in clinical practice.

Conclusion.—The evidence levels for diagnosis and treatment of ocular cGVHD are low, and most of the treatment options are based on empirical knowledge. Topical immunosuppression, for example, with cyclosporine, represents a promising strategy to reduce inflammation and dryness in ocular cGVHD. Further clinical trials are necessary to elucidate risk factors for eye manifestation, complications, and visual loss and to evaluate staging criteria and diagnostic and therapeutic measures for ocular cGVHD.

▶ Ocular graft-versus-host disease (GVHD) is an increasing problem for the ophthalmologist, as bone marrow and peripheral stem cell transplants are being performed more frequently and with more success, and GVHD is the most common cause of nonrelapse-related morbidity. Chronic GVHD is difficult to treat, as the patients often have severe ocular surface compromise, which greatly affects their quality of life. These patients are often quite conflicted—they are happy to have survived the cancer but frustrated by the chronic photophobia, variable vision, and pain.

This article reports the findings from a European consensus panel, comprising mostly German centers. The authors provide an evaluation of the current thinking in making the diagnosis of chronic ocular GVHD, which involves a full ophthalmic examination, not simply Schirmer testing (see Table 3 in the original article). They also evaluate the level of evidence of treatments and give recommendations based on those (see Table 5 in the original article). Topical cyclosporine, one of the therapies discussed, is under investigation in a National Eye Institute—sponsored study. One of the hopes in the treatment of these patients is that earlier cyclosporine therapy may improve outcomes in this condition. The authors make a short note regarding scleral lenses. In our practice, we have had very good success from the prosthetic replacement ocular surface ecosystem lens in returning these patients to a better quality of life. These remain expensive and with limited availability, but the centers offering this are increasing in the United States.

K. M. Hammersmith, MD

Treatment of Mucous Membrane Pemphigoid With Mycophenolate Mofetil
Nottage JM, Hammersmith KM, Murchison AP, et al (Thomas Jefferson Univ, Philadelphia, PA; Eye Consultants of Maryland, Owings Mills)
Cornea 32:810-815, 2013

Purpose.—To evaluate the clinical outcomes of mycophenolate mofetil (MMF) treatment of mucous membrane pemphigoid (MMP).

Methods.—This is a retrospective analysis of consecutive patients with clinical MMP seen in the Ocular Surface Disease Clinic at the Wills Eye Institute, between January 1, 2004, and December 31, 2010, treated with MMF.

The main outcomes measured were control of inflammation and discontinuation of MMF.

Results.—A total of 23 MMP patients taking MMF were identified. The median age of the MMF-treated patients was 77.0 years. Eleven of the 23 patients (47.8%) had biopsy-proven MMP. All patients were at least Foster grading system stage 2, with most stage 3 or 4. Eight patients (34.8%) failed previous treatments with dapsone, methotrexate, prednisone, azathioprine, cyclophosphamide, or 6-mercaptopurine. The average duration of MMF treatment was 23.32 ± 33.17 months (range 1-124.83 months, median 7.4 months). Of the 23 patients with MMP, control of inflammation was achieved with MMF within 3 months for 56.5% [95% confidence interval (CI) 54.5-59.6], within 6 months for 69.6% (95% CI 65.2-76.6), and within 12 months for 82.6% (95% CI 75.3-92.4) of the patients. Nineteen patients (82.4%) achieved control of inflammation, with 16 of the 19 (84.2%) achieving control of inflammation with MMF as monotherapy. Fifteen patients were treated with MMF as initial therapy. Twenty-one percent of patients (5 of 23) were taken off MMF for failure of inflammatory control (4) or an allergic reaction (1).

Conclusions.—Treatment of MMP with MMF in this uncontrolled case series resulted in control of inflammation in the majority of patients with minimal side effects. Our data support consideration of MMF as an initial treatment option for active ocular MMP.

▶ This report evaluates the use of mycophenolate mofetil (MMF) for the treatment of mucosal membrane pemphigoid (MMP). Our group started to use MMF as an initial treatment option in patients around 10 years ago, when results with dapsone and other agents were disappointing. It has been our experience that MMF has been a very good immunosuppressive agent in these patients, and this report was initiated to crystallize that experience. Prior reports on the treatment of MMP have had only a few patients treated with MMF for MMP. In fact, the Systemic Immunosuppressive Treatment (SITE) study, which compiled data from multiple centers, included only 18 patients. Using similar evaluation measures as the SITE study, we found in our 23 patients very good control of inflammation. By 6 and 12 months, ocular inflammation was controlled in 69.6% and 82.6%, respectively. Most of these patients were treated with MMF as a monotherapy. This medicine affords a favorable safety profiles, especially when compared with cyclophosphamide. The patients treated were mostly elderly, and the safer side-effect profile is very important with other comorbidities. One finding from this report was that we rarely were able to take patients off of the medicine. Others have reported good remission rates with cyclophosphamide, which we did not see with MMF. As such, when younger, healthier patients present with MMP, we are more likely to recommend cyclophosphamide therapy, with the hope that they will tolerate the medication better and have a higher chance of remission. However, in the elderly patient population we more often see, this remains a very attractive treatment option. The newer biologics, especially rituximab, may also be appealing treatments, but we await more data on their use.

K. M. Hammersmith, MD

Acanthamoeba **keratitis: The Persistence of Cases Following a Multistate Outbreak**
Yoder JS, Verani J, Heidman N, et al (Ctrs for Disease Control and Prevention, Atlanta, GA; ARUP Laboratories, Salt Lake City, UT; et al)
Ophthalmic Epidemiol 19:221-225, 2012

Purpose.—To describe the trend of *Acanthamoeba* keratitis case reports following an outbreak and the recall of a multipurpose contact lens disinfection solution. *Acanthamoeba* keratitis is a serious eye infection caused by the free-living amoeba *Acanthamoeba* that primarily affects contact lens users.

Methods.—A convenience sample of 13 ophthalmology centers and laboratories in the USA, provided annual numbers of *Acanthamoeba* keratitis cases diagnosed between 1999—2009 and monthly numbers of cases diagnosed between 2007—2009. Data on ophthalmic preparations of anti-*Acanthamoeba* therapies were collected from a national compounding pharmacy.

Results.—Data from sentinel site ophthalmology centers and laboratories revealed that the yearly number of cases gradually increased from 22 in 1999 to 43 in 2003, with a marked increase beginning in 2004 (93 cases) that continued through 2007 (170 cases; $p < 0.0001$). The outbreak identified from these sentinel sites resulted in the recall of a contact lens disinfecting solution. There was a statistically significant ($p \leq 0.0001$) decrease in monthly cases reported from 28 cases in June 2007 (following the recall) to seven cases in June 2008, followed by an increase ($p = 0.0004$) in reported cases thereafter; cases have remained higher than pre-outbreak levels. A similar trend was seen in prescriptions for *Acanthamoeba* keratitis chemotherapy. Cases were significantly more likely to be reported during summer than during other seasons.

Conclusion.—The persistently elevated number of reported cases supports the need to understand the risk factors and environmental exposures associated with *Acanthamoeba* keratitis. Further prevention efforts are needed to reduce the number of cases occurring among contact lens wearers.

▶ This study presents the epidemiology of *Acanthamoeba* keratitis (AK) over a 10-year period, which includes the years associated with the Complete Moisture-Plus outbreak. This study compiles data from 13 centers throughout the United States as well as data from a large compounding pharmacy to determine the number of prescriptions written for AK. AK cases increased from 1999 to 2003, with a marked increase from 2003 to 2007, commensurate with the outbreak. This is similar to the cases that we have seen at Wills. Also similar, the cases were more likely to present during the summer, which is not surprising given water exposure during that time. Unlike the outbreak associated with fungal keratitis and Fusarium MoistureLoc, the cases of AK did not see a dramatic decrease after the removal of the associated solution. The cases have remained significantly greater than the previous baseline. The authors postulate that one possible etiology of this is that more physicians are aware of AK and that recognition is more likely. However, in our practice, the same physicians have been involved with the care of patients during this entire study period. Certainly, AK remains persistently pesky, and we need better understanding about the pathogenesis and risk factors associated with its development.

K. M. Hammersmith, MD

***Pseudomonas aeruginosa* Keratitis: Outcomes and Response to Corticosteroid Treatment**
Sy A, Srinivasan M, Mascarenhas J, et al (Univ of California, San Francisco; Aravind Eye Care System, Madurai, India; et al)
Invest Ophthalmol Vis Sci 53:267-272, 2012

Purpose.—To compare the clinical course and effect of adjunctive corticosteroid therapy in *Pseudomonas aeruginosa* with those of all other strains of bacterial keratitis.

Methods.—Subanalyses were performed on data collected in the Steroids for Corneal Ulcers Trial (SCUT), a large randomized controlled trial in which patients were treated with moxifloxacin and were randomly assigned to 1 of 2 adjunctive treatment arms: corticosteroid or placebo (4 times a day with subsequent reduction). Multivariate analysis was used to determine the effect of predictors, organism, and treatment on outcomes, 3-month best-spectacle-corrected visual acuity (BSCVA), and infiltrate/scar size. The incidence of adverse events over a 3-month follow-up period was compared using Fisher's exact test.

Results.—SCUT enrolled 500 patients. One hundred ten patients had *P. aeruginosa* ulcers; 99 of 110 (90%) enrolled patients returned for follow-up at 3 months. Patients with *P. aeruginosa* ulcers had significantly worse visual acuities than patients with other bacterial ulcers ($P = 0.001$) but showed significantly more improvement in 3-month BSCVA than those with other bacterial ulcers, adjusting for baseline characteristics (-0.14 log-MAR; 95% confidence interval, -0.23 to -0.04; $P = 0.004$). There was no significant difference in adverse events between *P. aeruginosa* and other bacterial ulcers. There were no significant differences in BSCVA ($P = 0.69$), infiltrate/scar size ($P = 0.17$), and incidence of adverse events between patients with *P. aeruginosa* ulcers treated with adjunctive corticosteroids and patients given placebo.

Conclusions.—Although *P. aeruginosa* corneal ulcers have a more severe presentation, they appear to respond better to treatment than other bacterial ulcers. The authors did not find a significant benefit with corticosteroid treatment, but they also did not find any increase in adverse events. (ClinicalTrials.gov number, NCT00324168.) (Table 5).

▶ This is a subgroup analysis from the Steroids for Corneal Ulcers Trial (SCUT), which evaluated in a prospective, randomized, controlled study the addition of topical corticosteroids in the treatment of bacterial keratitis. Pseudomonas remains a very commonly encountered bacteria, especially in relation to contact lens use. A virulent organism, the addition of topical corticosteroids has always been controversial. Interestingly, the pseudomonas ulcers in this study, mostly

TABLE 5.—Comparison of Adverse Events in Placebo versus Corticosteroid Treatment Arms within the *P. aeruginosa* Subgroup

	Placebo $(n=51)^* n$ (%)	Corticosteroid $(n=59)^* n$ (%)	$P^\dagger$
Change in antibiotic/addition of other antibiotic[‡]	11 (22)	4 (7)	0.03
Corneal perforation	1 (2)	1 (2)	>0.99
Death	1 (2)	1 (2)	>0.99
IOP elevated >25 but ≤35 mm Hg with medications within 1 week of therapy[§]	3 (6)	1 (2)	0.34
Increase in infiltrate size (>50%) and >1 mm in maximum diameter	1 (2)	0 (0)	0.46
No resolution of epithelial defect at 21 days or later	6 (12)	13 (22)	0.21
Progressive corneal thinning ≥50% of enrollment thickness	1 (2)	0 (0)	0.46
Recurrence of epithelial defect	0 (0)	1 (2)	>0.99
Total subjects with any adverse events	12 (24)	15 (25)	>0.99

*Adverse events were recorded from enrollment until the 3-month follow-up. These values (*n*) reflect the number of cases at enrollment.
[†]Fisher's exact test.
[‡]Other antibiotics included gentamicin, ceftazidime, amikacin, doxycycline, tobramycin, and ciprofloxacin.
[§]IOP elevation >35 was considered a serious adverse event. There were no cases of IOP elevation >35 in SCUT.

out of India and not related to contact lens use, had more dramatic improvement than other forms of infectious keratitis. These ulcers started significantly worse but ended significantly better. The addition of steroids did not yield a significant benefit. The larger SCUT study did show a subgroup of "worse" ulcers, defined by size and poor vision, that seemed to benefit from the addition of steroids. When I read that study, I assumed that the "worse" ulcers were likely pseudomonas and that there may be benefit with those infections. However, this evaluation did not find that. The authors report that there were also no increased adverse events with these patients (Table 5). However, 22% of patients had a persistent epithelial defect at 21 days in the corticosteroid group vs 12% in the placebo. Although this did not reach statistical significance (it did in the larger study), it is concerning. In the past year or so since the SCUT trial was presented, I have tried steroids in some of these "worse" infections (several pseudomonas), feeling emboldened that there were no increased adverse events and that it may help the patient's pain and comfort. I have not been impressed and have felt on some occasions that it has hindered reepithelialization. With the findings of this subgroup that steroids did not significantly help, I am less likely to add early steroids at this point.

K. M. Hammersmith, MD

Pediatric Herpes Simplex of the Anterior Segment: Characteristics, Treatment, and Outcomes
Liu S, Pavan-Langston D, Colby KA (Schepens Eye Res Inst, Boston, MA)
Ophthalmology 119:2003-2008, 2012

Purpose.—To describe the clinical characteristics, treatment, and outcomes of herpes simplex virus (HSV) infections of the cornea and

TABLE 2.—Treatment and Prophylactic Dosages for Acyclovir in Children

Age	Treatment Dose Thrice Daily	Prophylactic Dose Twice Daily
Infants (up to 18 mos)	100 mg (2.5 ml)	100 mg (2.5 ml)
Toddlers (18 mos–3 yrs)	200 mg (5 ml)	200 mg (5 ml)
Young children (3–5 yrs)	300 mg (7.5 ml)	300 mg (7.5 ml)
Older children (6 yrs and older)	400 mg (10 ml)	400 mg (10 ml)

adnexae to raise awareness and to improve management of this important eye disease in children.

Design.—Retrospective case series.

Participants.—Fifty-three patients (57 eyes) 16 years of age or younger with HSV keratitis (HSK), HSV blepharoconjunctivitis (HBC), or both in an academic cornea practice.

Methods.—The following data were collected: age at disease onset, putative trigger factors, coexisting systemic diseases, duration of symptoms and diagnoses given before presentation, visual acuity, slit-lamp examination findings, corneal sensation, dose and duration of medications used, drug side effects, and disease recurrence.

Main Outcome Measures.—Presence of residual corneal scarring, visual acuity at the last visit, changes in corneal sensation, recurrence rate, and manifestations of HSK were assessed in patients receiving long-term prophylactic systemic acyclovir.

Results.—The median age at onset was 5 years. Mean follow-up was 3.6 years. Eighteen eyes had HBC only; 4 patients in this group had bilateral disease. Of 39 eyes with keratitis, 74% had stromal disease. Thirty percent of HSK cases were misdiagnosed before presentation. Seventy-nine percent of patients with keratitis had corneal scarring and 26% had vision of 20/40 or worse at the last visit. Eighty percent of patients had recurrent disease. Six of 16 patients (37%) receiving long-term oral acyclovir had recurrent HSV, at least one case of which followed a growth spurt that caused the baseline dosage of acyclovir to become subtherapeutic.

Conclusions.—In a large series, pediatric HSK had a high rate of misdiagnosis, stromal involvement, recurrence, and vision loss. Oral acyclovir is effective, but the dosage must be adjusted as the child grows (Table 2).

► This is an excellent review of the clinical characteristics and treatment of herpes simplex keratitis in children. Reviewing 10 years of data in the cornea practices at the Massachusetts Eye and Ear Infirmary, the authors identified 53 patients with herpes simplex virus. The clinical characteristics of these patients are described in Table 1 of the original article. Nearly 80% of the patients had recurrent disease, which is higher than in adults, underscoring the importance of antiviral prophylaxis. The authors also reinforce the importance of adjusting acyclovir dosing with growth and illustrate this with a case presentation. Many of the bilateral cases were dermatitis-only cases. Scarring was not uncommon in the population.

The authors include their recommendations for oral antiviral treatment and prophylactic dosing (Table 2).

K. M. Hammersmith, MD

Fungal Keratitis Responsive to Moxifloxacin Monotherapy
Matoba AY (Baylor College of Medicine, Houston, TX)
Cornea 31:1206-1209, 2012

Purpose.—To report 5 cases of culture-proven fungal keratitis that resolved with moxifloxacin monotherapy.

Methods.—Case reports and review of medical literature. Five patients with fungal keratitis were treated with topical moxifloxacin.

Results.—All 5 patients had resolution of their infection with topical moxifloxacin monotherapy.

Conclusions.—Topical fluoroquinolone agents may have significant antifungal properties. However, the vast majority of fungal keratitis patients cannot be cured with fluoroquinolone monotherapy. An initial response of keratitis to topical fluoroquinolone therapy should not lead to the assumption that the infection is bacterial because the possibility of fungal infection cannot be ruled out on that basis.

▶ This article presents information on 5 patients, with varied stories of corneal compromise, who responded to monotherapy with moxifloxacin and were subsequently cultured with fungal organisms. The article describes in some detail the clinical course and culture results (2 *Curvularia*, 1 *Aspergillus*, 1 *Paecilomyces* sp.) as well as pertinent literature. As I started reading this, I recalled a patient I treated in 2005, who initially responded to fluoroquinolone therapy for a contact lens keratitis. When he had some persistent inflammation, steroids were added, which led to significant worsening and the ultimate diagnosis of Fusarium keratitis. In fact, he was one of our group's first patients with fungal keratitis related to the ReNu with Moisture Loc outbreak. The following year at ARVO, I read with interest the poster out of Bascom Palmer (Munir et al[1]) that described 5 cases of fungal keratitis responsive to antibiotic therapy. Interestingly, since that time, 2 additional articles have discussed clinical responsiveness to antibiotic therapy with Fusarium cases related to the ReNu Moisture Loc solution (Khor, Rai[2,3]). Many fungal organisms have high levels of topoisomerase, which is inhibited by fluoroquinolones. Tobramycin has also been shown to have some antifungal effect. It does certainly lead one to wonder if the fluoroquinolones would have some role in enhancing the effects of antifungal therapy. But certainly, it reminds us that initial improvement on antibiotic therapy does not necessarily mean a bacterial etiology. As Matoba cautions, in general, corticosteroid therapy should be withheld until the organism is identified.

K. M. Hammersmith, MD

References

1. Munir WM, Rosenfeld SI, Udell I, Miller D, Karp CL, Alfonso EC. Clinical response of contact lens-associated fungal keratitis to topical fluoroquinolone therapy. *Cornea.* 2007;26:621-624.
2. Khor WB, Aung T, Saw SM, et al. An outbreak of Fusarium keratitis associated with contact lens wear in Singapore. *JAMA.* 2006;295:2867-2873.
3. Rai SK, Lam PT, Li EY, Yuen HK, Lam DS. A case series of contact lens-associated Fusarium keratitis in Hong Kong. *Cornea.* 2007;26:1205-1209.

5 Retina

Clinical outcomes of triamcinolone-assisted anterior vitrectomy after phacoemulsification complicated by posterior capsule rupture
Kasbekar S, Prasad S, Kumar BV (Arrowe Park Hosp, Wirral, UK)
J Cataract Refract Surg 39:414-418, 2013

Purpose.—To compare the clinical outcomes in patients who had triamcinolone acetate—assisted anterior vitrectomy and patients who had anterior vitrectomy without triamcinolone acetate after phacoemulsification complicated by posterior capsule rupture and vitreous loss.
Setting.—Arrowe Park Hospital, Wirral, United Kingdom.
Design.—Retrospective consecutive case note review.
Methods.—Consecutive case notes of patients who had anterior vitrectomy assisted by triamcinolone acetonide (triamcinolone group) or without triamcinolone acetate (no-triamcinolone group) after posterior capsule rupture between January 2007 and January 2011 were identified and examined. Data recorded at the clinic visit preoperatively and 1 day and 3 months postoperatively were collated. Information recorded on the pro forma included visual acuity, ocular comorbidities, intraocular pressure (IOP), vitreous strands in the anterior chamber, and other adverse events.
Results.—No statistically significant difference was found in the visual acuity or IOP between 17 patients in the triamcinolone group and 34 patients in the no-triamcinolone group at any time point. Vitreous strands in the anterior chamber were noted in 1 patient in the triamcinolone group and 7 patients in the no-triamcinolone group. Cystoid macular edema (CME) was present in 3 patients in the no-triamcinolone group, including 1 patient with vitreomacular traction.
Conclusions.—There was no significant increase in IOP after triamcinolone acetate—assisted anterior vitrectomy. Higher rates of CME and residual anterior chamber vitreous strands in the no-triamcinolone acetate group support the clinical use of triamcinolone acetate.

▶ Triamcinolone-assisted vitrectomy surgery has been well described and practiced routinely by some surgeons. Once the posterior capsule is ruptured, identification and removal of vitreous can be challenging. Often the inability to visualize vitreous is secondary to not having a tangential light source available in the operating room. Triamcinolone adheres to vitreous and can aid with vitreous removal.

This was a small study, but it highlights the potential advantages to this technique, which is not routinely used by all cataract surgeons. The use of triamcinolone was not shown to increase the intraocular pressure postoperatively. In addition, higher rates of cystoid macular edema were noted in patients who underwent vitrectomy without triamcinolone. This could be because the vitreous was not completely removed and there may have been some residual vitreous traction on the macula. In addition, patients in the triamcinolone-assisted vitrectomy group benefited from the anti-inflammatory properties of triamcinolone. There were no adverse side effects or apparent toxicity to the use of triamcinolone identified in the study. Given the fact that posterior capsular rupture is a relatively low-occurring event, cataract surgeons may not be routinely removing vitreous from the anterior chamber. This method has been demonstrated to be safe and effective in identifying vitreous. As this technique becomes more popular, outcomes of patients with posterior capsular rupture will continue to improve.

O. P. Gupta, MD

Cumulative Effect of Risk Alleles in *CFH, ARMS2*, and *VEGFA* on the Response to Ranibizumab Treatment in Age-related Macular Degeneration
Smailhodzic D, Muether PS, Chen J, et al (Radboud Univ Nijmegen Med Ctr, The Netherlands; Univ of Cologne, Germany; McGill Univ Health Centre, Montreal, Canada)
Ophthalmology 119:2304-2311, 2012

Purpose.—Intravitreal ranibizumab injections currently are the standard treatment for neovascular age-related macular degeneration (AMD). However, a broad range of response rates have been observed, the reasons for which are poorly understood. This pharmacogenetic study evaluated the impact of high-risk alleles in *CFH, ARMS2, VEGFA*, vascular endothelial growth factor (VEGF) receptor *KDR*, and genes involved in angiogenesis (*LRP5, FZD4*) on the response to ranibizumab treatment and on the age of treatment onset. In contrast to previous studies, the data were stratified according to the number of high-risk alleles to enable the study of the combined effects of these genotypes on the treatment response.

Design.—Case series study.

Participants.—A cohort of 420 eyes of 397 neovascular AMD patients.

Methods.—The change in visual acuity (VA) between baseline and after 3 ranibizumab injections was calculated. Genotyping of single nucleotide polymorphisms in the *CFH, ARMS2, VEGFA, KDR, LPR5*, and *FZD4* genes was performed. Associations were assessed using linear mixed models.

Main Outcome Measures.—The VA change after 3 ranibizumab injections and the age of neovascular disease onset.

Results.—After ranibizumab treatment, AMD patients without risk alleles in the *CFH* and *ARMS2* genes (4.8%) demonstrated a mean VA improvement of 10 Early Treatment Diabetic Retinopathy Study (ETDRS) letters, whereas no VA improvement was observed in AMD patients with 4 *CFH* and *ARMS2* risk alleles (6.9%; $P = 0.014$). Patients with 4 high-risk alleles in *CFH* and *ARMS2* were 5.2 years younger than patients with

1 or 2 risk alleles, respectively (63.5%; *P* < 0.0001). The mean age at which the first ranibizumab treatment was carried out among AMD patients with all 6 risk alleles in *CFH, ARMS2,* and *VEGFA* was 65.9 years (2%) versus 75.3 years in patients with 0 or 1 high-risk allele (8.8%; *P* = 0.001). After ranibizumab treatment, patients with 6 high-risk alleles demonstrated a mean VA loss of 10 ETDRS letters (*P* < 0.0001).

Conclusions.—This study evaluated the largest pharmacogenetic AMD cohort reported to date. A cumulative effect of high-risk alleles in *CFH, ARMS2,* and *VEGFA* seems to be associated with a younger age of onset in combination with poor response rates to ranibizumab treatment.

▶ The variable response to intravitreal ranibizumab in the setting of neovascular age-related macular degeneration (nAMD) has been associated with a variety of factors. Genetic susceptibility is the most promising and emerging variable. There are a number of high-risk alleles that have been identified. Not only does genetic analysis help identify high-risk patients early in the disease, but, as this article demonstrates, genetic analysis might also help predict response to treatment. Neovascular age-related macular degeneration patients with none of the high-risk alleles experienced a significant improvement in vision with intravitreal ranibizumab compared with some patients with high-risk alleles. In addition, these genetically high-risk patients were found to have a more aggressive form of nAMD. This study has started to scientifically prove that heterogeneity exists within AMD as a whole. As these types of studies continue, subgroup analysis will become more important. In the future, certain subtypes of nAMD may be treated very differently compared with the current practice in which nAMD is treated more uniformly.

O. P. Gupta, MD

A randomised double-masked trial comparing the visual outcome after treatment with ranibizumab or bevacizumab in patients with neovascular age-related macular degeneration
Krebs I, for the MANTA Research Group (The Ludwig Boltzmann Inst for Retinology and Biomicroscopic Laser Surgery, Vienna, Austria; et al)
Br J Ophthalmol 97:266-271, 2013

Aim.—The current accepted standard treatment for neovascular age-related macular degeneration (AMD) consists of antivascular endothelial growth factor agents including ranibizumab and bevacizumab. The aim of the study was to examine whether bevacizumab is inferior to ranibizumab with respect to maintaining/improving visual acuity.

Methods.—In this prospective randomised parallel group multicentre trial patients aged more than 50 years with treatment naive nAMD were included at 10 Austrian centres. Patients were randomised to treatment either with 0.5 mg ranibizumab or 1.25 mg bevacizumab. Both groups received three initial monthly injections and thereafter monthly evaluation of visual acuity and the activity of the lesion. Re-treatment was scheduled as needed. Outcome measures were early treatment of diabetic retinopathy visual acuity, retinal thickness, lesion size and safety evaluation.

Results.—A total of 321 patients were recruited of which four had to be excluded due to different reasons. Of the 317 remaining patients 154 were randomised into the bevacizumab group and 163 into the ranibizumab group. At month 12, there was a mean increase of early treatment of diabetic retinopathy visual acuity of 4.9 letters in the bevacizumab and 4.1 letters in the ranibizumab group ($p = 0.78$). Furthermore, there were no significant differences in the decrease of retinal thickness, change of lesion size and number of adverse events between the groups.

Conclusions.—Bevacizumab was equivalent to ranibizumab for visual acuity at all time points over 1 year. There was no significant difference of decrease of retinal thickness or number of adverse events.

▶ CATT and IVAN were 2 prospective trials that compared ranibizumab and bevacizumab in the treatment of neovascular age-related macular degeneration. Both studies reported some differences between these 2 groups, but in general, the results were comparable. Another very important question that was explored in these studies regarded different treatment regimens.

This article continues to address this question by exploring pro re nata (PRN) dosing. The CATT did not evaluate PRN dosing, but rather looked at monthly dosing and an as-needed regimen. The IVAN trial and this study designed similar dosing regimens. This study reemphasizes that monthly dosing still remains the gold standard. Although it is difficult to compare results between trials, PRN dosing seems to be inferior in terms of visual and anatomic outcomes. This study has a couple of limitations. It evaluated PRN dosing, but having an arm with monthly dosing would have added value to the validity of this dosing regimen. In addition, the anatomic outcomes were difficult to analyze because of the different optical coherence tomography (OCT) machines used in the study. Therefore, comparing OCT measurements even within the trial is flawed.

O. P. Gupta, MD

Optic Neuropathy after Vitrectomy for Retinal Detachment: Clinical Features and Analysis of Risk Factors
Bansal AS, Hsu J, Garg SJ, et al (Thomas Jefferson Univ, Philadelphia, PA)
Ophthalmology 119:2364-2370, 2012

Purpose.—To describe the clinical characteristics of and risk factors for the development of optic neuropathy after pars plana vitrectomy (PPV) for macula-sparing primary rhegmatogenous retinal detachment (RRD) repair.

Design.—Retrospective case-control study.

Participants.—Seven patients who underwent PPV for macula-sparing primary RRD with subsequent development of optic neuropathy and 42 age- and gender-matched control patients undergoing PPV for macula-sparing primary RRD.

Methods.—Retrospective chart review of medical and surgical records.
Main Outcome Measures.—Clinical features of patients who developed optic neuropathy after PPV for macula-sparing RRD and analysis of potential risk factors (age, gender, medical history, surgical technique, intraoperative ocular perfusion pressure [OPP], and operative time).

Results.—At last follow-up, all 7 patients with optic neuropathy had visual acuity less than 20/200, relative afferent pupillary defects, optic nerve pallor, and visual field defects. A total of 5 of 7 patients (71%) demonstrated intraoperative reduced OPP with associated systemic hypotension compared with 7 of 42 patients (17%) in the control cohort ($P = 0.01$).

Conclusions.—Optic neuropathy after PPV for macula-sparing primary RRD is a rare but potentially devastating complication. Although the cause is often unclear, reduced ocular perfusion due to intraoperative systemic hypotension may be a contributing risk factor in some eyes.

▶ Intraoperative and postoperative complications following pars plana vitrectomy (PPV) have been minimized with the advancement in surgical instrumentation. Although PPV has become safer, the basic steps of most procedures have not changed in many years. Optic neuropathy is one of the most devastating complications of PPV, especially in eyes with good visual potential.

These authors explored optic neuropathy following repair of macula-sparing rhegmatogenous retinal detachment. Potential causes such as mechanical trauma from the retrobulbar block, direction of the infusion cannula, and intraoperative manipulation of a variety of instruments have all been theorized to cause optic neuropathy after PPV. Although the results of this study are not definitive, one of the most important risk factors that was discussed was reduced ocular perfusion pressure (OPP). Increased intraocular pressure and reduced systemic blood pressure lead to reduced OPP. When the OPP is low, the optic nerve perfusion is compromised and potentially causes optic neuropathy. Perhaps an underappreciated risk factor, OPP requires surgeons to not only pay attention to the intraocular pressure but also to the systemic blood pressure. In addition to OPP, the authors identify many risk factors that can contribute to optic nerve injury during PPV. It is important to minimize all of these risk factors given how devastating its effect can be.

O. P. Gupta, MD

Intravitreal Aflibercept (VEGF Trap-Eye) in Wet Age-related Macular Degeneration

Heier JS, for the VIEW 1 and VIEW 2 Study Groups (Ophthalmic Consultants of Boston and Tufts Univ School of Medicine, MA; et al)
Ophthalmology 119:2537-2548, 2012

Objective.—Two similarly designed, phase-3 studies (VEGF Trap-Eye: Investigation of Efficacy and Safety in Wet AMD [VIEW 1, VIEW 2]) of neovascular age-related macular degeneration (AMD) compared monthly and every-2-month dosing of intravitreal aflibercept injection (VEGF Trap-Eye;

Regeneron, Tarrytown, NY, and Bayer HealthCare, Berlin, Germany) with monthly ranibizumab.

Design.—Double-masked, multicenter, parallel-group, active-controlled, randomized trials.

Participants.—Patients (n = 2419) with active, subfoveal, choroidal neovascularization (CNV) lesions (or juxtafoveal lesions with leakage affecting the fovea) secondary to AMD.

Intervention.—Patients were randomized to intravitreal aflibercept 0.5 mg monthly (0.5q4), 2 mg monthly (2q4), 2 mg every 2 months after 3 initial monthly doses (2q8), or ranibizumab 0.5 mg monthly (Rq4).

Main Outcome Measures.—The primary end point was noninferiority (margin of 10%) of the aflibercept regimens to ranibizumab in the proportion of patients maintaining vision at week 52 (losing <15 letters on Early Treatment Diabetic Retinopathy Study [ETDRS] chart). Other key end points included change in best-corrected visual acuity (BCVA) and anatomic measures.

Results.—All aflibercept groups were noninferior and clinically equivalent to monthly ranibizumab for the primary end point (the 2q4, 0.5q4, and 2q8 regimens were 95.1%, 95.9%, and 95.1%, respectively, for VIEW 1, and 95.6%, 96.3%, and 95.6%, respectively, for VIEW 2, whereas monthly ranibizumab was 94.4% in both studies). In a prespecified integrated analysis of the 2 studies, all aflibercept regimens were within 0.5 letters of the reference ranibizumab for mean change in BCVA; all aflibercept regimens also produced similar improvements in anatomic measures. Ocular and systemic adverse events were similar across treatment groups.

Conclusions.—Intravitreal aflibercept dosed monthly or every 2 months after 3 initial monthly doses produced similar efficacy and safety outcomes as monthly ranibizumab. These studies demonstrate that aflibercept is an effective treatment for AMD, with the every-2-month regimen offering the potential to reduce the risk from monthly intravitreal injections and the burden of monthly monitoring.

▶ This is an important article that presents the visual and anatomic outcomes of intravitreal aflibercept (Eylea) in the treatment of neovascular age-related macular degeneration (nAMD). Different doses and treatment intervals were explored. Monthly intravitreal ranibizumab served as the control arm. All treatment regimens demonstrated similar visual and anatomic outcomes. In addition, the ocular and systemic adverse events were not statistically different between the cohorts. The study demonstrated that intravitreal aflibercept dosed monthly or every 2 months after 3 monthly doses were similar to the visual and anatomic outcomes of monthly intravitreal ranibizumab. This is a relatively significant finding because this is the first time another drug has been shown to be equivalent to monthly ranibizumab in a double-masked, randomized, head-to-head trial for the treatment of nAMD. In addition, this was the first major trial that reported similar outcomes with treatment intervals every month and less than every month. This trial presented some compelling results but also created some concern for specific clinical scenarios. From a scientific and statistical standpoint, patients with monthly ranibizumab were similar to every 2-month dosing of aflibercept after the first 3 monthly injections. However, one might be tempted to continue to treat monthly with aflibercept in a patient with persistent exudation after the first 3 monthly injections. Since the protocol calls for a 2-month dose after every set of 3 monthly injections, continued monthly dosing after the first 3 monthly doses may present a reimbursement issue.

O. P. Gupta, MD

Interventions for Toxoplasma Retinochoroiditis: A Report by the American Academy of Ophthalmology
Kim SJ, Scott IU, Brown GC, et al (Vanderbilt Univ School of Medicine, Nashville, TN; Penn State College of Medicine, Herchey, PA; Ctr for Value Based Medicine, Flourtown, PA; et al)
Ophthalmology 120:371-378, 2013

Objective.—To evaluate the available evidence in peer-reviewed publications about the outcomes and safety of interventions for toxoplasma retinochoroiditis (TRC).

Methods.—Literature searches of the PubMed and the Cochrane Library databases were conducted last on July 20, 2011, with no date restrictions. The searches retrieved 275 unique citations, and 36 articles of possible clinical relevance were selected for full text review. Of these 36 articles, 11 were deemed sufficiently relevant or of interest, and they were rated according to strength of evidence.

Results.—Eight of the 11 studies reviewed were randomized controlled studies, and none of them demonstrated that routine antibiotic or corticosteroid treatment of TRC favorably affects visual outcomes or reduces lesion size. There is level II evidence from 1 study suggesting that long-term treatment with combined trimethoprim and sulfamethoxazole prevented recurrent disease in patients with chronic relapsing TRC. Adverse effects of antibiotic treatment were reported in as many as 25% of patients. There was no evidence supporting the efficacy of other nonmedical treatments such as laser photocoagulation.

Conclusions.—There is a lack of level I evidence to support the efficacy of routine antibiotic or corticosteroid treatment for acute TRC in immunocompetent patients. There is level II evidence suggesting that long-term prophylactic treatment may reduce recurrences in chronic relapsing TRC. Adverse effects of certain antibiotic regimens are frequent, and patients require regular monitoring and timely discontinuation of the antibiotic in some cases.

▶ This publication was an ophthalmic technology assessment that was organized by the American Academy of Ophthalmology. The overall goal was to propose a current, relevant question and explore the literature for the best evidence available. The treatment of toxoplasma retinochoroiditis (TRC) remains unclear. The pathogenesis and rather varied clinical presentations have been published in case reports, small series, and larger retrospective reports. Although antibiotic with or without corticosteroid treatment has been a popular option for treating either acute or chronic TRC, no randomized clinical trial to date has demonstrated favorable results in immunocompetent patients. This is known as level I evidence for well-designed and well-conducted clinical trials. There is 1 unmasked study where long-term treatment with trimethoprim and sulfamethoxazole prevented recurrence in chronic relapsing TRC. This was a level II study, which is designated for studies with well-designed case control or cohort studies or poorly designed randomized clinical trials. This study and a review of the literature are important for our understanding of the evidence or lack of evidence for the treatment of TRC. A larger, more coordinated clinical trial is difficult to perform because of its relatively low occurrence, wide variety of clinical presentations in the acute setting, and inability to quantify treatment response.

O. P. Gupta, MD

Intravitreal Aflibercept Injection for Macular Edema Secondary to Central Retinal Vein Occlusion: 1-Year Results From the Phase 3 COPERNICUS Study
Brown DM, Heier JS, Clark WL, et al (The Methodist Hosp, Houston, TX; Ophthalmic Consultants of Boston, MA; Palmetto Retina Ctr, West Columbia, SC; et al)
Am J Ophthalmol 155:429-437, 2013

- *Purpose.*—To evaluate intravitreal aflibercept injections (IAI; also called VEGF Trap-Eye) for patients with macular edema secondary to central retinal vein occlusion (CRVO).
- *Design.*—Randomized controlled trial.
- *Methods.*—This multicenter study randomized 189 patients (1 eye/patient) with macular edema secondary to CRVO to receive 6 monthly injections of either 2 mg intravitreal aflibercept (IAI 2Q4) (n = 115) or sham (n = 74). From week 24 to week 52, all patients received 2 mg intravitreal aflibercept as needed (IAI 2Q4 + PRN and sham + IAI PRN) according to retreatment criteria. The primary endpoint was the proportion of patients who gained ≥15 ETDRS letters from baseline at week 24. Additional endpoints included visual, anatomic, and quality-of-life NEI VFQ-25 outcomes at weeks 24 and 52.
- *Results.*—At week 24, 56.1% of IAI 2Q4 patients gained ≥15 letters from baseline compared with 12.3% of sham patients ($P < .001$). At week 52, 55.3% of IAI 2Q4 + PRN patients gained ≥15 letters compared with 30.1% of sham + IAI PRN patients ($P < .001$). At week 52, IAI 2Q4 + PRN patients gained a mean of 16.2 letters of vision vs 3.8 letters for sham + IAI PRN ($P < .001$). The most common adverse events for both groups were conjunctival hemorrhage, eye pain, reduced visual acuity, and increased intraocular pressure.
- *Conclusions.*—Monthly injections of 2 mg intravitreal aflibercept for patients with macular edema secondary to CRVO resulted in a statistically significant improvement in visual acuity at week 24, which was largely

maintained through week 52 with intravitreal aflibercept PRN dosing. Intravitreal aflibercept injection was generally well tolerated.

▶ Intravitreal aflibercept (Eylea) injection (IAI) was initially reported for the use of neovascular age-related macular degeneration. Similar to the application of other antivascular endothelial growth factor compounds, the use of IAI was applied to central retinal vein occlusion (CRVO). This study evaluated the use of IAI in a monthly fashion for 6 months followed by an as-needed treatment regimen for the remaining 6 months of the study. The sham arm received sham injections for the first 6 months and then received as-needed treatment with IAI for the remaining 6 months. This study was primarily conducted in the United States with a couple of international sites that collectively were named the COPERNICUS study cohort. The results of this trial are favorable for frequent dosing. There was a slight decline in the letters gained in the treatment arm once this group was treated as needed. In addition, there was a marked improvement in vision once patients in the sham group starting receiving treatment after the first 6 months of sham injections. One obvious limitation to this trial is that an appropriate control arm was not used. Both bevacizumab and ranibizumab have been widely used for the treatment of CRVO. The Study of the Efficacy and Safety of Ranibizumab Injection in Patients With Macular Edema Secondary to Central Retinal Vein Occlusion (CRUISE) trial had been previously published. Comparing the COPERNICUS to CRUISE results is not ideal because of the use of different methodologies.

O. P. Gupta, MD

Infliximab Treatment of Patients with Birdshot Retinochoroidopathy
Artornsombudh P, Gevorgyan O, Payal A, et al (Massachusetts Eye Res and Surgery Institution, Cambridge; Univ of Pennsylvania, Philadelphia)
Ophthalmology 120:588-592, 2013

Purpose.—To report the outcomes of infliximab treatment of birdshot retinochoroidopathy (BSRC) refractory to conventional immunomodulatory therapy.

Design.—Retrospective case series.

Participants.—Twenty-two refractory birdshot retinochoroidopathy patients (44 eyes) who received infliximab between July 2005 and June 2012 were identified by retrospective chart review.

Methods.—All patients received 4 to 5 mg/kg infliximab at 4- to 8-week intervals. Data regarding patient demographics, use of immunosuppressive drugs, biologic agents, and reason for conventional therapy discontinuation were gathered. Disease activity markers, including signs of ocular inflammation, fluorescein angiography evidence of retinal vasculitis or papillitis, indocyanine green angiography evidence of active choroiditis, electroretinography parameters indicative of stable or worsening of retinal functions, and optical coherence tomography findings indicative of static or worsening macular edema were recorded.

Main Outcome Measures.—Abolition of all evidence of active inflammation, visual acuity (VA), presence of cystoid macular edema at 6 months and 1 year, and adverse responses to infliximab.

Results.—Mean duration of disease before starting infliximab was 58.6 months. Before infliximab therapy, all patients received and failed conventional immunosuppressive therapy. Ten patients had received another biologic agent. After initiating infliximab, control of inflammation was achieved in 81.8% at 6 months and in 88.9% at the 1-year follow-up. Three patients had active inflammation during therapy. The rate of cystoid macular edema decreased from 22.7% at baseline to 13.9% at 6 months and 6.7% at 1 year after receiving the drug. Initial VA of 20/40 or better was found in 34 eyes (84.1%). At 6 months and 1 year, 91.7% and 94.4% of eyes, respectively, had VA of 20/40 or better. Six patients had adverse events; infliximab therapy was discontinued in these patients because of neuropathy, drug-induced lupus, allergic reaction, or fungal infection.

Conclusions.—The data suggest that infliximab is effective for controlling inflammation in otherwise treatment-refractory cases of BSRC.

▶ Steroid-sparing immunomodulatory therapy is becoming increasingly adopted as this large group of medicines becomes safer. For chronic inflammatory diseases, they are particularly attractive for long-term immunosuppression. Birdshot retinochoroidopathy (BSRC) is a slowly progressive, chronic inflammatory disease that leads to gradual visual loss. In this study, the investigators explored the use of infliximab (Remicade) for the treatment of refractory BSRC. Previous medications included mycophenolate mofetil, cyclosporine, sirolimus, methotrexate, and daclizumab. These patients were switched after persistent inflammation or side-effect intolerance. They had been on previous treatments a mean of almost 5 years before starting infliximab. In this high-risk, fairly aggressive group of patients with BSRC, control of inflammation, reduction of cystoid macular edema, and improvement of vision were noted in the majority of patients. Unfortunately, side effects are unavoidable with this medication and other immunomodulating agents. Almost 14% of patients experienced side effects and infliximab was discontinued. As we gain an understanding of the pathophysiology of this disease, our treatment options will become more targeted to the underlying cause. Some have implied that BSRC is a T-cell mediated disease and, therefore, infliximab is an appropriate agent.

O. P. Gupta, MD

Change in subfoveal choroidal thickness in central serous chorioretinopathy following spontaneous resolution and low-fluence photodynamic therapy
Kang NH, Kim YT (Ewha Womans Univ, Seoul, Republic of Korea)
Eye 27:387-391, 2013

Purpose.—To assess the change in subfoveal choroidal thickness (SFCT) in central serous chorioretinopathy (CSC) following spontaneous resolution and low-fluence photodynamic therapy (PDT) using the enhanced depth imaging optical coherence tomography (EDI-OCT).

Methods.—A total of 36 consecutive eyes of 36 patients were included in this retrospective study: 16 eyes with spontaneously resolved CSC and 20 eyes with PDT-treated CSC. Best-corrected visual acuity and SFCT were evaluated at each visit until complete absorption of the subretinal fluid. SFCT of 32 normal subjects were also measured, as the control group. Wilcoxon's singed-rank test was used to evaluate the effects of spontaneous resolution and PDT. To compare the SFCT of the eyes with resolved CSC with that of the normal eyes, Mann—Whitney U-test with Bonferroni correction was also employed.

Results.—SFCT of patients was $459.16 \pm 77.50\ \mu m$ at the baseline, and decreased to $419.31 \pm 54.49\ \mu m$ after a spontaneous resolution $(P = 0.015)$. However, SFCT was not normalized in comparison with that of the normal subjects $(P < 0.001)$. SFCT in PDT group was also reduced from 416.43 ± 74.01 to $349.50 \pm 88.99\ \mu m$ $(P < 0.001)$, with no significant difference with the normal value $(P = 0.087)$.

Conclusions.—SFCT in patients with CSC decreased both after spontaneous resolution and low-fluence PDT. However, only in the PDT group, after disappearance of subretinal fluid, did it decrease to that of normal subjects.

▶ The pathogenesis and treatment of central serous chorioretinopathy (CSC) is poorly understood. Through different diagnostic modalities, such as fluorescein angiography, indocyanine green angiography, and, most recently, optical coherence tomography (OCT), we have a better understanding of the role that the choroidal vasculature plays in this disease. More recent advancements in OCT technology have allowed the provider to evaluate structures deeper than the neurosensory retina. Enhanced-depth imaging OCT allows quantitative analysis of the choroidal vasculature thickness. Patients with CSC have already been found to have abnormally thick subfoveal choroidal vasculature. This study evaluates the choroidal thickness in patients with CSC who experience spontaneous resolution compared with those treated with photodynamic therapy (PDT). Patients with spontaneous resolution of subretinal fluid were found to have a persistently thick choroid. However, patients who underwent PDT were reported to have a reduced choroidal thickness with treatment. The choroidal thickness was not statistically different from that of the normal control group included in the study. Although the value of PDT has been already shown in the treatment of CSC, this study supports its use in restoring not only the retinal architecture but also the choroidal architecture. It also supports the use of half-fluence PDT, which was used in this study. Although anatomic restoration after PDT has scientific merits, evaluation of the long-term recurrence rate between these 2 groups still remains unclear.

O. P. Gupta, MD

A Longitudinal Analysis of Risk Factors Associated with Central Retinal Vein Occlusion

Stem MS, Talwar N, Comer GM, et al (Univ of Michigan Med School, Ann Arbor)

Ophthalmology 120:362-370, 2013

Purpose.—To identify risk factors associated with central retinal vein occlusion (CRVO) among a diverse group of patients throughout the United States.

Design.—Longitudinal cohort study.

Participants.—All beneficiaries aged ≥ 55 years who were continuously enrolled in a managed care network for at least 2 years and who had ≥2 visits to an eye care provider from 2001 to 2009.

Methods.—Insurance billing codes were used to identify individuals with a newly diagnosed CRVO. Multivariable Cox regression was performed to determine the factors associated with CRVO development.

Main Outcome Measures.—Adjusted hazard ratios (HRs) with 95% confidence intervals (CIs) of being diagnosed with CRVO.

Results.—Of the 494 165 enrollees who met the study inclusion criteria, 1302 (0.26%) were diagnosed with CRVO over 5.4 (± 1.8) years. After adjustment for known confounders, blacks had a 58% increased risk of CRVO compared with whites (HR, 1.58; 95% CI, 1.25−1.99), and women had a 25% decreased risk of CRVO compared with men (HR, 0.75; 95% CI, 0.66−0.85). A diagnosis of stroke increased the hazard of CRVO by 44% (HR, 1.44; 95% CI, 1.23−1.68), and hypercoagulable state was associated with a 145% increased CRVO risk (HR, 2.45; 95% CI, 1.40−4.28). Individuals with end-organ damage from hypertension (HTN) or diabetes mellitus (DM) had a 92% (HR, 1.92; 95% CI, 1.52−2.42) and 53% (HR, 1.53; 95% CI, 1.28−1.84) increased risk of CRVO, respectively, relative to those without these conditions.

Conclusions.—This study confirms that HTN and vascular diseases are important risk factors for CRVO. We also identify black race as being associated with CRVO, which was not well appreciated previously. Furthermore, we show that compared with patients without DM, individuals with end-organ damage from DM have a heightened risk of CRVO, whereas those with uncomplicated DM are not at increased risk of CRVO. This finding may provide a potential explanation for the conflicting reports in the literature on the association between CRVO and DM. Information from analyses such as this can be used to create a risk calculator to identify possible individuals at greatest risk for CRVO.

▶ It is important to identify and control risk factors contributing to central retinal vein occlusions (CRVO). Modifiable risk factors often lead to an increased risk of morbidity and mortality. This study identified risk factors that have an increased risk for CRVO. The authors analyzed data from a very large managed care database. African-Americans and men were identified as having nonmodifiable risk factors. Patients who have a history of stroke, hypercoagulable state, atherosclerosis, end-organ damage from hypertension, or diabetes mellitus (DM) were found to have an increased risk of CRVO. This is different from previous reports and the conflicting findings regarding the relationship between CRVO and diabetes mellitus. Patients with uncomplicated DM did not have an increased risk of CRVO, but those with more advanced DM showed a higher hazard ratio. One of the major limitations of this study is that the analysis was based on claims data, not clinical data. The diagnosis that was coded may not always be consistent with the clinical picture. In addition, a certain proportion was likely misdiagnosed and miscoded.

O. P. Gupta, MD

VEGF Trap-Eye for macular oedema secondary to central retinal vein occlusion: 6-month results of the phase III GALILEO study
Holz FG, Roider J, Ogura Y, et al (Univ of Bonn, Germany; Univ of Kiel, Germany; Nagoya City Univ Graduate School of Med Science, Japan; et al)
Br J Ophthalmol 97:278-284, 2013

Aim.—To evaluate intravitreal VEGF Trap-Eye (VTE) in patients with macular oedema secondary to central retinal vein occlusion (CRVO).

Methods.—In this double-masked study, 177 patients were randomised (3:2 ratio) to intravitreal injections of VTE 2 mg or sham procedure every 4 weeks for 24 weeks. Best-corrected visual acuity was evaluated using the Early Treatment Diabetic Retinopathy Study chart. Central retinal thickness (CRT) was measured with optical coherence tomography.

Results.—From baseline until week 24, more patients receiving VTE (60.2%) gained ≥ 15 letters compared with those receiving sham injections (22.1%) ($p < 0.0001$). VTE patients gained a mean of 18.0 letters compared with 3.3 letters with sham injections ($p < 0.0001$). Mean CRT decreased by 448.6 and 169.3 μm in the VTE and sham groups ($p < 0.0001$). The most frequent ocular adverse events in the VTE arm were typically associated with the injection procedure or the underlying disease, and included eye pain (11.5%), increased intraocular pressure (9.6%) and conjunctival haemorrhage (8.7%).

Conclusions.—VTE 2 mg every 4 weeks was efficacious in CRVO with an acceptable safety profile. Vision gains with VTE were significantly higher than with observation/panretinal photocoagulation if needed. Based on these data, VTE may provide a new treatment option for CRVO.

▶ Intravitreal aflibercept, or VEGF Trap, has been evaluated for neovascular age-related macular degeneration (nAMD). This study cohort was a group of international sites that was termed the *GALILEO study group*. The COPERNICUS study cohort was essentially the same trial predominately conducted in the United States with some international sites. This study reported the initial 6-month results of the use of VEGF Trap. There will be a 6-month extension in which both treatment arms (intervention and sham) receive injections as needed as well as another 6-month extension in which patients receive an injection every 2 months. This study was well conducted and supports the use of VEGF Trap for macular edema secondary to central retinal vein occlusion (CRVO). However, the authors also make comparisons between this trial and the Study of the Efficacy and Safety of Ranibizumab Injection in Patients with Macular Edema Secondary to Central Retinal Vein Occlusion trial, which can be misleading. Direct comparisons among these cohorts and the visual and anatomic outcomes cannot be made in a rigorous fashion. The inclusion and exclusion criteria were different and resulted in different study cohorts. Although this comparison is tempting, a more appropriate way of comparing these 2 groups would involve using ranibizumab as the control arm. There are many reasons this did not happen and most likely will not happen with industry-sponsored research. A federally funded trial like the Comparison of Age-related Macular Degeneration Treatments Trials would need to be performed, but, unfortunately, CRVO is not as large a public health problem as nAMD.

O. P. Gupta, MD

Intravitreal bevacizumab plus grid laser photocoagulation or intravitreal bevacizumab or grid laser photocoagulation for diffuse diabetic macular edema: Results of the Pan-American Collaborative Retina Study Group at 24 Months

Arevalo JF, for the Pan-American Collaborative Retina Study Group (PACORES) (Johns Hopkins Univ School of Medicine, Baltimore, MD; et al)
Retina 33:403-413, 2013

Purpose.—To evaluate the anatomical and functional outcomes at 24 months in patients with diffuse diabetic macular edema treated with primary intravitreal bevacizumab (IVB) plus grid laser photocoagulation (GLP) or primary IVB alone or GLP alone.

Methods.—Retrospective, interventional, comparative, multicenter study. We included in this analysis 141 eyes of 120 patients with diffuse diabetic macular edema treated with primary IVB alone (Group A), 120 eyes of 94 patients with GLP therapy (Group B), and 157 eyes of 104 patients treated with IVB plus GLP (Group C).

Results.—In all 3 groups, the authors observed improvement of Early Treatment Diabetic Retinopathy Study best-corrected visual acuity from baseline to 24-month follow-up ($P < 0.0001$). The improvement rate in Group A was statistically significantly better than in Group B (analysis of variance, $P = 0.013$). The authors also found a decrease in central macular thickness in all groups from baseline to the 24-month follow-up ($P < 0.0001$). The comparison among 3 groups showed higher central macular thickness decrease in Group A than in Groups B and C (analysis of variance, $P < 0.001$).

Conclusion.—The study provides evidence to support the use of primary IVB with or without GLP as treatment of diffuse diabetic macular edema. Primary IVB without GLP seems to be superior to GLP alone to provide stability or improvement in best-corrected visual acuity in patients with diffuse diabetic macular edema at 24 months.

▶ Along with the work produced by the Diabetic Retinopathy Clinical Research Network, the Pan-American Collaborative Retina Study Group has also been evaluating new treatment algorithms for fovea-involving diabetic macular edema. This study re-emphasizes the importance of antivascular endothelial growth factor medications in the management of this disease. Intravitreal bevacizumab (IVB) was used in this multicenter, retrospective trial. The investigators found that focal laser was not shown to be as effective without the use of IVB. Intravitreal bevacizumab plus laser was statistically better than IVB alone. This study is one of many that resulted in fairly similar conclusions. Focal laser photocoagulation still plays a role in the management of fovea-involving macular edema, but as monotherapy it is no longer the best option. As we gain a better understanding of these treatment algorithms, a more standardized approach might emerge. For now, even though this and other studies have guided our treatment, there is much left to the provider's discretion.

O. P. Gupta, MD

Comparison of Vitrectomy with Brilliant Blue G or Indocyanine Green on Retinal Microstructure and Function of Eyes with Macular Hole

Baba T, Hagiwara A, Sato E, et al (Chiba Univ Graduate School of Medicine, Japan)

Ophthalmology 119:2609-2615, 2012

Purpose. To evaluate the microstructure of the inner and outer retina and the visual function after macular hole (MH) surgery using brilliant blue G (BBG) or indocyanine green (ICG) to make the internal limiting membrane (ILM) more visible.

Design.—Comparative, retrospective, interventional case series.

Participants.—Sixty-three eyes of 63 consecutive cases with MH were studied. Thirty-five eyes of 35 cases were treated with BBG between January and August 2011. Twenty-eight eyes of 28 MH cases were treated with ICG from April 2009 through April 2010.

Methods.—Vitrectomy was performed with a 23-gauge system and 0.25 mg/ml BBG or with 0.125% ICG.

Main Outcome Measures.—The best-corrected visual acuity (BCVA) and the microperimetry-determined retinal sensitivity were measured at baseline and at 3 and 6 months after surgery. The length of the defect of the photoreceptor inner segment/outer segment (IS/OS) junction and external limiting membrane (ELM), the central foveal thickness (CFT), and the thickness of the ganglion cell complex (GCC) were measured in the spectral-domain optical coherence tomographic images.

Results.—The average BCVA was significantly better in the BBG group than in the ICG group at 3 months ($P = 0.021$) and 6 months ($P = 0.045$) after surgery. The mean retinal sensitivity in the BBG group was improved significantly in the central 2° at 3 and 6 months ($P = 0.001$ and $P = 0.030$, respectively), but was not significantly improved in the adjacent 10°. The length of IS/OS junction defect was significantly shorter in the BBG group at 3 months ($P = 0.048$), but was not significantly different at 6 months ($P = 0.135$). The length of ELM defect and the GCC thickness were not significantly different between the 2 groups at 3 and 6 months. The CFT was significantly thinner in the ICG group than in the BBG group at 3 and 6 months ($P = 0.013$ and $P = 0.001$, respectively).

Conclusions.—The postoperative BCVA and retinal sensitivity in the central 2° were better in eyes after BBG-assisted vitrectomy. The restoration of IS/OS junction was faster in the BBG group, and the CFT was significantly thinner in eyes after ICG. Brilliant blue G may be a better agent than ICG to make the ILM more visible.

▶ Toxicity of surgical adjuncts in the setting of macular hole repair has been debated in the literature. Some of the original literature regarding toxicity has been described with in vitro experiments, while more recent studies have attempted to evaluate the safety and efficacy of surgical adjuncts with in vivo experiments.

This retrospective study suggests that brilliant blue G (BBG) is superior to indocyanine green (ICG) in terms of safety and outcomes. The safety endpoint was retinal sensitivity measured with microperimetry, and their surgical outcomes were visual acuity and optical coherence tomography analysis. At 6 months postoperatively, the central 2° retinal sensitivity was statistically better in the BBG group compared with the ICG group. In terms of surgical outcomes at 6 months postoperatively, the best-corrected visual acuity, restoration of the inner segment or outer segment junction, and central foveal thickness were superior in the BBG group. This is a small (63 eyes) retrospective study with significant limitations. The sample size may not be powered to demonstrate statistical significance. Although the surgical technique was similar, 3 surgeons were involved in the study. Among other subtle differences in technique, the exposure and the surgical adjunct may be different. Lastly, almost all the cases were combined with cataract extraction. This is a confounding variable when interpreting the results, especially when comparing preoperative and postoperative data.

O. P. Gupta, MD

Long-term Use of Aspirin and Age-Related Macular Degeneration
Klein BEK, Howard KP, Gangnon RE, et al (Univ of Wisconsin School of Medicine and Public Health, Madison)
JAMA 308:2469-2478, 2012

Context.—Aspirin is widely used for relief of pain and for cardioprotective effects. Its use is of concern to ophthalmologists when ocular surgery is being considered and also in the presence of age-related macular degeneration (AMD).

Objective.—To examine the association of regular aspirin use with incidence of AMD.

Design, Setting, and Participants.—The Beaver Dam Eye Study, a longitudinal population-based study of age-related eye diseases conducted in Wisconsin. Examinations were performed every 5 years over a 20-year period (1988-1990 through 2008-2010). Study participants (N = 4926) were aged 43 to 86 years at the baseline examination. At subsequent examinations, participants were asked if they had regularly used aspirin at least twice a week for more than 3 months.

Main Outcome Measure.—Incidence of early AMD, late AMD, and 2 subtypes of late AMD (neovascular AMD and pure geographic atrophy), assessed in retinal photographs according to the Wisconsin Age-Related Maculopathy Grading System.

Results.—The mean duration of follow-up was 14.8 years. There were 512 incident cases of early AMD (of 6243 person-visits at risk) and 117 incident cases of late AMD (of 8621 person-visits at risk) over the course of the study. Regular aspirin use 10 years prior to retinal examination was associated with late AMD (hazard ratio [HR], 1.63 [95% CI, 1.01-2.63]; $P = .05$), with estimated incidence of 1.76% (95% CI, 1.17%-2.64%) in regular users and 1.03% (95% CI, 0.70%-1.51%) in nonusers. For subtypes of late AMD, regular aspirin use 10 years prior to retinal examination was significantly associated with neovascular AMD (HR, 2.20 [95% CI, 1.20-4.15]; $P = .01$) but not pure geographic atrophy (HR, 0.66 [95% CI, 0.25-1.95]; $P = .45$). Aspirin use 5 years (HR, 0.86 [95% CI, 0.71-1.05]; $P = .13$) or 10 years (HR, 0.86 [95% CI, 0.65-1.13]; $P = .28$) prior to retinal examination was not associated with incident early AMD.

Conclusions.—Among an adult cohort, aspirin use 5 years prior to observed incidence was not associated with incident early or late AMD. However, regular aspirin use 10 years prior was associated with a small but statistically significant increase in the risk of incident late and neovascular AMD.

▶ The relationship of aspirin (ASA) to age-related macular degeneration (AMD) has been debated in the literature for many years. Some studies have statistically demonstrated an association between ASA and AMD, while others report there is no association. This study used the Beaver Dam Eye database, which was a large population-based longitudinal study. Regular ASA use, which was defined as at least twice a week for more than 3 months, was associated with a small increased risk of development of late dry AMD and neovascular AMD. In addition, this correlation was only found among patients with 10 years of ASA use and not those with 5 years of ASA use. Because of the high prevalence of the use of ASA and AMD, these data are compelling. However, these results are not convincing. One of the major issues with this investigation is that it is very difficult to determine association or causation. The recommendation to reduce ASA use among patients with AMD is predicated on proving causation. In other words, patients with AMD should not take ASA only if it can be proven that ASA causes progression of AMD. One confounding factor when interpreting the results in this study is that patients with cardiovascular risk factors have a high rate of AMD. In addition, these patients often present with aggressive AMD subtypes. Because of their cardiovascular risk factors, they are more commonly recommended to take ASA. Consequently, the higher rate of progression to late dry AMD and neovascular AMD among ASA users might be because this is an inherently higher risk pool.

O. P. Gupta, MD

Clinical Classification of Age-related Macular Degeneration
Ferris FL III, on behalf of the Beckman Initiative for Macular Research Classification Committee (Natl Eye Inst, Bethesda, MD; et al)
Ophthalmology 120:844-851, 2013

Objective.—To develop a clinical classification system for age-related macular degeneration (AMD).

Design.—Evidence-based investigation, using a modified Delphi process.

Participants.—Twenty-six AMD experts, 1 neuro-ophthalmologist, 2 committee chairmen, and 1 methodologist.

Methods.—Each committee member completed an online assessment of statements summarizing current AMD classification criteria, indicating agreement or disagreement with each statement on a 9-step scale. The group met, reviewed the survey results, discussed the important components of a clinical classification system, and defined new data analyses needed to refine a classification system. After the meeting, additional data analyses from large studies were provided to the committee to provide risk estimates related to the presence of various AMD lesions.

Main Outcome Measures.—Delphi review of the 9-item set of statements resulting from the meeting.

Results.—Consensus was achieved in generating a basic clinical classification system based on fundus lesions assessed within 2 disc diameters of the fovea in persons older than 55 years. The committee agreed that a single term, *age-related macular degeneration*, should be used for the disease. Persons with no visible drusen or pigmentary abnormalities should be considered to have no signs of AMD. Persons with small drusen (<63 μm), also termed *drupelets*, should be considered to have normal aging changes with no clinically relevant increased risk of late AMD developing. Persons with medium drusen (≥63-<125 μm), but without pigmentary abnormalities thought to be related to AMD, should be considered to have early AMD. Persons with large drusen or with pigmentary abnormalities associated with at least medium drusen should be considered to have intermediate AMD. Persons with lesions associated with neovascular AMD or geographic atrophy should be considered to have late AMD. Five-year risks of progressing to late AMD are estimated to increase approximately 100 fold, ranging from a 0.5% 5-year risk for normal aging changes to a 50% risk for the highest intermediate AMD risk group.

Conclusions.—The proposed basic clinical classification scale seems to be of value in predicting the risk of late AMD. Incorporating consistent nomenclature into the practice patterns of all eye care providers may improve communication and patient care.

▶ Classification of disease is helpful for communication among providers and between providers and patients. It also provides a systematic method for risk-stratifying patients. In this study, the committee developed a clinical classification system for age-related macular degeneration (AMD). The stratification based on drusen size has been widely published. In particular, the classification of small drusen (< 63 μm), medium drusen (≥63 to < 125 μm), and large drusen (> 125 μm) has been used since the original Age-Related Eye Disease Study (AREDS) trials. Although pigmentary changes alone were not enough to be classified as AMD, they did dramatically change the stratification in conjunction with 1 or more large drusen. The patient severity score was then determined based on the presence or absence of these 2 clinical features. For example, if a patient had a large drusen in 1 eye and pigmentary changes in the other eye, then the patient severity score was a total of 2. To simplify the 5-year risk of developing advanced AMD (geographic atrophy or neovascular AMD), the conversion rates were rounded to more easily remembered numbers. Patients with a severity score of 0 had a 5-year risk of developing late AMD of 0%, those with a score of 1 had a 0.5% risk, those with a score of 2 had a 12% risk, those with a score of 3 had a 25% risk, and those with a score of 4 had a 50% risk. This grading methodology can serve as a powerful tool for management of dry AMD patients and provide patients with an accurate idea of what their future may hold.

O. P. Gupta, MD

Epimacular Brachytherapy for Neovascular Age-related Macular Degeneration: A Randomized, Controlled Trial (CABERNET)
Dugel PU, for the CABERNET Study Group (Retinal Consultants of Arizona, Phoenix; et al)
Ophthalmology 120:317-327, 2013

Purpose.—To evaluate the safety and efficacy of epimacular brachytherapy (EMBT) for the treatment of neovascular age-related macular degeneration (AMD).

Design.—Multicenter, randomized, active-controlled, phase III clinical trial.

Participants.—Four hundred ninety-four participants with treatment-naïve neovascular AMD.

Methods.—Participants with classic, minimally classic, and occult lesions were randomized in a 2:1 ratio to EMBT or a ranibizumab monotherapy control arm. The EMBT arm received 2 mandated, monthly loading injections of 0.5 mg ranibizumab. The control arm received 3 mandated, monthly loading injections of ranibizumab then quarterly injections. Both arms also received monthly as needed (pro re nata) retreatment.

Main Outcome Measures.—The proportion of participants losing fewer than 15 Early Treatment Diabetic Retinopathy Study (ETDRS) letters from baseline visual acuity (VA) and the proportion gaining more than 15 ETDRS letters from baseline VA.

Results.—At 24 months, 77% of the EMBT group and 90% of the control group lost fewer than 15 letters. This difference did not meet the prespecified 10% noninferiority margin. This end point was noninferior using a 20% margin and a 95% confidence interval for the group as a whole and for classic and minimally classic lesions, but not for occult lesions. The EMBT did not meet the superiority end point for the proportion of participants gaining more than 15 letters (16% for the EMBT group vs. 26% for the control group): this difference was statistically significant (favoring controls) for occult lesions, but not for predominantly classic and minimally classic lesions. Mean VA change was −2.5 letters in the EMBT arm and +4.4 letters in the control arm. Participants in the EMBT arm received a mean of 6.2 ranibizumab injections versus 10.4 in the control arm. At least 1 serious adverse event occurred in 54% of the EMBT arm, most commonly postvitrectomy cataract, versus 18% in the control arm. Mild, nonproliferative radiation retinopathy occurred in 3% of the EMBT participants, but no case was vision threatening.

Conclusions.—The 2-year efficacy data do not support the routine use of EMBT for treatment-naïve wet AMD, despite an acceptable safety profile. Further safety review is required.

▶ Although the results of this trial were not favorable for the use of epimacular brachytherapy (EMBT) in the treatment of neovascular age-related macular degeneration (nAMD), this study reminds us of the importance of clinical trials. Different modalities of radiation have been described for the treatment of nAMD for over a decade. This exact technology was used overseas with rave reviews. During the early stages of the clinical trials, US investigators were optimistic regarding its value. The CABERNET trial evaluated the use of this technology, which was a hand-held β-radiation device that was held over the macula during pars plana vitrectomy. The device was only unshielded once it was in the eye and over the macula. It delivered a very controlled and concentrated amount of radiation to the macula and significantly less radiation to the optic nerve and even less to the lens and external environment. This was compared with ranibizumab monotherapy in treatment-naïve patients with nAMD over 2 years. The hope was that this technology would reduce the burden of frequent injections in exchange for a one-time surgical procedure with less frequent injections. However, compared with ranibizumab monotherapy, patients in the EMBT arm on average lost more lines of vision, and a smaller proportion gained more than 15 letters and had a higher rate of serious adverse events. Although there might be a future application of radiation in the treatment of nAMD, this study clearly demonstrates that EMBT does not meet the current standard of care. Moreover, this study reemphasizes that anecdotal case reports, retrospective studies, and uncontrolled clinical trials need to be supported with larger, more rigorous studies to validate safety and efficacy.

O. P. Gupta, MD

Intravitreal Ranibizumab for Diabetic Macular Edema with Prompt Versus Deferred Laser Treatment: Three-Year Randomized Trial Results

Diabetic Retinopathy Clinical Research Network (Elman Retina Group, Baltimore, MD; Jaeb Ctr for Health Res, Tampa, FL; Harvard Med School, Boston, MA; et al)
Ophthalmology 119:2312-2318, 2012

Objective.—To report the 3-year follow-up results within a previously reported randomized trial evaluating prompt versus deferred (for ≥24 weeks) focal/grid laser treatment in eyes treated with intravitreal 0.5 mg ranibizumab for diabetic macular edema (DME).

Design.—Multicenter, randomized clinical trial.

Participants.—Three hundred sixty-one participants with visual acuity of 20/32 to 20/320 (approximate Snellen equivalent) and DME involving the fovea.

Methods.—Ranibizumab every 4 weeks until no longer improving (with resumption if worsening) and random assignment to prompt or deferred (≥24 weeks) focal/grid laser treatment.

Main Outcome Measures.—Best-corrected visual acuity and safety at the 156-week (3-year) visit.

Results.—The estimated mean change in visual acuity letter score from baseline through the 3-year visit was 2.9 letters more (9.7 vs. 6.8 letters; mean difference, 2.9 letters; 95% confidence interval, 0.4-5.4 letters; $P = 0.02$) in the deferral group compared with the prompt laser treatment group. In the prompt laser treatment group and deferral group, respectively, the percentage of eyes with a ≥10-letter gain/loss was 42% and 56% ($P = 0.02$), whereas the respective percentage of eyes with a ≥10-letter gain/loss was 10% and 5% ($P = 0.12$). Up to the 3-year visit, the median numbers of injections were 12 and 15 in the prompt and deferral groups, respectively ($P = 0.007$), including 1 and 2 injections, respectively, from the 2-year up to the 3-year visit. At the 3-year visit, the percentages of eyes with central subfield thickness of 250 μm or more on time-domain optical coherence tomography were 36% in both groups ($P = 0.90$). In the deferral group, 54% did not receive laser treatment during the trial. Systemic adverse events seemed to be similar in the 2 groups.

Conclusions.—These 3-year results suggest that focal/grid laser treatment at the initiation of intravitreal ranibizumab is no better, and possibly worse, for vision outcomes than deferring laser treatment for 24 weeks or more in eyes with DME involving the fovea and with vision impairment. Some of the observed differences in visual acuity at 3 years may be related to fewer cumulative ranibizumab injections during follow-up in the prompt laser treatment group. Follow-up through 5 years continues.

▶ The treatment of fovea-involving diabetic macular edema has radically changed over the last several years. Focal laser photocoagulation has been the mainstay for treatment. Because the visual outcome in these patients was not extremely favorable, other options have been explored, including intravitreal triamcinolone. Although this has been found to be more effective than focal laser alone, side effects, including cataract and intraocular pressure elevation, limited its use. That study, as well as this study, was performed by the Diabetic Retinopathy Clinical Research Network. This study explores the use of intravitreal ranibizumab with focal laser. This is the 3-year follow-up to the previously reported studies. The authors report that deferring laser for the first 6 months is superior to more prompt laser. For the first 6 months, patients received monthly ranibizumab for at least 4 doses and then only when patients showed signs of exudation or decline in vision. Starting at month 6, patients received focal laser for persistent diabetic macular edema or no improvement with the injection alone. Interestingly, more than half of the eyes did not receive focal laser in the deferred group, and 100% of eyes in the prompt group received laser at the 3-year time point. Patients received an average of 15 injections in the deferred laser arm and 12 injections in the prompt laser arm over the 3 years.

O. P. Gupta, MD

Baseline Predictors for One-Year Visual Outcomes with Ranibizumab or Bevacizumab for Neovascular Age-related Macular Degeneration
Ying G-S, on behalf of the Comparison of Age-related Macular Degeneration Treatments Trials Research Group (Univ of Pennsylvania, Philadelphia; et al)
Ophthalmology 120:122-129, 2013

Objective.—To determine the baseline predictors of visual acuity (VA) outcomes 1 year after treatment with ranibizumab or bevacizumab for neovascular age-related macular degeneration (AMD).

Design.—Cohort study within the Comparison of Age-related Macular Degeneration Treatments Trials (CATT).

Participants.—A total of 1105 participants with neovascular AMD, baseline VA 20/25 to 20/320, and VA measured at 1 year.

Methods.—Participants were randomly assigned to ranibizumab or bevacizumab on a monthly or as-needed schedule. Masked readers evaluated fundus morphology and features on optical coherence tomography (OCT). Visual acuity was measured using electronic VA testing. Independent predictors were identified using regression techniques.

Main Outcome Measures.—The VA score, VA score change from baseline, and ≥3-line gain at 1 year.

Results.—At 1 year, the mean VA score was 68 letters, mean improvement from baseline was 7 letters, and 28% of participants gained ≥ 3 lines. Older age, larger area of choroidal neovascularization (CNV), and elevation of retinal pigment epithelium (RPE) were associated with worse VA (all $P < 0.005$), less gain in VA (all $P < 0.02$), and a lower proportion gaining ≥ 3 lines (all $P < 0.04$). Better baseline VA was associated with better VA at 1 year, less gain in VA, and a lower proportion gaining ≥ 3 lines (all $P < 0.0001$). Predominantly or minimally classic lesions were associated with worse VA than occult lesions (66 vs. 69 letters; $P = 0.0003$). Retinal angiomatous proliferans (RAP) lesions were associated with more gain in VA (10 vs. 7 letters; $P = 0.03$) and a higher proportion gaining ≥ 3 lines (odds ratio, 1.9; 95%

confidence interval, 1.2—3.1). Geographic atrophy (GA) was associated with worse VA (64 vs. 68 letters; $P = 0.02$). Eyes with total foveal thickness in the second quartile (325—425 μm) had the best VA ($P = 0.01$) and were most likely to gain ≥ 3 lines ($P = 0.004$). Predictors did not vary by treatment group.

Conclusions.—For all treatment groups, older age, better baseline VA, larger CNV area, predominantly or minimally classic lesion, absence of RAP lesion, presence of GA, greater total fovea thickness, and RPE elevation on optical coherence tomography were independently associated with less improvement in VA at 1 year.

▶ The Comparison of Age-Related Macular Degeneration Treatments Trials (CATT) was an important federally funded trial that compared ranibizumab and bevacizumab with monthly and as-needed dosing in neovascular age-related macular degeneration (nAMD). Over the next several years, subsequent analysis of this rich dataset will be equally important. In this study, risk factors were identified for both favorable and unfavorable visual outcome primarily using regression analysis. The predictors for favorable visual outcome included better baseline visual acuity, predominately or minimally classic choroidal neovascular (CNV) lesions, and retinal angiomatous proliferation (RAP) lesions. Eyes with a foveal thickness on presentation of 325 to 425 μm experienced the most significant gain in vision and were the highest proportion of ≥3 line gainers. This is likely because these patients had a moderate amount of macular edema without significant fibrosis as determined by optical coherence tomography (OCT). Predictors of poor visual outcome included older age, larger CNV size, elevation of retinal pigment epithelial detachment, occult CNV, and the presence of geographic atrophy. This study is important because it reemphasizes the importance of fluorescein angiograms in the evaluation of patients with nAMD. Currently, the main diagnostic and management tool for nAMD is OCT. This has revolutionized the detection of activity. It has rendered fluorescein angiograms almost obsolete by some providers who treat nAMD. As more data analysis is performed on the CATT cohort, we will learn more about the treatment of nAMD and perhaps the subtle differences between ranibizumab and bevacizumab.

O. P. Gupta, MD

6 Oculoplastic Surgery

Long-term outcomes of pegged and unpegged bioceramic orbital implants
Karslıoğlu S, Buttanrı IB, Fazıl K, et al (Oculoplastic Surgery and Ocular
Oncology Ctr, Istanbul, Turkey)
Ophthal Plast Reconstr Surg 28:264-267, 2012

Purpose.—To evaluate the long-term outcomes of pegged and unpegged
bioceramic orbital implants.

Methods.—A retrospective analysis of 101 cases of evisceration, enucleation, or secondary implant surgery with placement of a bioceramic porous
implant was conducted. Type of surgery, existence of a peg, peg system used,
time of pegging, problems encountered before and after pegging, treatment
methods, and final status were recorded.

Results.—Evisceration was performed on 74, enucleation on 16, and
secondary implant surgery on 11 patients. The patients were observed
for a mean of 68.4 months (3 months-12 years). Fifty-three of the 101
patients were pegged. Patients were pegged at a mean of 9.3 months (6-
23 months). Hydroxyapatite-coated, titanium-sleeved, titanium pegs were
used in 43 patients, and titanium peg and sleeve system was used in 10
patients. Major complications were exposure and infection. Three patients
presented with early exposure and late exposure developed in 14 of pegged
and 4 of unpegged patients. The difference in late-exposure rates between
pegged and unpegged group was statistically significant ($p < 0.05$). Implant
infection developed in 9 of the pegged and in 1 of the unpegged patients.
Implant exposure was noted in 6 of these 10 patients with infection. The
difference in infection rates between the pegged and unpegged patients was
statistically significant ($p < 0.05$). In 2 of the pegged patients, removal of bioceramic implant was required and after resolution of infection, another type
of porous implant was implanted and repegged. The peg system was removed
in 6 patients for the management of either exposure, infection, extrusion,
hypermobility of sleeve, or peg falling out. Four patients were repegged.
The time period between peg insertion and development of complications
ranged from 15 days to 10 years. 86.8% of pegged patients were free of
major complications and satisfied with the result at the last follow-up visit.

Conclusion.—Despite potential complications that can occur as late as
10 years, bioceramic porous implants yield satisfactory long-term results.
Existence of a peg system appears to play a role in the increased rate of

late-onset complications. Further investigations on new and safer pegging systems should be conducted.

▶ The practice of placing a motility peg in a porous orbital implant has become a rare event in my practice and at Wills Eye Institute as well. The exact reason for this may be multifactorial, but this article points out a strong reason to think twice about risks before placing a motility peg in a porous implant.

This article is a retrospective analysis of 101 patients who had their eye removed by enucleation or evisceration with placement of a bioceramic porous implant. Fifty-three of those patients had placement of a titanium motility peg at a mean of 9.3 months after eye removal. Seventeen of 53 (32%) patients with pegs had implant exposure vs 4 of 48 (8.3%) of unpegged implants. Because exposure often leads to implant infection, it is not surprising that 9 of 53 (17%) implants with pegs became infected vs 1 of 48 (2%) of the unpegged implants. These numbers are not only statistically significant but, to me, they certainly make a case for not placing a motility peg. It is also important to note exposures occurred as long as 10 years after peg placement.

It must be pointed out that these were all bioceramic implants, and this information may not be the same for other implant materials. At Wills Eye Institute, we use hydroxyapatite and porous polypropylene implants, and currently no one uses bioceramic implants. I would agree that there are significantly more problems with a pegged implant, such as more mucous discharge and giant papillary conjunctivitis, to more serious problems like exposure. In my practice, I will continue to discourage peg placement, and for those who really desire improved motility, this report must be discussed.

R. B. Penne, MD

Botulinum toxin-A-induced protective ptosis in the treatment of lagophthalmos associated with facial paralysis

Yücel OE, Artürk N (Ondokuz Mayıs Univ, Samsun, Turkey)
Ophthal Plast Reconstr Surg 28:256-260, 2012

Purpose.—To evaluate the safety and efficacy of the protective ptosis created by botulinum neurotoxin type-A in lagophthalmos cases due to peripheral facial paralysis.

Methods.—Protective ptosis was induced by 7.5 U botulinum neurotoxin type-A injection into levator muscles in 15 patients with peripheral facial paralysis and lagophthalmos. Its efficacy and safety were evaluated prospectively. Complete ophthalmological examinations were performed before and after injections; interpalpebral fissure, upper eyelid margin reflex distance, and levator muscle function were measured. In control visits, degree and duration of ptosis and side effects of the drug were evaluated.

Results.—The mean age of the patients was 55 ± 14.28 years (22-78 years). Ptosis created by botulinum neurotoxin type-A injection was severe in 12 patients (80%), moderate in 2 patients (13.3%), and mild in 1 patient (6.7%). The effect of botulinum neurotoxin type-A began in

2.33 ± 1.44 days and peaked in 5.73 ± 2.63 days. No patient needed a second injection. The mean duration for ptosis was 10.53 ± 2.89 weeks. After development of ptosis, statistically significant improvement in corneal symptoms ($p < 0.01$) and decrease in daily artificial tear requirement ($p < 0.01$) were detected. Local or systemic side effects were not observed in any of the patients.

Conclusion.—In patients with peripheral facial paralysis and lagophthalmos, protective ptosis created by botulinum neurotoxin type-A injection into the levator muscle is a reliable and effective technique for the protection of the ocular surface and treatment of existing corneal complications. It represents an alternative treatment modality in cases requiring surgery.

▶ The use of Botox to create a paralytic tarsorrhaphy is not a new concept, but for various reasons it has not become a mainstay of treatment. This article looks at 15 patients with a facial palsy and corneal exposure who received a Botox injection to the levator muscle. They all received 7.5 units of Botox injected through the upper eyelid skin placed over the levator muscle with a 27-gauge needle. This resulted in a protective ptosis in all 15 patients, had its onset in an average of 2 days, and lasted an average of 10.5 weeks.

This technique is useful, but in select patients only, and even then it has its difficulties. This is a temporary procedure but one that lasts 10 weeks. For the patient who has a permanent facial palsy, this will protect the eye for 10 weeks but then the same problem will still be present. Unless there is some other issue that suggests the corneal exposure is only temporary, selecting a more permanent treatment is preferable. In patients with a temporary problem, the downside of Botox is it is going to last 10 weeks. If the corneal exposure is better after 1 week there is no way to reverse the ptosis. If you have placed a suture tarsorrhaphy, it can be removed and the eye will be open. Another issue is the cost of the Botox. The amount of Botox required is not large, but it is not covered by insurance. Opening a new bottle of Botox is cost-prohibitive for those who do not use it on a regular basis and do not have an open bottle to use.

Despite all these issues, this is a nice procedure for select patients and should be kept in mind.

R. B. Penne, MD

Periocular Abscesses Following Brow Epilation
Elmann S, Pointdujour R, Blaydon S, et al (SUNY Downstate Med Ctr, Brooklyn, NY; Texas Oculoplastic Consultants, Austin)
Ophthal Plast Reconstr Surg 28:434-437, 2012

Purpose.—The aim of this article was to report the clinical presentation, radiography, culture results, treatment modalities, and outcomes of periocular abscesses associated with brow epilation.

Methods.—This was a retrospective case series including 26 patients referred for periocular abscess following brow epilation.

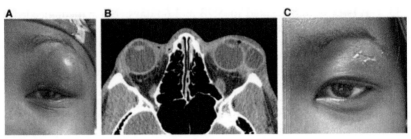

FIGURE 1.—A, Clinical photograph of a young female patient with a left lateral subbrow abscess and associated upper eyelid preseptal cellulitis 2 days after brow epilation. B, Axial orbital CT image demonstrating the preseptal abscess. C, Complete resolution 1 week following incision and drainage and systemic antibiotics. CT, computed tomography. (Reprinted from Elmann S, Pointdujour R, Blaydon S, et al. Periocular abscesses following brow epilation. *Ophthal Plast Reconstr Surg.* 2012;28:434-437, with permission from The American Society of Ophthalmic Plastic and Reconstructive Surgery, Inc.)

Results.—Twenty-six female patients with a median age of 20.5 (range, 12–73) years were referred for oculoplastic evaluation of periocular abscesses related to recent brow epilation. All patients were treated with incision and drainage along with systemic antibiotics. Culture results revealed 16 cases of methicillin-resistant *Staphylococcus aureus*, 3 of methicillin-sensitive *Staphylococcus aureus*, and 7 cultures that showed no growth. All patients had resolution of their abscesses at 1-month follow-up visits without progression to orbital cellulitis.

Conclusions.—Periocular abscess formation after brow epilation has been previously described in only a single case report in the literature. The authors believe this entity is underreported given their current report describing 26 such cases. Given the high prevalence of cosmetic brow epilation in females, the authors believe a careful history regarding brow epilation in any patient presenting with a periocular abscess or preseptal cellulitis is essential to explore the possible cause of their infection. The majority of patients in the current study's cohort had methicillin-resistant *Staphylococcus aureus*-related abscesses, and treatment with antibiotics with methicillin-resistant *Staphylococcus aureus* coverage may be a prudent first line choice in such patients (Fig 1).

▶ This is a retrospective case series that identifies 26 cases of periocular abscesses from brow hair epilation. The value of this article is two-fold. First, with only one previous such case in the literature, this establishes that the occurrence of a brow abscess after epilating or waxing brow hairs is not rare. Second, the article identifies methicillin-resistant *Staphylococcus aureus* (MRSA) as being the most common pathogen causing the abscess.

With this information, the suspicion of an abscess in the appropriate patient is warranted. This would be someone with swelling and pain in the brow area when hair has been removed by epilation or waxing in the previous 2–10 days. These patients need to be seen emergently and if an abscess is suspected, it needs to be drained. In addition, although cultures are pending, the appropriate antibiotic coverage needs to cover MRSA. Oral treatment may include doxycycline, clindamycin, or trimethoprim/sulfamethoxazole antibiotics.

R. B. Penne, MD

Does Upper Lid Blepharoplasty Improve Contrast Sensitivity?
Rogers SAG, Khan-Lim D, Manners RM (Southampton Univ Hosp, Hampshire, UK)
Ophthal Plast Reconstr Surg 28:163-165, 2012

Purpose.—To assess the effect of upper eyelid blepharoplasty surgery on contrast sensitivity.

Methods.—A prospective study was performed. Pre- and postoperative contrast sensitivity measurements were taken on patients undergoing routine upper eyelid blepharoplasty surgery. The patients were selected for surgery on the basis of a functional visual field effect from dermatochalasis. Contrast sensitivity was measured using a Pelli-Robson chart, read at 1 m under standard lighting conditions. This produces a result in log contrast sensitivity. Other data collected included visual acuity and an automated 60:4 visual field. A paired t test was used to assess the change in contrast sensitivity.

Results.—28 eyes of 14 patients underwent upper eyelid blepharoplasty surgery. The mean preoperative log contrast sensitivity was 1.49, and the mean postoperative log contrast sensitivity was 1.64. The mean increase in log contrast sensitivity was 0.14 (range 0-0.45). The increase in log contrast sensitivity was statistically significant ($p = 0.00002$).

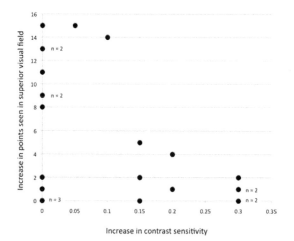

FIGURE 3.—A chart comparing the changes in visual field with the change in contrast sensitivity. (Reprinted from Rogers SAG, Khan-Lim D, Manners RM. Does upper lid blepharoplasty improve contrast sensitivity? *Ophthal Plast Reconstr Surg.* 2012;28:163-165, with permission from The American Society of Ophthalmic Plastic and Reconstructive Surgery, Inc.)

Conclusions.—Dermatochalasis is well known to cause visual field defects in many patients. Anecdotally, patients often report that their vision is brighter following upper eyelid blepharoplasty. The authors have demonstrated a significant increase in contrast sensitivity in patients who have undergone upper eyelid blepharoplasty surgery. This information may be of use in justifying blepharoplasty surgery in the future (Fig 3).

▶ This is a prospective study looking at how contrast sensitivity is affected by upper eyelid blepharoplasty. The traditional measure of visual function improvement used in upper lid ptosis or dermatochalasis surgery is a taped and untaped automated visual field. That is what insurance companies use to decide whether upper lid surgery is covered by insurance or considered cosmetic.

This study demonstrates that there is a statistically significant improvement in contrast sensitivity after upper eyelid blepharoplasty. However, the improvement was not universal, with 12 of the 28 eyes showing no improvement in contrast sensitivity. Visual fields were also done pre- and postoperatively, and 6 of 28 eyes showed no improvement in visual field after surgery. Three patients showed no improvement in the field or in contrast sensitivity.

This is a small study and, when the numbers are looked at, there were a lot of eyes with no improvement. There is no obvious reason for this. Nor was there any attempt to correlate the amount of skin with the change in contrast sensitivity. This study does offer an objective reason through contrast sensitivity improvement for patients' perception that thing are brighter after upper eyelid surgery. Before contrast sensitivity has any chance of being used as a way to prove the value of ptosis surgery on the quality of vision, more studies are needed.

R. B. Penne, MD

Giant Fornix Syndrome: A Case Series
Turaka K, Penne RB, Rapuano CJ, et al (Thomas Jefferson Univ, Philadelphia, PA)
Ophthal Plast Reconstr Surg 28:4-6, 2012

Purpose.—To describe the demographics, characteristics, and treatment of giant fornix syndrome, a rare cause of chronic purulent conjunctivitis in the elderly.

Methods.—Retrospective chart review of five patients with giant fornix syndrome evaluated by the Cornea Service, Oculoplastics and Orbital Surgery Service and the Department of Pathology at the Wills Eye Institute.

Results.—The median age of the 5 female patients was 75 years (mean 80, range 70—95). The median duration of eye symptoms before presentation was 2 years (mean 2.4, range 1—4). Before referral, the chronic conjunctivitis was treated with topical antibiotics in all 5 cases and with additional dacryocystorhinostomy in one case. The right eye was affected in 2 cases, and the left eye was affected in the other 3 cases. Floppy eyelids were present in 2 cases. The superior fornix was involved in 4 cases, and the inferior fornix was involved in one case. Pseudomembranes and superficial punctate

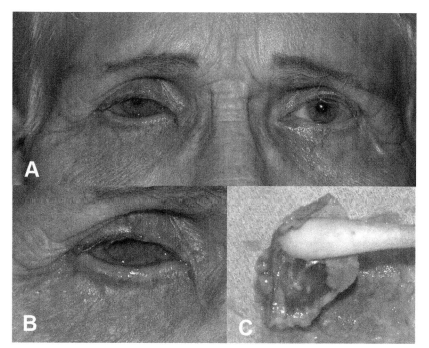

FIGURE 1.—A 75-year-old woman with giant fornix syndrome of the right eye. A–C, Clinical external photograph showing blepharitis (A) and conjunctival chemosis and deep superior sulcus of the right eye (B). The soft contact lens removed from the superior fornix was surrounded by the thick mucous discharge and a pseudomembrane (C). (Reprinted from Turaka K, Penne RB, Rapuano CJ, et al. Giant fornix syndrome: a case series. *Ophthal Plast Reconstr Surg.* 2012;28:4-6, with permission from The American Society of Ophthalmic Plastic and Reconstructive Surgery, Inc.)

keratitis (SPK) were seen in 3 cases. Diagnosis of giant fornix syndrome was made in all 5 cases. Conjunctival culture grew methicillin-resistant *Staphylococcus aureus* (MRSA), *Pseudomonas aeruginosa*, and *S. aureus* in singular cases. Case 1 was treated with topical moxifloxacin, Case 2 was treated with topical vancomycin and repair of the upper eyelid, Case 3 was treated with topical besifloxacin, and Case 4 was treated with dacryocystorhinostomy and topical vancomycin. Case 5 was treated with reconstruction of the left upper eyelid. The median duration of follow up was 4 months (mean 21.6, range 1–84).

Conclusions.—Giant fornix syndrome can lead to chronic relapsing conjunctivitis in the elderly. Deep conjunctival fornices in affected patients can be a site for prolonged sequestration of bacteria causing recurrent infections. Removing the infected debris from the superior fornix and reconstruction of the upper eyelid may prevent the recurrent chronic persistent infection (Fig 1).

▶ This is a retrospective chart review of 5 patients with giant fornix syndrome (GFS). The real importance of this article is to remind us to keep this in the differential diagnosis when confronted with a patient with a chronic mucopurulent conjunctivitis. If this is considered, and if on examination the superior fornix is evaluated, the diagnosis, although rare, is straightforward. These patients have high eyelid creases and often have ptosis on external examination. It is important to take the time to look into the superior fornix to see if there is an accumulation of debris. This is not easy and may require double lid eversion. Making it more difficult is that patients with GFS are frequently tender in this area, so this process can be uncomfortable. If you cannot see the superior extent of the superior fornix, you can sweep it with a moist cotton tip to make the diagnosis.

Dacryostenosis with dacryocystitis and canaliculitis is by far a more common reason that I see for undiagnosed chronic mucopurulent conjunctivitis. However, I have seen a few patients who underwent DCRs for lacrimal obstruction in the setting of chronic mucopurulent conjunctivitis who did not get better. They later had GFS diagnosed and were cured by simply cleaning out the superior fornix.

R. B. Penne, MD

Thyroid Volume and Severity of Graves' Orbitopathy
Profilo MA, Sisti E, Marcocci C, et al (Univ Hosp of Pisa, Italy)
Thyroid 23:97-102, 2013

Background.—Graves' orbitopathy (GO) is thought to be related to one or more autoantigens present in the thyroid and in orbital tissues. Although this may not imply a quantitative relation between thyroid antigens and degree of GO, which in turn is a risk factor for a more pronounced GO, we postulated that the severity of GO may parallel the amount of thyroid tissue, namely, the size of the thyroid gland. This hypothesis is also based on the observation that patients with Graves' disease presenting with large goiters tend to have more severe hyperthyroidism. Thus, we evaluated retrospectively whether there is a correlation between the degree of GO at its first observation and, among other parameters, the thyroid volume.

Methods.—Eighty-six consecutive patients with untreated GO lasting for no longer than 24 months underwent an endocrinological and an ophthalmological evaluation, the latter including: exophthalmometry, eyelid width, clinical activity score (CAS), diplopia, and visual acuity. The overall degree of GO was ranked using the NOSPECS score as well as a modification of the NOSPECS score. The following parameters were considered for correlations: time since GO appearance, time since detection of hyperthyroidism, FT3, anti-thyrotropin receptor antibodies, thyroid volume, and cigarette-years.

Results.—Thyroid volume, but not the other parameters, correlated significantly by simple regression with exophthalmometry ($p = 0.02$) and CAS ($p = 0.02$). The standard NOSPECS score correlated with FT3 ($p = 0.05$), thyroid volume ($p = 0.02$), and cigarette-years ($p = 0.03$), by simple, but not by multiple regression analysis. The modified NOSPECS score correlated with thyroid volume ($p = 0.007$) and cigarette-years ($p = 0.04$) by simple regression, and with thyroid volume also by multiple regression analysis ($p = 0.05$).

Conclusions.—Thyroid volume correlates with the severity of GO at its first observation, especially with exophthalmometry and CAS. The finding

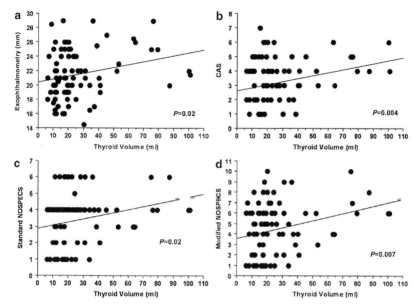

FIGURE 1.—Correlation between thyroid volume and (a) exophthalmometry, (b) clinical activity score (CAS), (c) standard NOSPECS score, or (d) modified NOSPECS score, at the first observation in patients with untreated Graves' orbitopathy. All findings refer to 86 patients. Dots may seem fewer than 86 because of overlaps. (Reprinted from Profilo MA, Sisti E, Marcocci C, et al. Thyroid volume and severity of graves' orbitopathy. *Thyroid.* 2013;23:97-102, Copyright 2013, with permission from Mary Ann Liebert, Inc.)

is in line with a possible pathogenetic role of antigens shared by the thyroid and orbital tissues. Nevertheless, other mechanisms may explain this observation, including an overall more reactive immune system in patients with a large goiter, resulting in more severe thyroid and eye disease, regardless of the nature of the autoantigen, or whether it is shared by the thyroid and the orbit (Fig 1).

▶ As the medical community continues to try to elucidate the exact etiology of Graves orbitopathy (GO) and the relationship to the thyroid gland, we often are left with more correlations and few answers. This article is an example of finding another relationship between GO and the thyroid gland.

The authors found that the larger the thyroid gland is by ultrasound scan, the more severe the GO is. The specific factors that were found to be worse (and were clinically significant) in patients with the larger thyroid glands were clinical activity score (CAS), exophthalmometry, and NOSPECS score (Fig 1).

This is something that I have never considered and have never asked the treating endocrinologist about the size of the thyroid gland. From this article, a larger gland would imply worse GO and may influence decisions on how to treat patients. The real problem with this study is that there was only one eye examination done, and there is no information about progression or stability. Did a larger gland mean a longer period of activity? It would have been nice to have longer eye follow-up to see if these observations on the severity of GO changed.

As with many studies on GO, as many questions are brought out as are answered in this report. I do think it is worth considering the size of the thyroid gland as a possible factor to consider when discussing the potential course of GO with an individual patient. More studies are needed to confirm this.

R. B. Penne, MD

Eyebrow Tissue Expansion: An Underappreciated Entity in Thyroid-Associated Orbitopathy
Savar LM, Menghani RM, Chong KK, et al (Jules Stein Eye Inst, Los Angeles, CA)
Arch Ophthalmol 130:1566-1569, 2012

Objectives.—To report photographic evidence of eyebrow tissue expansion in patients with thyroid-associated orbitopathy (TAO) and to demonstrate consistency in grading through the use of standardized photographs.

Methods.—A retrospective cohort study of patients referred for evaluation of TAO in an orbitofacial tertiary care center between January 1, 2000, and December 31, 2010. A grading key was produced with representative views of each of 4 grades (0 [no expansion] to 3 [severe expansion]), corresponding to increasing severity of eyebrow tissue expansion. Photographs of each study patient, including both premorbid and morbid photographs, were retrieved from an electronic medical record system and graded by 6 independent, masked observers using this 4-point system.

Results.—Seventy-five patients with TAO were identified for inclusion. The average grade was 0.3 for premorbid eyes and 1.1 for morbid eyes. Intraclass correlation coefficients for the premorbid photographs were 0.705 and 0.632 for the right and left eyes, respectively. Intraclass correlation coefficients for the morbid photographs were 0.921 and 0.916 for the right and left eyes, respectively.

Conclusions.—Eyebrow tissue expansion is a common manifestation in TAO. Comparison of premorbid and morbid photographs is a useful means to identify and characterize the extent of brow involvement. The use of a grading key improves the consistency of identifying and grading eyebrow tissue expansion. Recognition of the eyebrow tissue as distinct anatomically in TAO may be crucial to rehabilitation of these patients, which may entail multiple surgical procedures.

▶ The observation of the eyebrow expansion in thyroid-associated orbitopathy (TAO) is something about which most people who see a lot of TAO patients can sit back and say "yes, patients with bad TAO do often have enlarged, thick eyebrows." The importance of this report is that the authors have identified another manifestation of TAO. This tends to be something that occurs with more advanced TAO, so it may not be useful as a sign to make the initial diagnosis of TAO (Fig 1 in the original article).

The authors looked at 150 eyes in 75 patients. Photos were obtained when the TAO was mild and then when the disease was more advanced. These photos were graded by 6 independent, masked observers on a grade of 0 to 4 for eyebrow tissue expansion. This showed a significant expansion of eyebrow tissue as the TAO became more severe.

Unfortunately, the authors are not able to offer advice on how to treat this or exactly why it occurs. Identifying the problem is the first step, and hopefully the future will offer treatment options. Although there is no follow-up to see if eyebrow tissue expansion improves when the TAO quiets down, my impression is it may get slightly better but is a change in the patients' periocular area that will remain.

R. B. Penne, MD

A Randomized Trial Comparing the Cost-Effectiveness of 2 Approaches for Treating Unilateral Nasolacrimal Duct Obstruction

Pediatric Eye Disease Investigator Group (Jaeb Ctr for Health Res, Tampa, FL)
Arch Ophthalmol 130:1525-1533, 2012

Objective.—To compare the cost-effectiveness of 2 approaches for treating unilateral nasolacrimal duct obstruction (NLDO).

Methods.—One hundred sixty-three infants aged 6 to less than 10 months with unilateral NLDO were randomly assigned to receive immediate office-based nasolacrimal duct probing (n = 82) or 6 months of observation/nonsurgical management (n = 81) followed by probing in a facility for persistent symptoms.

Main Outcome Measures.—Treatment success was defined as the absence of clinical signs of NLDO (epiphora, increased tear lake, mucous discharge) on masked examination at age 18 months. Cost of treatment between randomization and age 18 months included costs for all surgical procedures and medications.

Results.—In the observation/deferred facility-probing group, NLDO resolved within 6 months without surgery in 44 of the 67 patients (66%; 95% CI, 54% to 76%) who completed the 6-month visit. Twenty-two (27%) of the 81 patients in the observation/deferred facility-probing group underwent surgery, 4 of whom were operated on within the initial 6 months. At age 18 months, 69 of 75 patients (92%) in the immediate office-probing group were treatment successes, compared with 58 of 71 observation/deferred facility-probing group patients (82%) (10% difference in success; 95% CI, −1% to 21%). The mean cost of treatment was $562 in the immediate office-probing group compared with $701 in the observation/deferred facility-probing group (difference, −$139; 95% CI, −$377 to $94). The immediate office-probing group experienced 3.0 fewer months of symptoms (95% CI, −1.8 to −4.0).

Conclusions.—The immediate office-probing approach is likely more cost-effective than observation followed by deferred facility probing if needed. Adoption of the immediate office-probing approach would result in probing in approximately two-thirds of infants whose obstruction would have resolved within 6 months of nonsurgical management, but would largely avoid the need for probing under general anesthesia.

Application to Clinical Practice.—Although unilateral NLDO often resolves without surgery, immediate office probing is an effective and potentially cost-saving treatment option.
Trial Registration.—clinicaltrials.gov Identifier: NCT00780741 (Table 2).

▶ This is an interesting prospective, randomized study of the cost of 2 different approaches to the time of probing for unilateral congenital nasolacrimal duct obstruction (NLDO). There were 163 children age 6 to 10 months enrolled. One group had probing in the office on presentation, and the other group was observed for 6 months. Those who still had NLDO after 6 months had probing in a surgical facility.

The results were interesting and also bring up ethical questions. In the observation group, 67% had resolution of the NLDO in 6 months and 27% required surgery. At 18 months, 92% of the immediate probing group had treatment success, and 82% of the observation/deferred surgery group had success. The mean cost of treatment was $562 in the immediate probing group and $701 in the deferred surgery group.

This brings up an interesting situation. By both cost and overall success as a group, the immediate probing is superior. However, by probing early, on

TABLE 2.—Outcomes at Age 18 Months Primary Outcome Visit[a]

Outcome	Immediate Office Probing Group (n = 75)	Observation/Deferred Facility-Probing Group (n = 71)
Clinical outcome and No. of surgical procedures at age 18 mo		
Success	69 (92)	58 (82)
No surgery	1	43
Initial surgery	62	15
Reoperation	6	0
Failure	6 (8)	13 (18)
No surgery	0	7
Initial surgery	5	5
Reoperation	1	1
Duration of symptoms between randomization and age 18 mo, mo		
< 1	58 (77)	0
1 to <3	1 (1)	27 (38)
3 to <6	3 (4)	18 (25)
6 to <9	5 (7)	17 (24)
9 to 12	8 (11)	9 (13)
Mean	1.8	4.8
Median (range)	0 (0.0-12.0)	4.5 (1.5-12.0)
Total estimated costs for surgical procedures and medications between randomization and age 18 mo, $		
101 to 250	1 (1)	46 (65)
251 to 500	67 (89)	5 (7)
501 to 1000	0	1 (1)
1001 to 1500	0	4 (6)
1501 to 2000	1 (1)	2 (3)
2001 to 2500	5 (7)	11 (15)
2501 to 3000	1 (1)	2 (3)
Mean	562	701
Median (range)	385 (141-2597)	237 (141-2794)

[a]Data are given as number (percentage) unless otherwise noted.

presentation, 66% of those patients underwent a procedure that they would not have needed if they had been observed. I personally don't do probing in the office and will continue to observe until 12 months of age as long as the parents are agreeable. This study makes arguments for both approaches, and which to choose continues to be an individualized decision.

R. B. Penne, MD

Pushed monocanalicular intubation: An alternative stenting system for the management of congenital nasolacrimal duct obstructions
Fayet B, Katowitz WR, Racy E, et al (Univ of Paris, France; The Children's Hosp of Philadelphia and the Univ of Pennsylvania; Clinique Saint-Jean-de-Dieu, Paris, France)
J AAPOS 16:468-472, 2012

Purpose.— To present our experience with a "pushed" monocanalicular nasolacrimal intubation device in the management of nasolacrimal duct obstruction in children.

Methods.—The cases of consecutive patients with nasolacrimal duct obstruction who were treated with primary probing and intubation with the Masterka were reviewed retrospectively. The Masterka includes a metal guide placed inside a silicone tube for "pushed" intubation as opposed to material attached at the distal end of the silicone for intranasal retrieval ("pulled" intubations). All procedures were accomplished with the patients receiving masked airway anesthesia; neither laryngeal mask airway nor endotracheal intubation was necessary. Only patients noted to have a membranous (mucosal) obstruction were considered for treatment with the Masterka. The duration of operation, duration of stent intubation, and

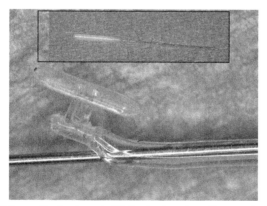

FIGURE 1.—High magnification image (×10) showing how the guide enters the lumen of the Masterka just below the punctual plug of the device. There are 3 lengths: 30, 35, and 40 mm. Inset, Masterka with guide in place. (Reprinted from Journal of AAPOS. Fayet B, Katowitz WR, Racy E, et al. Pushed monocanalicular intubation: an alternative stenting system for the management of congenital nasolacrimal duct obstructions. *J AAPOS.* 2012;16:468-472, Copyright 2012, with permission from the American Association for Pediatric Ophthalmology and Strabismus.)

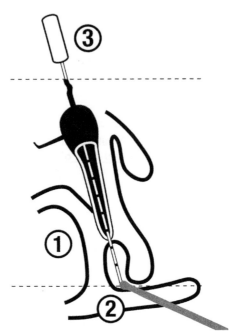

FIGURE 2.—Proper patient selection and Masterka length measurement is accomplished by determining the presence of distal membranous stenosis (1) and confirming intranasal passage with metal-on-metal contact (2). The newer probe with markings allows for greater ease of duct measurement and stent length selection (3). (Reprinted from Journal of AAPOS. Fayet B, Katowitz WR, Racy E, et al. Pushed monocanalicular intubation: an alternative stenting system for the management of congenital nasolacrimal duct obstructions. *J AAPOS*. 2012;16:468-472, Copyright 2012, with permission from the American Association for Pediatric Ophthalmology and Strabismus.)

severity of symptoms on follow-up were noted. Success was defined as absence of symptoms after stent removal or loss.

Results.—A total of 110 eyes of 88 patients were included (average age, 2.4 years; range, 1-8 years). The average operating time was 3 minutes (range, 2-9 minutes). Persistent tearing on follow-up with the stent in place was noted in 26 eyes (24%); tearing resolved after stent removal in 19 eyes (73%). Success was achieved in 94 eyes (85%). with an average follow-up of 33.7 weeks (range, 4-139). Keratitis was noted in 2 eyes (2%). Early stent loss occurred in 17 ducts (15%).

Conclusions.—The Masterka was an effective primary treatment for nasolacrimal duct obstruction associated with mucosal obstructions in this small series of patients (Figs 1-3).

▶ This is a retrospective review of 110 eyes in 88 patients who underwent primary treatment of congenital nasolacrimal duct obstruction (CNLDO) with a new type of stenting system called a *Masterka*. The study finds an 85% success rate using this tube. One question that must be asked is whether placement of any tube should be the first treatment for CNLDO. Traditionally, probing alone has been

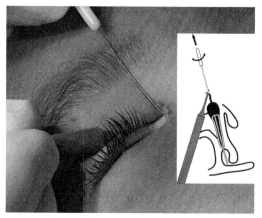

FIGURE 3.—While holding the plug of the stent in place against the eyelid with the inserting device (clinical photograph), the physician retracts the guide gently with a back-and-forth rotation of the probe (drawing). (Reprinted from Journal of AAPOS. Fayet B, Katowitz WR, Racy E, et al. Pushed monocanalicular intubation: an alternative stenting system for the management of congenital nasolacrimal duct obstructions. *J AAPOS.* 2012;16:468-472, Copyright 2012, with permission from the American Association for Pediatric Ophthalmology and Strabismus.)

the initial treatment with tube placement being a second step. This study does not address that.

The reason I included this article is to be sure everyone is aware of a new type of stenting system that is now available called the *Masterka*. This system has the advantage of mono canalicular fixation like a Monoka tube but is able to be pushed through the lacrimal sac and duct via a probe incorporated into the tube, and then the probe is removed after placement. This assures the tube extends fully through the lacrimal system and into the nose. My experience with this stent at this time is limited, because it has not been available until recently. The Masterka has the potential to be used in many cases of lacrimal surgery not just CNLDO, but time and experience will determine how useful it is.

R. B. Penne, MD

Public Health Relevance of Graves' Orbitopathy
Ponto KA, Merkesdal S, Hommel G, et al (Johannes Gutenberg Univ Med Centre, Mainz, Germany; Hannover Med School, Germany)
J Clin Endocrinol Metab 98:145-152, 2013

Context.—Disfiguring proptosis and functional impairment in patients with Graves' orbitopathy (GO) may lead to impaired earning capacity and to considerable indirect/direct costs.

Objective.—The aim of the study was to investigate the public health relevance of GO.

Design and Setting.—This cross-sectional study was performed between 2005 and 2009 at a multidisciplinary university orbital center.

TABLE 2.—Indirect Costs in 215 Employed Patients with GO

	Mean± SD		Range	
	Euros	U.S. Dollars	Euros	U.S. Dollars
Work disability				
HCA	4,086 ± 5,986	5,140 ± 7,530	0–24,288	0–30,554
HCA + friction method	666 ± 975	878 ± 1,227	0–3,947	0–4,965
Sick leave	2,652 ± 6,933	3,336 ± 8,722	0–28,500	0–35,853
Total				
HCA	6,738 ± 10,978	8,476 ± 13,810	0–40,308	0–50,707
HCA + friction method	3,318 ± 7,415	4,174 ± 9,328	0–30,433	0–38,2847

The human capital approach (HCA) and the human capital approach applying a friction cost period of 58 d (friction method) were performed.
Costs were given in euros and U.S. dollars (exchange rate 1.258, May 28, 2012).

TABLE 3.—Direct Costs in Patients with GO

	Regular Costs Per Patient (mean ± SD)		Frequency in 310 GO
Therapy	Euros	U.S. Dollars	Patients, n (%)
Outpatient treatment			
Ophthalmologist	110 ± 7.0	138 ± 8.8	310 (100)
Endocrinologist	117 ± 6.9	147 ± 8.7	310 (100)
Intravenous steroids (methylprednisolone, 6 wk 500 mg weekly, followed by 6 wk 250 mg weekly)	384 ± 1.8	438 ± 2.3	214 (69)
Cyclosporine therapy (body weight adapted)	1,215 ± 258.7	1,528 ± 325.4	52 (17)
Orbital radiotherapy	2,840 ± 0	3,573 ± 0	95 (31)
Squint surgery	4,621 ± 0	5,813 ± 0	17 (6)
Eyelid surgery	4,621 ± 0	5,813 ± 0	16 (5)
Orbital fat resection	10,212 ± 0	12,847 ± 0	6 (2)
Orbital decompression	14,953 ± 0	18,811 ± 0	45 (15)

Costs were given in euros and U.S. dollars (exchange rate 1.258, May 28, 2012).

Patients.—A total of 310 unselected patients with GO of various degrees of severity and activity participated in the study.

Interventions.—We conducted an observational study.

Main Outcome Measures.—We measured work disability and sick leave as well as the resulting indirect/direct costs of GO-specific therapies.

Results.—Of 215 employed patients, 47 (21.9%) were temporarily work disabled, and 12 (5.6%) were permanently work disabled. Five (2.3%) had lost their jobs, and nine (4.2%) had retired early. The mean duration of sick leave was 22.3 d/yr. Compared with the German average of 11.6 d/yr, 32 (15%) patients had taken longer sick leaves. The duration of sick leave correlated with the disease severity ($P = 0.015$), and work disability correlated with diplopia ($P < 0.001$). Multivariable analysis identified diplopia as the principal predictor for work disability (odds ratio, 1.7; $P < 0.001$). The average costs due to sick leave and work disability ranged between 3,301€ (4,153$) and 6,683€ (8,407$) per patient per year. Direct costs were 388 ± 56€ (488 ± 70$) per patient per year and per year were higher in sight-threatening GO (1,185 ± 2,569€; 1,491 ± 3,232$) than in moderate-to-severe (373 ± 896€; 469 ± 1,127$; $P = 0.013$) or in mild GO (332 ± 857€; 418 ± 1,078$; $P = 0.016$). Total indirect costs ranged between 3,318€ (4,174$) (friction cost method) and 6,738€ (8,476$) (human capital approach). Work impairment as well as direct and indirect costs of GO significantly correlated with the scores of the internationally standardized and specific GO quality-of-life questionnaire.

Conclusions.—Productivity loss and a prolonged therapy for GO incur great indirect and direct costs (Tables 2 and 3).

▶ This article provides financial evidence of how costly Graves orbitopathy (GO) is to a patient and to society in general. This study was done in Germany, so the exact cost may vary in the United States because the health care system and disability compensation are not the same.

The study looked at 215 patients with GO who were employed and compared them with a control group who did not have GO. The study looked at work disability, sick leave, and direct and indirect cost of GO-specific treatment.

As expected, the costs associated with having GO were significant. Loss of work costs were from $4153 to $8407. Indirect costs averaged from $4174 to $8476 (range 0—$50 707; Table 2), and direct costs were as high as $4723 (Table 3). All these were per year. The cost and loss of work correlated well with severity of disease with patients who had the more severe clinical disease being out of work more and spending more financial resources on their disease.

This is the first article to attempt to quantify the cost of having GO. From these figures, the average person's disease can cost as much as $63 837 per year in the most severe form. Once again, that amount may not be accurate in the United States for many reasons. This study does show that having GO not only has significant physical and emotional impacts, but the financial costs are great.

R. B. Penne, MD

Upper-Eyelid Wick Syndrome: Association of Upper-Eyelid Dermatochalasis and Tearing

Avisar I, Norris JH, Selva D, et al (Queen Victoria Hosp, East Grinstead, England; Univ of Adelaide, South Australia, Australia)

Arch Ophthalmol 130:1007-1012, 2012

Objective.—To highlight a case series of patients manifesting epiphora and misdirection of tears laterally or along the upper-eyelid skin crease. This association has been termed *upper-eyelid wick syndrome.* We describe the clinical features and outcomes of management of these patients.

Methods.—A retrospective review of patients referred to 2 oculoplastic centers during a 6-year period for epiphora, who were considered to have misdirection of tears related in some way to upper-eyelid dermatochalasis.

Results.—Nine patients (7 women and 2 men; mean [SD] age, 61.2 [11.3] years, range, 41-76 years) with bilateral epiphora and lateral spillover

(100%), occasionally combined with upper-eyelid wetting (n = 2). All patients had upper-eyelid dermatochalasis. Five patients had upper-eyelid skin obscuring and in contact with the lateral canthus (type 1), and in 4 the lateral canthus was only partially obscured by upper-eyelid skin (type 2). Five patients (56%) had linear excoriation of skin in the lateral canthus. All patients underwent upper-eyelid blepharoplasty, 3 combined with ptosis repair and 3 combined with eyebrow-lift. All patients achieved 80% to 100% improvement in epiphora following surgical intervention to the upper eyelid. The mean (range) follow-up was 2.8 (1-6) years.

Conclusions.—We defined *upper-eyelid wick syndrome* as the misdirection of tears laterally or along the upper-eyelid skin crease causing epiphora, related in some way to upper-eyelid dermatochalasis. In all cases, epiphora improved with treatment of upper-eyelid dermatochalasis. Although recognized among physicians, this has never been formally described in the ophthalmic literature, to our knowledge.

▶ This article proposes a relatively unknown (in the literature) cause for tearing and one that is hard to not believe as real. The authors note that some patients with epiphora, an open lacrimal drainage system, and no lower lid malposition may have upper lid dermatochalasis as the cause of the tearing. These patients have skin that overhangs the entire upper lid or the lateral canthal area, and this skin touching the lateral canthus wicks the tears from the canthal area up under the excess upper eyelid skin. The tears then accumulate under the upper lid skin and may run laterally (Figs 1 and 2 in the original article).

The authors have shown this mechanism in 2 ways. One by placing fluorescein dye in the eye and showing it accumulated under the overhanging upper lid skin. They then mechanically lift the skin, and the dye no longer accumulates. Ultimately, in the 9 patients who had this, the authors performed an upper lid blepharoplasty, and the symptoms resolved.

This is a mechanism for tearing that I do not generally think of, and must be considered, but only after ruling out all other causes. These patients may be the same patients we see who get upper eyelid dermatitis from dermatochalasis. It must be emphasized, that this is a rare cause of tearing. Lacrimal obstruction, dry eyes, blepharitis, and lower eyelid malposition must all be eliminated as causes before this should be considered. Most patients with dermatochalasis do not have tearing, but it is something to keep in mind in the differential diagnosis of epiphora.

R. B. Penne, MD

Primary endoscopic dacryocystorhinostomy with or without silicone tubing: A prospective randomized study
Al-Qahtani AS (King Khalid Univ, Abha, Kingdom of Saudi Arabia)
Am J Rhinol Allergy 26:332-334, 2012

Background.—Endoscopic dacryocystorhinostomy (DCR) is an effective surgical procedure to treat saccal and postsaccal stenosis or nasolacrimal duct obstruction. The use of silicone tube after endoscopic DCR is still controversial. A prospective randomized study was conducted to compare the success rate between the use of silicone stent and no use of silicone stent in endoscopic DCR.

Methods.—A prospective randomized study was conducted at Aseer Central Hospital and Abha Private Hospital, Abha, Kingdom of Saudi Arabia, on all patients undergoing endoscopic DCR between July 1, 2006 and 30 June 30, 2010. Patients were allocated randomly for endoscopic DCR with or without stent. The data collection included age, sex, diagnosis, method, and duration of surgery. Patients were followed up postoperatively at 1 week, 1 month, and then every 3 months for 1 year.

Results.—During the period of the study a total of 173 cases of postsaccal stenosis underwent endoscopic DCR (67 male and 106 female subjects). The mean age was 51.8 years (range, 18–72 years). A stent was used in 92 patients (53.2%) and not used in 81 patients (46.8%). With silicone tubing the success rate was 96%, and without silicone tubing it was 91%, an overall success rate of 94%. The odds ratio of failure without a silicone tube was 3.25 but confidence interval was from 0.84 to 12.60 and the difference between these two groups was statistically not significant ($p = 0.117$).

Conclusion.—In this study, there was no statistically significant advantage of using endoscopic DCR with stent over the endoscopic DCR without stent (Table 3).

▶ Endoscopic dacryocystorhinostomy (DCR) has become more popular recently and offers the advantage of no external incision, less postoperative swelling and bruising, and a similar success rate compared with external DCRs (Table 3). The downside, at least at Wills Eye Institute, is it is done together with otolaryngology, so the fact that 2 doctors are involved and the equipment required (including a computed tomography for navigation) make this more costly. This report looks at the need for silicone intubation as part of the procedure.

This is a prospective, randomized study that used a silicone tube as part of the endoscopic DCR in 92 patients and no silicone tube in 81 patients. The tube was removed at 4 months, and patients were followed up for 1 year. Success was defined as no complaints of tearing, no dacryocystitis, and endoscopic visualization

TABLE 3.—Review of the Literature on Success Rate with or without Stent on Endoscopic DCR Techniques

Source	No. of Patients	Technique	Success Rate (%) With Stent	Success Rate (%) Without Stent
Mortimore *et al.*[18]	15	Endonasal	89.0	87.0
Halis *et al.*[19]	21	Endonasal	NA	90.5
Halis *et al.*[17]	30	Endonasal	85.7	81.3
Smirnov *et al.*[11]	42	Endonasal	89.0	75.0
Smirnov *et al.*[16]	46	Endonasal	78.0	100
Saeed[3]	35	Endonasal	NA	100
Ramakrishnan *et al.*[20]	27	Endonasal	93	NA

DCR = dacryocystorhinostomy.
Editor's Note: Please refer to original journal article for full references.

of the neo-ostium. Lacrimal irrigation was not done. The surgery was successful in 96% of the patients with silicone tubes and 91% of those without. There was no statistically significant difference between the 2 groups.

This makes me ask whether tubes are really needed in endoscopic DCRs. The study is not enough to make me quit using tubes. I would like to see a study in which patency of the lacrimal system is verified with irrigation before I might consider no tubes. Even though there is no statistical difference between the groups, I can't help seeing the 91% with no tube and the 96% with tube and asking, why not place a tube?

R. B. Penne, MD

Brow Ptosis After Temporal Artery Biopsy: Incidence and Associations
Murchison AP, Bilyk JR (Wills Eye Inst, Philadelphia, PA)
Ophthalmology 119:2637-2642, 2012

Objective.—Temporal artery biopsy (TAB), performed for the diagnosis of giant cell arteritis, has a low reported rate of complications. One complication is damage to the facial nerve branches, which can result in brow ptosis and/or orbicularis oculi weakness. However, the incidence of facial nerve damage after TAB is unknown.

Design.—Prospective, institutional review board-approved study of all TABs performed by 2 surgeons over a 17-month period.

Participants.—Seventy patients undergoing 77 TABs.

Methods.—Demographic data, including age, gender, and race/ethnicity, were collected for all patients. Frontalis and orbicularis oculi muscle function were evaluated pre- and postoperatively in all patients. The use of blood thinners, location of the incision, length of incision and biopsy, biopsy results, and procedure difficulty were recorded. Incidence of postoperative facial nerve damage, other complications, and rates of facial nerve recovery were evaluated. Analysis of variables was performed for any potential correlation with facial nerve damage.

Main Outcome Measures.—Incidence of facial nerve damage.

Results.—Analysis included 75 biopsies performed in 68 patients. The majority of the patients were white (75.0%) and female (67.6%). The mean age was 72.6 years (range, 51−96). Postoperative facial nerve damage was found in 12 patients (16.0%) and 58.3% of these fully resolved at an average of 4.43 months (range, 1−6). Two patients (2.7%) had postoperative infections. There was no correlation with facial nerve damage and use of blood thinners, biopsy result, surgeon, procedure difficulty, incision length, or specimen length. The distance from the incision to both the orbital rim and the brow was significant: Incisions farther from the orbital rim and brow were less likely to have postoperative facial nerve damage.

Conclusions.—There is a 16.0% incidence of postoperative facial nerve damage with TABs, which recovers fully in over half of patients. Incisions closer to the orbital rim and brow were more likely to have postoperative facial nerve dysfunction. Incisions >35 mm from both the orbital rim and

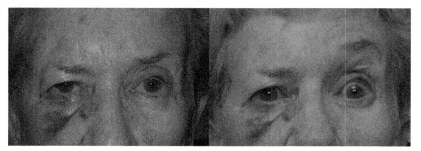

FIGURE 2.—Postoperative photos of patient demonstrating right-sided brow ptosis. Left, at rest, note brow asymmetry. Right, with frontalis activation, note complete lack of right brow elevation. (Reprinted from Murchison AP, Bilyk JR. Brow ptosis after temporal artery biopsy: incidence and associations. *Ophthalmology.* 2012;119:2637-2642, Copyright 2012, with permission from the American Academy of Ophthalmology.)

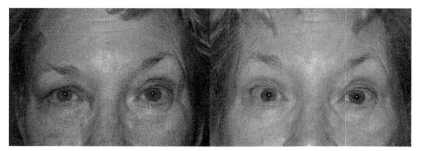

FIGURE 3.—Postoperative clinical photos of patient after temporal artery biopsy on the right. Left, note right brow ptosis with frontalis weakness 1 week after biopsy. Right, 6 months after surgery, frontalis function has fully recovered. (Reprinted from Murchison AP, Bilyk JR. Brow ptosis after temporal artery biopsy: incidence and associations. *Ophthalmology.* 2012;119:2637-2642, Copyright 2012, with permission from the American Academy of Ophthalmology.)

brow or above the brow were less likely to have postoperative brow ptosis (Figs 2-4).

▶ This is a nice prospective study looking at the incidence of brow ptosis after temporal artery biopsy (TAB). The relatively high incidence of brow ptosis (16%) (Fig 2) was surprising to me. I have not had a patient complain of this, nor have I noted it postoperatively. As noted in the article, these patients often have their biopsy and then follow up with the referring neuro-ophthalmologist who requested the temporal artery biopsy. I would estimate that I see fewer than 50% of these patients back postoperatively, and I will admit brow ptosis is not something I look for. Many times at 5 to 7 days postop, they have swelling and bruising, and any brow ptosis may be blamed on that. This article will make me look for this, and I will consider seeing all patients back in my office postoperatively to look for this.

Another important contribution this report makes is identifying the factors that increase the risk of a brow ptosis after TAB. The position of the incision seemed to be the one variable that made a difference. If the incision is above the brow, the risk

Brow Ptosis Incidence and Recovery

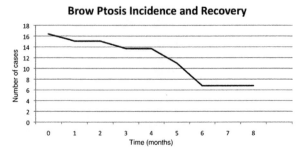

FIGURE 4.—Incidence of brow ptosis after temporal artery biopsy and recovery over time. (Reprinted from Murchison AP, Bilyk JR. Brow ptosis after temporal artery biopsy: incidence and associations. *Ophthalmology.* 2012;119:2637-2642, with permission from the American Academy of Ophthalmology.)

of brow ptosis was zero in this study. If the incision was more lateral to the brow, the farther it is from the lateral brow/lateral orbital rim, the lower the chance of brow ptosis. The problem with this is that the artery is where it is in each individual patient. Thus, if the artery is located in an area with higher risk of brow ptosis, you have to go there to do the biopsy, but this higher risk needs to be discussed with the patient before surgery.

The good news is only 4% of the patients undergoing TAB have a residual brow ptosis at 6 months, so most do resolve with time (Figs 3 and 4). This is a complication that needs to be included in the preoperative discussion for patients undergoing a TAB.

R. B. Penne, MD

Symptomatic Relief Associated With Eyelid Hygiene in Anterior Blepharitis and MGD
Guillon M, Maissa C, Wong S (OTG Res and Consultancy, London, UK)
Eye Contact Lens 38:306-312, 2012

Objective.—The principal objective of this investigation was to assess the symptomatic relief associated with eyelid hygiene using Blephaclean eye pads, a cosmetic product, to manage anterior blepharitis or Meibomian gland dysfunction (MGD) associated with dry eye complaints.

Method.—The investigation was a bilateral, prospective, interventional open label investigation of 3-month duration. The test population was made up of dry eye sufferers with at least mild symptoms (Ocular Surface Disease Index [OSDI] $\geq$ 13) who presented with mild to moderate anterior blepharitis or MGD. Eyelid hygiene was intensive (twice a day) for the initial 3 weeks and a maintenance regimen (once a day) for the remainder of the study. At each visit, a detailed assessment of symptomatology was carried out. The assessment included the reporting of overall symptomatology with the OSDI questionnaire, of comfort and specific symptoms at the end of the day on 100-point visual analog scales and of specific MGD-related symptoms on forced choice 5-point scales.

TABLE 3.—Anterior Blepharitis and MGD Patient Reported Signs and Symptoms Classification

Crusts or flakes on the eyelashes
The subject was asked to indicate how often crusts or flakes were noted on the eyelashes when waking up. The rating scale were as below:
0=Never
1=Some mornings
2=Half of the mornings
3=Most of the mornings
4=Every morning
5=Do not know
Eyelids stuck together on waking
The subjects were asked to indicate how often their eyelids were stuck together when waking up. The rating scale was as below:
0=Never
1=Some mornings
2=Half of the mornings
3=Most of the mornings
4=Every morning
5=Do not know
Eyelids red on waking
The subjects were asked to indicate how often their eyelids were red when waking up. The rating scale was as below:
0=Never
1=Some mornings
2=Half of the mornings
3=Most of the mornings
4=Every morning
5=Do not know
Eyelids heavy and/or puffy at any time of the day
The subjects were asked to indicate how often their eyelids were heavy and/or puffy anytime of the day The rating scale will be as below:
0=Never
1=Some of the time
2=Half of the time
3=Most of the time
4=All the time
5=Do not know

Result.—Forty subjects aged 22 to 74 years (54 ± 15 years) were enrolled, of whom 39 completed the investigation. The product usage revealed good overall compliance throughout the study. The results revealed significant improvement in symptomatology. A significant ($P < 0.001$) decrease in overall symptomatology was recorded (Mean OSDI: baseline = 30, day 21 = 18, day 90 = 19; Symptomatic status: baseline 100%, day 21 55%, day 90 54%) associated with significant ($P < 0.001$) increase in the end of day comfort (Mean score: baseline = 56, day 21 = 67, day 90 = 67) and decrease in end of day dryness (Mean score: baseline = 55, day 21 = 42, day 90 = 41).

Conclusions.—The results showed that eyelid hygiene with Blephaclean wipes by subjects with anterior blepharitis or MGD significantly decreased their associated symptomatology and increased their ocular comfort. The data confirmed the efficiency of the clinical methodology, put forward of 3 weeks of intensive use (twice a day) of eyelid wipes followed by maintenance use (once a day); that approach achieved a rapid symptomatic improvement that was maintained over time (Table 3).

▶ This was a study of a very simple eyelid treatment, eyelid hygiene, which is commonly used to treat meibomian gland dysfunction (MGD). In the study, it was used in patients who had both dry eyes and MGD. The conclusion was that eyelid hygiene using a specific type of eyelid scrub (Blephaclean wipes) improved dry eye symptoms. This conclusion was based on questionnaires (Table 3) filled out before starting treatment, at 3 weeks, and at 3 months after treatment initiation. The improvement reported by study participants was statistically significant.

It is unfortunate that the study did not go a step further and grade the severity of the blepharitis before and after treatment. The patients had grading done before the study to be sure they qualified to be in the study. The entire study would be more impressive if the physical signs went along with the patients' symptomatic improvements. Often, a patient's symptoms are what drive our treatment in both MGD and dry eyes. Thus, the fact the patients reported improvement is positive. However, it is a study in which patients really can't have a placebo because they are applying the scrub, and there may be some bias in the results in that patients who invest the time to treat themselves want to be better. The other issue is how other types of commercially available lid scrubs compare with this type. I believe they would be similar. I find the old fashioned baby shampoo and wash cloth is often irritating for patients and may not have the same results or frequency of use as commercial lid scrubs.

Ultimately, this study could have been much stronger with physical evidence of improvement in MGD. The fact that eyelid hygiene has no risk and is inexpensive makes it a good choice. This study at least suggests patients with MGD and dry eyes will feel better using eyelid hygiene.

R. B. Penne, MD

7 Pediatric Ophthalmology

Incidence and clinical characteristics of periocular infantile hemangiomas
Alniemi ST, Griepentrog GJ, Diehl N, et al (Mayo Clinic College of Medicine, Rochester, MN)
Arch Ophthalmol 130:889-893, 2012

Objective.—To report the incidence, demographics, and clinical findings among a population-based cohort of children with periocular infantile hemangiomas.

Methods.—The medical records of all patients (<19 years of age) diagnosed as having periocular infantile hemangiomas while residing in Olmsted County, Minnesota, from January 1, 1965, through December 31, 2004, were retrospectively reviewed.

Results.—Forty-three children were diagnosed as having periocular infantile hemangiomas during the 40-year period, yielding an incidence of 5.4 per 100,000 individuals younger than 19 years (95% CI, 3.8-7.1) or a birth prevalence of 1 in 1586 live births. Thirty children (70%) were female (*P* < .001). There was a history of maternal infertility in approximately 1 in 5 children and premature birth in 1 in 8 children. Twenty-six children (61%) had other abnormalities, including secondary hemangiomas in 9 (21%). Forty-one patients (95%) had unilateral disease, and 37 hemangiomas (86%) were located on the upper eyelid.

Conclusions.—In this population-based study, periocular infantile hemangiomas occurred in 1 in 1586 live births and were most prevalent on the unilateral upper eyelid of white female patients. Prevalent associations included maternal infertility and premature birth. Other abnormalities, including secondary hemangiomas in 1 in 5 children, were common in this cohort.

▶ Periocular hemangiomas are relatively common, occurring in 1 in 1586 live births. It is unclear to me why there is a female predominance and why girls are more likely to have larger periocular hemangiomas and more severe amblyopia than boys with periocular hemangiomas. In the findings of 5 patients with periocular hemangiomas, there was a history of maternal infertility, and 1 in 8 were born prematurely, suggesting that perhaps infertility drugs could be a factor. The authors emphasize the importance of a careful follow-up of all children with periocular hemangiomas for the possible development of amblyopia.

L. B. Nelson, MD, MBA

Clinical Course and Characteristics of Acute Presentation of Fourth Nerve Paresis

Khaier A, Dawson E, Lee J

J Pediatr Ophthalmol Strabismus 49:1-4, 2012

Purpose.—Many cases of acute-onset cranial nerve paresis have benign etiologies such as microvascular occlusion. Most will resolve completely and neuroimaging is usually unnecessary. Few reports exist on acute fourth nerve paresis.

Methods.—A retrospective review was conducted of all patients presenting with diplopia to the emergency department for 1 year caused by isolated fourth cranial nerve paresis from any cause including trauma.

Results.—Thirty-two patients met the criteria, 26 (81%) males and 6 (19%) females, with an average age of 59.5 years (range: 14 to 80 years). Eighteen (56%) had a microvascular etiology with diabetes mellitus, hypertension, or both; 6 were already taking medication. Six (19%) had decompensating fourth nerve paresis (2 had hypertension and 1 had recent head trauma). Closed head trauma accounted for 2 patients, migraine and herpes zoster virus accounted for one each, and 4 remained unknown. Nineteen patients (59%) were prescribed prisms and 2 patients were given occlusion. Diplopia resolved without treatment in 23 patients (72%) within 2 weeks to 10 months, but 89% of patients with microvascular etiology resolved spontaneously. Three patients continued with prisms, one patient underwent surgery.

Conclusion.—The prognosis for complete and spontaneous resolution of microvascular fourth nerve paresis was excellent, with 89% completely resolved within 10 months.

► Acute fourth nerve paresis is probably the most frequent cause of acquired vertical diplopia. The authors of this article found that many cases of acute fourth nerve paresis have a benign etiology and clinical course. Although the most common cause of vertical diplopia related to a fourth nerve palsy has been thought to be a decompensation of a congenital condition, the authors in this study found microvascular disease to be the most common cause. However, acute fourth nerve paresis can be an early clinical sign of a serious intracranial abnormality. The authors suggest that because they found a benign etiology and clinical course for most acute fourth nerve paresis, there is no need for hasty neuroimaging. This recommendation is predicated on a normal neurologic assessment, and the clinical presentation is compatible with a benign etiology. Because a normal neurologic assessment in a patient with an acute fourth nerve palsy does not completely rule out a serious intracranial abnormality, neurologic imaging prior to a 3-month observation period, as recommended by these authors, may be a better course of action.

L. B. Nelson, MD, MBA

Twelve-year review of pediatric traumatic open globe injuries in an urban U.S. population
Lesniak SP, Bauza A, Son JH, et al (New Jersey Med School, Newark)
J Pediatr Ophthalmol Strabismus 49:73-79, 2012

Purpose.—To evaluate the epidemiology, anatomical characteristics, and clinical outcomes of pediatric traumatic open globe injuries and to compare the observed final visual acuity to the expected visual acuity as predicted by the Ocular Trauma Score (OTS).
Methods.—Retrospective chart review of 89 pediatric patients (89 eyes) with open globe injury presenting between 1997 and 2008.
Results.—Sixty-five patients (73%) were male, average age was 9.7 years, and mean follow-up was 22.6 months. The most common causes of trauma were: accidents (79%), violence (10%), and motor vehicle accidents (9%). Penetrating ocular injury was the most common trauma (54%), followed by blunt rupture (34%). Zone 1 injuries represented 49% of cases, and zones 2 and 3 represented 29% and 21%, respectively. No patient developed endophthalmitis. The average presenting and final visual acuities were logarithm of the minimum angle of resolution 1.927 and 1.401, respectively. Lens trauma was noted in 44 (49%) eyes. Twenty-eight patients (31%) had retinal detachment within 6 months of presentation. Total retinal attachment was achieved in 12 (63%) of 19 eyes undergoing repair. Enucleation was performed in 9 (10%) patients. Final visual acuities were not statistically different from visual acuities predicted by OTS (*P* > .05).
Conclusions.—The visual prognosis in pediatric open globe injury is poor. The zone of injury may correlate with poor final visual acuity, risk of retinal detachment, and subsequent need for an enucleation. The final predicted visual acuity correlated well with the observed final visual acuity in these patients.

▶ Ocular trauma is a significant cause of visual loss in children. The socioeconomic cost related to pediatric ocular trauma is staggering. Therefore, prevention of eye injuries in children is paramount. Children should be educated about the dangers of ocular trauma. Parents should set a positive example by wearing protective eyewear while doing risky tasks or being involved in sports. Children need to be encouraged to wear safety glasses under similar circumstances. Because many eye injuries in children can occur in the home setting, it is important to make homes a safer place (ie, cushion sharp corners and edges in furniture and fixtures and keep all chemicals and tools out of the reach of children). Parents should avoid having children play with potentially dangerous toys.

Legislation should also be passed to improve toy safety standards. This should include placing warning labels on toys that have the potential to cause eye injuries. Parents should be alerted to the potential risks in order to prevent pediatric eye injuries.

L. B. Nelson, MD, MBA

Suture contamination in strabismus surgery
Eustis HS, Rhodes A
J Pediatr Ophthalmol Strabismus 49:206-209, 2012

Purpose.—To document the contamination rate of sutures used in strabismus surgery and evaluate the reduction of contamination using antibiotic-coated and antiseptic/antibiotic-coated sutures.

Methods.—This was a prospective randomized analysis of suture contamination and potential prophylaxis measures after strabismus surgery. Muscle sutures (6-0 polyglactin) used in 302 consecutive cases of strabismus from October 2008 to May 2009 were collected and randomly assigned to three groups: (1) a control without pretreatment sutures (61); (2) antibiotic/steroid-coated sutures (200); and (3) antiseptic-soaked and antibiotic/steroid-coated sutures (141). The sutures were used under sterile conditions and then cut into pieces and transferred to blood agar plates, which were incubated for 48 hours and then checked for growth.

Results.—Group 1 had bacterial growth in 17 of 61 (28%) sutures; group 2 had growth in 44 of 200 (22%) sutures; and group 3 had growth in 12 of 141 (9%) sutures. The reduction in bacterial growth using the antibiotic/antiseptic coating was significant ($P = .006$). One patient developed coagulase-negative Staphylococcus epidermidis endophthalmitis 1 week after surgery, which was promptly diagnosed and successfully treated. No complications from the antibiotic-coated or antiseptic-soaked sutures were noted.

Conclusions.—Although endophthalmitis after strabismus surgery is rare, estimated at 1 in 35,000 to 1 in 185,000, visual outcome is uniformly poor. The authors hypothesize that strabismus sutures can be contaminated via contact with the eyelashes and skin, providing a possible conduit for endophthalmitis. Bacterial contamination of strabismus sutures is high (28%) and can be reduced significantly if sutures are soaked in antiseptic before use.

► The incidence of perioperative inflammation after strabismus surgery is uncommon. Many of these cases may be related to when there is prolongation of the suture material dissolving, creating conjunctival injection around the suture. This phenomenon is more common in adult strabismus surgery patients. The incidence of endophthalmitis after strabismus surgery is extremely rare. These authors estimate the incidence rate as 1 in 35 000 to 1 in 185 000 cases following strabismus surgery. These authors also note in a prospective, randomized analysis that the contamination rate of suture material use in strabismus surgery was least when the suture was presoaked with antiseptic and an antibiotic—steroid combination compared with sutures without pretreatment or soaked just with an antibiotic—steroid combination. Unfortunately, the authors did not identify the pathogen contaminating the sutures. Many of the pathogens were most likely normal flora. Because the incidence of endophthalmitis following strabismus surgery is rare and no specific pathogens were identified in this study, further prospective studies may help to determine whether presoaking sutures prior to strabismus surgery is appropriate.

L. B. Nelson, MD, MBA

Effect of age on response to amblyopia treatment in children
Holmes JM, Pediatric Eye Disease Investigator Group (Mayo Clinic, Rochester, MN)
Arch Ophthalmol 129:1451-1457, 2011

Objective.—To determine whether age at initiation of treatment for amblyopia influences the response among children 3 to less than 13 years of age with unilateral amblyopia who have 20/40 to 20/400 amblyopic eye visual acuity.

Methods.—A meta-analysis of individual subject data from 4 recently completed randomized amblyopia treatment trials was performed to evaluate the relationship between age and improvement in logMAR amblyopic eye visual acuity. Analyses were adjusted for baseline amblyopic eye visual acuity, spherical equivalent refractive error in the amblyopic eye, type of amblyopia, prior amblyopia treatment, study treatment, and protocol. Age was categorized (3 to <5 years, 5 to <7 years, and 7 to <13 years) because there was a nonlinear relationship between age and improvement in amblyopic eye visual acuity.

Results.—Children from 7 to less than 13 years of age were significantly less responsive to treatment than were younger age groups (children from 3 to <5 years of age or children from 5 to <7 years of age) for moderate and severe amblyopia ($P < .04$ for all 4 comparisons). There was no difference in treatment response between children 3 to less than 5 years of age and children 5 to less than 7 years of age for moderate amblyopia ($P = .67$), but there was a suggestion of greater responsiveness in children 3 to less than 5 years of age compared with children 5 to less than 7 years of age for severe amblyopia ($P = .09$).

Conclusions.—Amblyopia is more responsive to treatment among children younger than 7 years of age. Although the average treatment response is smaller in children 7 to less than 13 years of age, some children show a marked response to treatment.

▶ The shortest duration in which a medical condition that requires treatment is actually treated usually gives the best result. It is not surprising that children less than 7 years of age tend to have a better response to amblyopia treatment. Also, in the case of amblyopia, the closer a child is to age 9, the end of the sensitive period of visual development, the less likelihood that treatment will be successful. In children with amblyopia who were not diagnosed early there was poor compliance; however, even in children over the age of 9, amblyopia treatment should be instituted. In many of these cases, a moderate response to amblyopia treatment may occur.

L. B. Nelson, MD, MBA

Optical Treatment of Strabismic and Combined Strabismic–Anisometropic Amblyopia

Writing Committee for the Pediatric Eye Disease Investigator Group (Southern California College of Optometry, Fullerton, CA; Jaeb Ctr for Health Res, Tampa, FL; Mayo Clinic, Rochester, MN; et al)
Ophthalmology 119:150-158, 2012

Objective.—To determine visual acuity improvement in children with strabismic and combined strabismic–anisometropic (combined-mechanism) amblyopia treated with optical correction alone and to explore factors associated with improvement.

Design.—Prospective, multicenter, cohort study.

Participants.—We included 146 children 3 to <7 years old with previously untreated strabismic amblyopia (n = 52) or combined-mechanism amblyopia (n = 94).

Methods.—Optical treatment was provided as spectacles (prescription based on a cycloplegic refraction) that were worn for the first time at the baseline visit. Visual acuity with spectacles was measured using the Amblyopia Treatment Study HOTV visual acuity protocol at baseline and every 9 weeks thereafter until no further improvement in visual acuity. Ocular alignment was assessed at each visit.

Main Outcome Measures.—Visual acuity 18 weeks after baseline.

Results.—Overall, amblyopic eye visual acuity improved a mean of 2.6 lines (95% confidence interval [CI], 2.3–3.0), with 75% of children improving ≥2 lines and 54% improving ≥3 lines. Resolution of amblyopia occurred in 32% (95% CI, 24%–41%) of the children. The treatment effect was greater for strabismic amblyopia than for combined-mechanism amblyopia (3.2 vs 2.3 lines; adjusted $P = 0.003$). Visual acuity improved regardless of whether eye alignment improved.

Conclusions.—Optical treatment alone of strabismic and combined-mechanism amblyopia results in clinically meaningful improvement in amblyopic eye visual acuity for most 3- to <7-year-old children, resolving in at least one quarter without the need for additional treatment. Consideration should be given to prescribing refractive correction as the sole initial treatment for children with strabismic or combined-mechanism amblyopia before initiating other therapies.

▶ It is reasonable to try glasses initially without amblyopia treatment in patients with strabismus or combined strabismic-anisometropia amblyopia. These patients should be evaluated within 1 month to determine the alignment and the visual acuity improvement. It is imperative that in both types of strabismus and amblyopia patients that the alignment is controlled with optical correction. If the strabismus is controlled with glasses, then unless there is a substantial improvement in the vision in the amblyopic eye, further treatment of the amblyopia should be instituted at that time. It is not surprising that these authors found that optical correction alone improved the vision with strabismus and amblyopia vs combined strabismus-anisometropia amblyopia patients.

L. B. Nelson, MD, MBA

Cerebral damage may be the primary risk factor for visual impairment in preschool children born extremely premature
Slidsborg C, Bangsgaard R, Fledelius HC, et al
Arch Ophthalmol 130:1410-1417, 2012

Objectives.—To investigate the importance of cerebral damage and retinopathy of prematurity (ROP) for visual impairment in preschool children born extremely premature and to determine the primary risk factor of the two.

Methods.—A clinical follow-up study of a Danish national cohort of children born extremely premature (gestational age, <28 weeks). The study sample consisted of 262 extremely preterm children born between February 13, 2004, and March 23, 2006, of whom 178 children (67.9%) participated. A matched control group consisted of 56 term-born children (gestational age, 37 to <42 weeks). All participants were identified through the National Birth Register and invited to participate in a clinical examination. The children were evaluated with regard to visual acuity, foveal sequelae, and maximum ROP stage and the presence of global developmental deficits (an indicator for cerebral damage) that was measured by the Ages and Stages Questionnaire.

Results.—Global developmental deficits and foveal sequelae occurred more often in extremely preterm children than in term-born control children and increased with ROP severity (χ^2 test; $P = .11$ and $P < .001$, respectively). Global developmental deficits, moderate to severe foveal abnormality, and ROP treatment were independently associated with visual impairment ($P < .05$, for better and worse eyes). A stepwise multiple logistic regression for better-eye logarithmic visual acuities of 0.3 or greater (Snellen scale, ≤0.5) yielded an odds ratio of 8.7 (95% CI, 3.0-25.2; $P < .001$) for global developmental deficit and 6.3 (95% CI, 2.2-18.5; $P < .001$) for moderate to severe foveal sequelae.

Conclusion.—Cerebral damage and ROP are independent risk factors for visual impairment in children born extremely premature, and cerebral damage may be the primary risk factor.

▶ Although retinopathy of prematurity is an important cause of visual impairment in severely preterm infants, cerebral damage does have a great impact on the visual development of these infants. Pediatric ophthalmologists and pediatricians should strongly consider cerebral damage to be a primary cause of blindness or visual impairment in all premature infants. I agree with the authors of this article about the need to determine how severe visual impairment, regardless of the cause, in premature infants impacts the degree of developmental deficits.

L. B. Nelson, MD, MBA

Laser In Situ Keratomileusis for the Treatment of Refractive Accommodative Esotropia

Brugnoli de Pagano OM, Pagano GL (Natl Univ of Cuyo, Mendoza, Argentina; Centrovision Mendoza Eye Clinic, Argentina)
Ophthalmology 119:159-163, 2012

Purpose.—To demonstrate the effectiveness of refractive surgery with an excimer laser to correct hyperopia and convergent strabismus caused by compensatory accommodation of refractive error.

Design.—Prospective, interventional, noncomparative case series.

Participants.—Forty-six eyes of 23 patients with hyperopia and fully or partially refractive accommodative esotropia.

Methods.—Patients were treated with an excimer laser and the LASIK technique between 2000 and 2010.

Main Outcome Measures.—Preoperative and postoperative refractive spherical equivalent and ocular alignment.

Results.—Mean age ± standard deviation [SD] was 25 ± 12.6 years. Mean hyperopia ± SD was 3.67 ± 1.28 diopters (D) before surgery and 0.21 ± 0.59 D after surgery ($P < 0.001$). The mean angle of deviation without correction was 21.0 prism diopters (Δ) before surgery and 3.7 Δ after surgery ($P < 0.001$).

Conclusions.—Refractive surgery with excimer laser is a promising option for the treatment of refractive accommodative esotropia.

▶ I was surprised at how successful laser treatment for accommodative and partially accommodative esotropia was in reducing the esotropia while eliminating the hyperopic correction. In patients with accommodative esotropia, the hyperopic correction reduces the accommodative effort and, in turn, reduces the esotropia. By eliminating the hyperopic correction of these patients when they accommodate, why does the esotropia not occur? In patients who have accommodative esotropia and undergo bilateral cataract surgery that eliminates their hyperopic correction, esotropia may continue. What is the clinical difference in the laser and cataract patients who have accommodative esotropia and have their hyperopic correction eliminated? Further studies will hopefully answer these questions.

L. B. Nelson, MD, MBA

Optic Disc Change with Incipient Myopia of Childhood

Kim TW, Kim M, Weinreb RN, et al (Seoul Natl Univ Bundang Hosp, Seongnam, Korea; Univ of California San Diego, La Jolla)
Ophthalmology 119:21-26, 2012

Purpose.—To describe progressive tilting of the optic nerve head (ONH) and development/enlargement of parapapillary atrophy (PPA) observed in children with incipient myopia and to investigate factors associated with such changes.

Design.—Retrospective, observational study.

Participants.—This study included 118 eyes of 118 Korean children who were assessed by serial disc photography at intervals of 1 year or more.

Methods.—All disc photographs were reviewed by 2 experienced ophthalmologists, and eyes were classified into 2 groups with respect to the change in the ONH appearance and development/enlargement of β-zone PPA: (1) ONH/PPA changed group and (2) ONH/PPA unchanged group. To quantify the ONH/PPA changes, the ratio of the horizontal to vertical disc diameter (HVDR) and the ratio of the maximum PPA width to vertical disc diameter (PVDR) were measured. Factors associated with ONH/PPA changes were evaluated using logistic regression analysis. Refractive errors were measured with cycloplegic refraction.

Main Outcome Measures.—Morphologic changes of the ONH/PPA as observed in serial disc photographs and its association with myopic shift.

Results.—Mean subject age and refractive error at the time of initial fundus examination were 7.3 ± 3.7 years (range, $1-17$ years) and -0.9 ± 1.9 diopters (range, -5.9 to $+3.0$ diopters), respectively. Mean follow-up period was 38.1 ± 19.6 months (range, $12-88$ months). Fifty-one eyes (43%) were classified as the ONH/PPA change group. In the ONH/PPA change group, HVDR decreased from the initial value of 0.92 ± 0.08 to the final value of 0.86 ± 0.11, and the PVDR increased from the initial value of 0.08 ± 0.07 to the final value of 0.20 ± 0.11. The ONH/PPA changes were most remarkable in subjects between 7 and 9 years of age (odds ratio [OR] = 6.698; 95% confidence interval [CI], 2.296—19.546) and were associated with greater myopic shift during the follow-up period (OR − 0.483; 95% CI, 0.345—0.676).

Conclusions.—We demonstrate progressive tilting of the ONH, which was observed with development/enlargement of PPA in children who exhibited myopic shift. These findings suggest that tilted disc, as well as PPA, may be an acquired feature in myopic eyes, arising from scleral stretching.

▶ This study confirms my own observation that in some children with increasing myopia, tilting of the optic disc develops. The ratio of the parapapillary atrophy to the optic nerve head was associated with a change in myopia, although the horizontal-to-vertical disc diameter was not correlated to the degree of myopic shift. I agree with the authors' suggestion that factors other than a noted change in myopia must play a more significant factor in the development of the tilting. A correlation between the acquired tilting of the optic nerve and a possible change in corrected vision was not documented in this study. Because less-than-normal vision is associated with tilting of the optic nerve, further studies evaluating the acquired tilting and its possible effect on the vision should be done.

L. B. Nelson, MD, MBA

Resolution of congenital nasolacrimal duct obstruction with nonsurgical management

Pediatric Eye Disease Investigator Group
Arch Ophthalmol 130:730-734, 2012

Objective.—To determine how often nasolacrimal duct obstruction (NLDO) resolves with 6 months of nonsurgical management in infants aged 6 to less than 10 months.

Methods.—As part of a randomized trial evaluating the cost-effectiveness of immediate office probing vs observation with deferred probing for unresolved cases, 107 infants aged 6 to less than 10 months who had NLDO and no history of nasolacrimal duct surgery were prescribed 6 months of nasolacrimal duct massage and topical antibiotics as needed. Resolution of the NLDO was assessed 6 months after study entry and was defined as the absence of all clinical signs of NLDO (epiphora, increased tear lake, or mucous discharge) and not having undergone NLDO surgery. Exploratory analyses assessed whether baseline characteristics, including age, sex, laterality, and prior treatment, were associated with the probability of NLDO resolving without surgery.

Results.—At the 6-month examination, which was completed for 117 of the 133 eyes (88%), the NLDO had resolved without surgery in 77 eyes (66% [95% CI, 56%-74%]). None of the baseline characteristics we evaluated were found to be associated with resolution.

Conclusions.—In infants 6 to less than 10 months of age, more than half of eyes with NLDO will resolve within 6 months with nonsurgical management. Knowledge of the rate of NLDO resolution in infancy without surgery will help clinicians and parents effectively discuss treatment options.

▶ Because there have been a number of reports documenting the high resolution rate of congenital nasolacrimal duct obstruction (NLDO) at less than 1 year of age, a better-designed study would have evaluated the resolution rate beyond age one. This study had several factors that were pointed out by the authors and may have affected the results. The retention rate was lower than expected. The study did not assess the compliance of the parents with lacrimal massage. Without a control group, it is difficult to determine the extent of resolution with and without treatment.

L. B. Nelson, MD, MBA

A Randomized Trial Comparing the Cost-effectiveness of 2 Approaches for Treating Unilateral Nasolacrimal Duct Obstruction
Pediatric Eye Disease Investigator Group
Arch Ophthalmol 130:1525-1533, 2012

Objective.—To compare the cost-effectiveness of 2 approaches for treating unilateral nasolacrimal duct obstruction (NLDO).

Methods.—One hundred sixty-three infants aged 6 to less than 10 months with unilateral NLDO were randomly assigned to receive immediate office-based nasolacrimal duct probing (n = 82) or 6 months of observation/nonsurgical management (n = 81) followed by probing in a facility for persistent symptoms.

Main Outcome Measures —Treatment success was defined as the absence of clinical signs of NLDO (epiphora, increased tear lake, mucous discharge) on masked examination at age 18 months. Cost of treatment between randomization and age 18 months included costs for all surgical procedures and medications.

Results.—In the observation/deferred facility-probing group, NLDO resolved within 6 months without surgery in 44 of the 67 patients (66%; 95% CI, 54% to 76%) who completed the 6-month visit. Twenty-two (27%) of the 81 patients in the observation/deferred facility-probing group underwent surgery, 4 of whom were operated on within the initial 6 months. At age 18 months, 69 of 75 patients (92%) in the immediate office-probing group were treatment successes, compared with 58 of 71 observation/deferred facility-probing group patients (82%) (10% difference in success; 95% CI, −1% to 21%). The mean cost of treatment was $562 in the immediate office-probing group compared with $701 in the observation/deferred facility-probing group (difference, −$139; 95% CI, −$377 to $94). The immediate office-probing group experienced 3.0 fewer months of symptoms (95% CI, −1.8 to −4.0).

Conclusions.—The immediate office-probing approach is likely more cost-effective than observation followed by deferred facility probing if needed. Adoption of the immediate office-probing approach would result in probing in approximately two-thirds of infants whose obstruction would have resolved within 6 months of nonsurgical management, but would largely avoid the need for probing under general anesthesia.

Application to Clinical Practice.—Although unilateral NLDO often resolves without surgery, immediate office probing is an effective and potentially cost-saving treatment option.

Trial Registration.—clinicaltrials.gov Identifier: NCT00780741.

▶ Most nasolacrimal duct obstructions (NLDO) resolve by 1 year of age without the need for probing. Although the mean cost of treatment in the immediate office-probing group was slightly less costly ($562 vs $701) than the facility-probing group, many of the patients who were probed early would have improved without the need for a probing at all. Although the immediate office-probing patient is at least as successful as those in the observation/deferred facility-probing group, in the end much of the early probing ultimately was unnecessary, as these patients would have improved on their own. Most probings in an outpatient facility usually take less than 10 minutes and are performed without intubation but rather with mask anesthesia. Most parents, in my experience, will usually accept observation and proper massage, as most of the patients with an NLDO will improve and not need a probing by 1 year of age.

L. B. Nelson, MD, MBA

Ocular Motor and Sensory Function in Parkinson's Disease
Almer Z, Klein KS, Marsh L, et al (Johns Hopkins Med Institutions, Baltimore, MD)
Ophthalmology 119:178-182, 2012

Purpose.—To evaluate the effect of dopaminergic medication and deep brain stimulation on ocular function in Parkinson's disease (PD) and to measure vision-related quality of life in subjects with PD.

Design.—Prospective, comparative case series.

Participants and Controls.—Twenty-seven PD and 16 control subjects were recruited.

Methods.—Visual acuity, ocular motor function, convergence, and vision-related quality of life using the 25-item National Eye Institute Visual Function Questionnaire (VFQ-25) were measured. Visual sensory and motor measurements were obtained during the on and off states of PD dopaminergic treatment.

Main Outcome Measures.—Convergence ability and vision-related quality of life.

Results.—The PD subjects had a mean age of 58.8 years; 30% were female. Their mean duration of PD was 10.9 ± 6.8 years. The control subjects had a mean age of 61.6 years; 56% were female. There was no difference in visual acuity, contrast sensitivity, or color vision of the PD subjects in their on state compared with controls. Convergence amplitudes measured with base-out prism were significantly poorer in PD subjects in their on state compared with controls (24.1 ± 8 Δ vs. 14.8 ± 10.3 Δ; $P = 0.003$). The mean composite VFQ-25 score was significantly worse in the PD subjects compared with the controls (87.1 ± 8.69 vs. 96.6 ± 3.05; $P = 0.0001$). Comparing the PD subjects in their on with their off states, there was no difference in distance exodeviation, near exodeviation, or ocular ductions. Mean convergence amplitudes and near point of convergence were better in the on state compared with the off state: 14.8 ± 10.3 Δ versus 10.7 ± 9.0 Δ ($P = 0.0006$) and 13.1 ± 9.1 cm versus 18.1 ± 12.2 cm ($P = 0.002$), respectively.

Conclusions.—Convergence ability is significantly poorer in PD subjects in both the on and off states compared with controls, but improves significantly with systemic dopaminergic treatment. Ocular motor function in PD subjects fluctuates in response to treatment, which complicates ophthalmic management. Parkinson's disease subjects have a significant reduction in vision-related quality of life, especially with near activities, that is not associated with visual acuity.

▶ Parkinson disease (PD) is a progressive, neurodegenerative disorder of the brain with associated ocular motility findings including convergence insufficiency. Although the convergence insufficiency may temporarily improve with systemic dopaminergic treatment, it may continue to fluctuate as the medicine wears off prior to the next dose. The variability of the near exodeviation throughout the day makes it difficult to treat with base-in prisms. Adult patients with PD who have convergence insufficiency must wear a patch over one eye when they read.

L. B. Nelson, MD, MBA

Congenital Esotropia and the Risk of Mental Illness by Early Adulthood
Olson JH, Louwagie CR, Diehl NN, et al (Mayo Clinic and Mayo Foundation, Rochester, MN; Mayo Clinic Jacksonville, FL)
Ophthalmology 119:145-149, 2012

Objective.—The purpose of this study is to investigate whether children with congenital esotropia (CET) are more likely than controls to develop mental illness by early adulthood.

Design.—Retrospective, population-based cohort.

Participants.—Children (aged <19 years) diagnosed with CET while residing in Olmsted County, Minnesota, from January 1, 1965, to December 31, 1994, and their 1-to-1 non-strabismic birth- and gender-matched controls.

Methods. The medical records of patients with esotropia and their controls were retrospectively reviewed for the subsequent development of psychiatric disease.

Main Outcome Measures.—The development of mental illness and associated comorbidities among patients with CET and their controls.

Results.—A mental health disorder was diagnosed in 42 (33%) of the 127 patients with CET followed to a mean age of 20.4 years compared with 16% of controls ($P = 0.002$). Congenital esotropia increased the odds of developing a psychiatric illness 2.6 times (confidence interval, 1.5–4.8) compared with controls. The number of mental health diagnoses ($P = 0.019$) and the use of psychotropic medications ($P = 0.015$) were significantly more common among esotropic patients compared with non-strabismic controls.

Conclusions.—Congenital esotropia, similar to those with intermittent exotropia or convergence insufficiency, increases the odds of developing mental illness by early adulthood 2.6 times compared with controls. The cause of this association does not seem to be associated with premature birth.

▶ Psychosocial aspects of patients with strabismus in general have been previously described by numerous investigators. Therefore, it should not be surprising that there may be mental disorders in adults who had congenital esotropia as children. It is unclear from this study whether early surgery to correct the esotropia had an effect on the possibility of developing mental illness in an adult. As the authors point out, this study was performed in an ethnically homogenous population of a single geographic area and may not be representative of other population groups.

L. B. Nelson, MD, MBA

The prevalence of ocular structural disorders and nystagmus among preschool-aged children
Repka MX, Friedman DS, Katz J, et al (Johns Hopkins Univ School of Medicine, Baltimore, MD; Wilmer Eye Inst, Baltimore, MD)
J AAPOS 16:182-184, 2012

Purpose.—To describe the prevalence of structural disorders of the eye and nystagmus in preschoolaged children.

Methods.—Population-based evaluation of children 6 months through 71 months of age in Baltimore, Maryland, United States.

Results.—Among 4,132 children identified from 54 census tracts, 3,990 eligible children (97%) were enrolled and 2,546 children (62%) were examined. Structural disorders were found in 41 children and nystagmus in 9 children for an overall prevalence of 1.96% (95% CI, 1.46%-2.59%). Only 11 (0.43%; 95% CI, 0.22%-0.77%) had vision loss in at least one eye, most often due to posterior segment disease.

Conclusions.—Structural ocular abnormalities and nystagmus combined are present in nearly 2% of preschool-aged children in this population-based study. Vision loss due to these abnormalities is uncommon.

▶ Vision screening programs are extremely important in detecting visual abnormalities in children. Amblyopia, especially anisometropia amblyopia, is an asymptomatic condition. Therefore, a vision screening test is necessary to determine whether a child has poor vision in one or both eyes. In this present population-based study, the majority of ocular disorders that affect vision could have been detected by the present standard vision screening tests. Although a rare ocular abnormality may not be detected by the present vision screening, most of the abnormal ocular findings will not be visually significant.

L. B. Nelson, MD, MBA

8 Neuro-ophthalmology

VZV ischemic optic neuropathy and subclinical temporal artery infection without rash
Nagel MA, Russman AN, Feit H, et al (Univ of Colorado School of Medicine, Aurora; Henry Ford Hosp, Detroit, MI; et al)
Neurology 80:220-222, 2013

Background.—Clinicians have speculated that varicella zoster virus (VZV) may be a cause of giant cell arteritis (GCA). VZV reactivates most in elderly persons, which is the same patient group in whom GCA is found predominantly. A case report detailed a patient who developed symptoms consistent with GCA and VZV infection.

Case Report.—Woman, 75, developed periorbital pain and blurred vision of her left eye. Her visual acuity (VA) was 20/40 in her right eye and 20/400 in her left eye with mild left relative afferent pupillary defect (APD). Other signs and symptoms included swollen, hyperemic left optic nerve with peripapillary flame hemorrhages. She was given intravenous methylprednisolone 250 mg every 6 hours, and her headache and vision improved 3 days later. On the fourth day of treatment a left temporal artery biopsy uncovered thickened intima and intact internal elastic lamina, but no medial necrosis, which is characteristic of GCA. Based on tests of the temporal artery, the steroid treatment was changed to oral prednisone 60 mg daily. A brain magnetic resonance imaging (MRI) scan was normal, but 2 days later the patient had increased pain and vision problems. Orbital computed tomography (CT) and head CT angiography were negative. On the seventeenth day, the patient's left eye became blind and lacked direct pupillary light reaction. The fundus was obscured by vitreous hemorrhage. The asymptomatic temporal artery biopsy was negative for GCA, so VZV ischemic optic neuropathy (ION) was diagnosed. Treatment with intravenous acyclovir 10 mg/kg every 8 hours was prescribed for 7 days. Thirty-one days after her initial appearance for treatment, the patient's cerebrospinal fluid contained anti-VZV IgG but not anti-herpes simplex virus IgG antibody. Immunohistochemical and pathologic analysis revealed VZV antigen and neutrophils in the original left temporal artery specimen. The patient was given oral valacyclovir 1 gram three times a day for 6 weeks, with her prednisone dose reduced to 20 mg daily and tapered 5 mg each week. Her pain resolved over the next 6 weeks, and VA improved to finger accounting. The left optic nerve was no longer hemorrhagic.

Conclusions.—This case expands the spectrum of disease that may be produced by VZV without rash to ION, documents ipsilateral GCA-negative temporal artery VZV infection that can guide diagnosis, and confirmed early VZV infection of the adventitia in VZV vasculopathy. It shows that extracranial arteries can be infected transaxonally after VZV reactivation. The headache, vision loss, and elevated erythrocyte sedimentation rate (ESR) found in both VZV and GCA can complicate diagnosis.

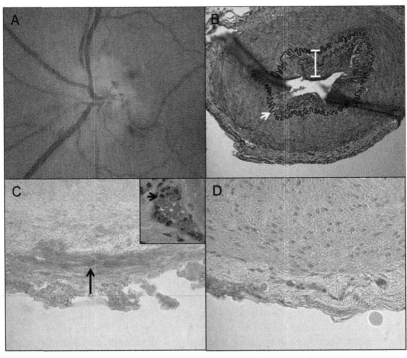

FIGURE.—Fundus examination, histology, and immunohistochemistry on temporal artery biopsy of varicellazoster virus ischemic optic neuropathy. (A) Fundus photograph of the left eye reveals a swollen elevated optic disc with blurred margins and peripapillary flame hemorrhages. (B) Histologic and immunohistochemical analysis of the left temporal artery biopsy obtained 4 days after the patient's onset of loss of vision. Modified Movat pentachrome stain of a formalin-fixed paraffin-embedded section of the temporal artery demonstrates a thickened intima (white bar) and nearly intact internal elastic lamina (white arrow). Original magnification 3200. Note the presence of varicella-zoster virus (VZV) antigen in the adventitia of the temporal artery stained with anti-VZV antibody (C, black arrow, pink, ×600 magnification), but not with normal rabbit serum (D), and an abundance of neutrophils in the adventitia around the vaso vasorum vessels (C, inset, black arrow, hematoxylin & eosin, ×600 magnification). For interpretation of the references to color in this figure legend, the reader is referred to web version of this article. (Reprinted from Nagel MA, Russman AN, Feit H, et al. VZV ischemic optic neuropathy and subclinical temporal artery infection without rash. *Neurology.* 2013;80:220-222, with permission from American Academy of Neurology.)

Giving long-term steroid therapy based on a possible diagnosis of GCA can aggravate VZV, making it especially important to obtain an accurate diagnosis. Virologic confirmation requires either the detection of VZV DNA or anti-VZV antibody in the CSF or the identification of VZV antigen in a temporal artery biopsy. Because VZV can be found in GCA-negative temporal artery samples in ION, even in the absence of a rash, it is wise to examine temporal artery biopsies for VZV antigen, especially because antiviral therapy is effective against VZV infections (Fig).

▶ This is a fascinating case report illustrating how varicella zoster infection can mimic giant cell arteritis (GCA). In cases of anterior ischemic optic neuropathy (ION) in elderly patients, in which the clinical presentation suggests GCA but the temporal artery biopsy is negative, this entity should be considered. As the authors state in the last sentence of their article, clinicians should consider the following: "Finally, because VZV [varicella zoster virus] can be found in GCA-negative temporal artery in ION, even without rash, it would be prudent to examine GCA-negative temporal artery biopsies for VZV antigen, particularly since VZV infections respond to antiviral therapy."

R. C. Sergott, MD

VZV multifocal vasculopathy with ischemic optic neuropathy, acute retinal necrosis and temporal artery infection in the absence of zoster rash
Mathias M, Nagel MA, Khmeleva N, et al (Univ of Colorado School of Medicine, Aurora)
J Neurol Sci 325:180-182, 2013

We describe a 54-year-old diabetic woman who developed ischemic optic neuropathy followed by acute retinal necrosis and multiple areas of focal venous beading. Vitreous fluid contained amplifiable VZV DNA but not HSV-1, CMV or toxoplasma DNA. The clinical presentation was remarkable for jaw claudication and intermittent scalp pain, prompting a temporal artery biopsy that was pathologically negative for giant cell arteritis, but notable for VZV antigen. The current case adds to the clinical spectrum of multifocal VZV vasculopathy. The development of acute VZV retinal necrosis after ischemic optic neuropathy supports the notion that vasculitis is an important additional mechanism in the development of VZV retinal injury (Figs 1-3).

▶ This is another important case about the sequelae of varicella zoster infection mimicking giant cell arteritis; however, the patient progressed to the devastating complication of acute retinal necrosis syndrome rather than ischemic optic neuropathy. Varicella zoster virus antigen was found in the temporal artery as with the previous case report. As a new general clinical rule, clinicians need to be aware of the wide spectrum of findings possible with varicella zoster infection

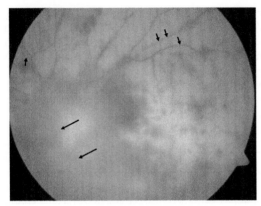

FIGURE 1.—Fundus photo of the left eye demonstrates extensive retinal necrosis with intraretinal hemorrhage, overlying vitreitis (long arrows) and focal beading in multiple retinal veins (short arrows). (Reprinted from Journal of the Neurological Sciences. Mathias M, Nagel MA, Khmeleva N, et al. VZV multifocal vasculopathy with ischemic optic neuropathy, acute retinal necrosis and temporal artery infection in the absence of zoster rash. *J Neurol Sci.* 2013;325:180-182, Copyright 2013, with permission from Elsevier.)

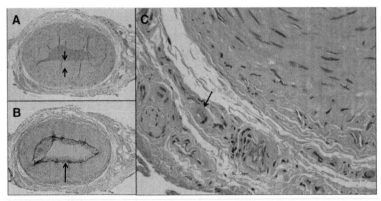

FIGURE 2.—Cross-sections of the temporal artery showed mild intimal thickening (short arrows) and an intact internal elastic lamina (long arrow) (A, H&E; B, Van Gieson stain, respectively; magnification 100×). Hyalinization of vasa vasorum arterioles was noted (C, long arrows), consistent with diabetic vasculopathy. No evidence of inflammation was noted, particularly in the adventitial connective tissue or in association with vasa vasorum or vasa nervosum structures (H&E,magnification 400×). CD45 immunohistochemistry, as previously described, confirmed the absence of an inflammatory cell infiltrate (not shown). (Reprinted from Journal of the Neurological Sciences. Mathias M, Nagel MA, Khmeleva N, et al. VZV multifocal vasculopathy with ischemic optic neuropathy, acute retinal necrosis and temporal artery infection in the absence of zoster rash. *J Neurol Sci.* 2013;325:180-182, Copyright 2013, with permission from Elsevier.)

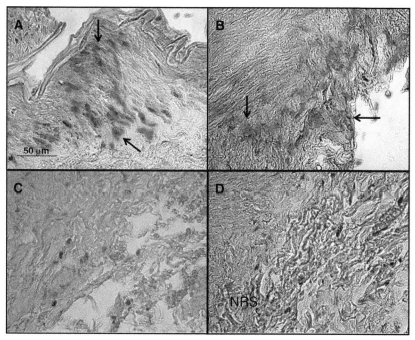

FIGURE 3.—The left temporal artery in a patient with multifocal vasculopathy was analyzed for the presence varicella zoster virus (VZV) antigen as previously described. A positive control cadaveric cerebral artery 14 days after VZV infection in vitro (A, pink color, arrows). VZV antigen was seen in the adventitia of the left temporal artery of the subject after staining with anti-VZV antibody (B, pink color, arrows), but not after staining adjacent sections with anti-HSV antibody (C) or normal rabbit serum (D). Magnification 200×. For interpretation of the references to color in this figure legend, the reader is referred to web version of this article. (Reprinted from Journal of the Neurological Sciences. Mathias M, Nagel MA, Khmeleva N, et al. VZV multifocal vasculopathy with ischemic optic neuropathy, acute retinal necrosis and temporal artery infection in the absence of zoster rash. *J Neurol Sci.* 2013;325:180-182, Copyright 2013, with permission from Elsevier.)

and search for this entity when the patient presentation suggests giant cell arteritis but the temporal artery biopsy is negative.

R. C. Sergott, MD

Downbeat nystagmus associated with damage to the medial longitudinal fasciculus of the pons: A vestibular balance control mechanism via the lower brainstem paramedian tract neurons
Nakamagoe K, Fujizuka N, Koganezawa T, et al (Univ of Tsukuba, Ibaraki, Japan)
J Neurol Sci 328:98-101, 2013

The paramedian tract (PMT) neurons, a group of neurons associated with eye movement that project into the cerebellar flocculus, are present in or near the medial longitudinal fasciculus (MLF) in the paramedian region of the lower brainstem. A 66-year-old man with multiple sclerosis in whom

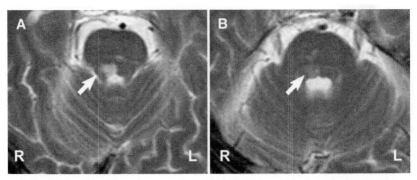

FIGURE 1.—Cranial MRI images. Axial T2-weighted images from the abducens nucleus of the ponto-medullary sulcus to the rostral pons. A shows the pons at the level of the superior cerebellar peduncle. B shows the pons at the level of the inferior cerebellar peduncle. A high-intensity plaque lesion is evident in the right paramedian region adjacent to the fourth ventricle of the pontine tegmentum. This lesion includes the MLF. R: right, L: left. (Reprinted from Journal of the Neurological Sciences. Nakamagoe K, Fujizuka N, Koganezawa T, et al. Downbeat nystagmus associated with damage to the medial longitudinal fasciculus of the pons: a vestibular balance control mechanism via the lower brainstem paramedian tract neurons. *J Neurol Sci.* 2013;328:98-101, Copyright 2013, with permission from Elsevier.)

downbeat nystagmus appeared along with right MLF syndrome due to a unilateral pontomedullary lesion is described. In light of these findings, a possible schema for the vestibular balance control mechanism circuit of the PMT neurons via the flocculus is presented. Damage to the PMT neurons impaired the elective inhibitory control mechanism of the anterior semicircular canal neural pathway by the flocculus. This resulted in the appearance of anterior semicircular canal-dominant vestibular imbalance and the formation of downbeat nystagmus.

From the pathogenesis of this vertical vestibular nystagmus, the action of the PMT neurons in the vestibular eye movement neuronal pathway to maintain vestibular balance was conjectured to be as follows. PMT neurons transmit vestibular information from the anterior semicircular canals to the cerebellum, forming a cerebellum/brainstem feedback loop. Vestibular information from that loop is integrated in the cerebellum, inhibiting only the anterior semicircular canal neuronal pathway via the flocculus and controlling vestibular balance (Fig 1).

▶ No topic engenders more discomfort in ophthalmologists than nystagmus. Although downbeat nystagmus has traditionally been localized to the cervico-medullary junction, this well-documented case report clearly defines another location for this process—the pontine medial longitudinal fasciculus in association with lower brainstem neurons. The magnetic resonance image (Fig 1) is exquisitely localizing. The authors' anatomic diagram is quite comprehensive and helps explain the clinical findings. In the future, when evaluating a patient with downbeat nystagmus, clinicians will need to image both the cervico-medullary junction and the pons.

R. C. Sergott, MD

Adult Horner's syndrome: A combined clinical, pharmacological, and imaging algorithm

Davagnanam I, Fraser CL, Miszkiel K, et al (Moorfields Eye Hosp, London, UK)
Eye 27:291-298, 2013

The diagnosis of Horner's syndrome (HS) can be difficult, as patients rarely present with the classic triad of ptosis, miosis, and anhydrosis. Frequently, there are no associated symptoms to help determine or localise the underlying pathology. The onset of anisocoria may also be uncertain, with many cases referred after incidental discovery on routine optometric assessment. Although the textbooks discuss the use of cocaine, apracloni-dine, and hydroxyamphetamine to diagnose and localise HS, in addition to reported false positive and negative results, these pharmacological agents are rarely available during acute assessment or in general ophthalmic departments. Typically, a week is required between using cocaine or apraclonidine for diagnosis and localisation of HS with hydroxyamphetamine, leaving the clinician with the decision of which investigations to request and with what urgency. Modern imaging modalities have advanced significantly and become more readily available since many of the established management algorithms were written. We thus propose a practical and safe combined

TABLE 1.—Anatomical Pathway, Pathological Processes, and Localising Clinical Features

Neuronal Order	Location	Pathology	Associated Clinical Signs
First order (central)	Posterior hypothalamus Brainstem	Pituitary tumour Stroke—Wallenberg syndrome, pontine haemorrhage Demyelination	Vertigo Altered facial sensation Contralateral CN IV palsy Crossed motor/sensory signs
	C-spine Intermediolateral grey substance C8-T2	Arnold-chiari Cervical spondylosis Syringomyelia Neck trauma	Radicular signs
Second order (intermediate)	C8–T2 ventral nerve roots Apex of the lung	Cervical rib Brachial plexus injury Tumours - Pancoast tumour - mesothelioma	Neck/arm pain and weakness Signs of lung disease
	Mediastinum	Cardiothoracic procedure Aortic aneurysm or dissection	
	Cervical sympathetic chain	Subclavian artery aneurysm Thyroid tumour Post neck dissection	Vocal cord paralysis Anhydrosis of face and neck
Third order (post ganglionic)	Superior cervical ganglion at C2-3 Carotid artery	Jugular venous ectasia Carotid - Dissection - aneurysm - arteritis	Facial pain Stroke Ocular ischaemia
	Cavernous sinus Orbit	Base of skull tumours Inflammatory mass Herpes zoster	Abducens palsy

clinical and radiological diagnostic protocol for HS that can be applied in most clinical settings (Table 1).

▶ Patients with Horner syndrome with either an acute or insidious presentation will often present to comprehensive ophthalmologists. Clinicians must be adept at establishing the diagnosis as well as having a systematic approach to defining the cause. This article provides a valuable framework for both approaching the diagnosis and the etiology. The tables (Table 1) and the figures in the original article are excellent examples.

R. C. Sergott, MD

Optic Neuropathy after Vitrectomy for Retinal Detachment: Clinical Features and Analysis of Risk Factors
Bansal AS, Hsu J, Garg SJ, et al (Thomas Jefferson Univ, Philadelphia, PA)
Ophthalmology 119:2364-2370, 2012

Purpose.—To describe the clinical characteristics of and risk factors for the development of optic neuropathy after pars plana vitrectomy (PPV) for macula-sparing primary rhegmatogenous retinal detachment (RRD) repair.

Design.—Retrospective case-control study.

Participants.—Seven patients who underwent PPV for macula-sparing primary RRD with subsequent development of optic neuropathy and 42 age- and gender-matched control patients undergoing PPV for macula-sparing primary RRD.

Methods.—Retrospective chart review of medical and surgical records.

Main Outcome Measures.—Clinical features of patients who developed optic neuropathy after PPV for macula-sparing RRD and analysis of potential risk factors (age, gender, medical history, surgical technique, intraoperative ocular perfusion pressure [OPP], and operative time).

Results.—At last follow-up, all 7 patients with optic neuropathy had visual acuity less than 20/200, relative afferent pupillary defects, optic nerve pallor, and visual field defects. A total of 5 of 7 patients (71%) demonstrated intraoperative reduced OPP with associated systemic hypotension compared with 7 of 42 patients (17%) in the control cohort ($P = 0.01$).

Conclusions.—Optic neuropathy after PPV for macula-sparing primary RRD is a rare but potentially devastating complication. Although the cause is often unclear, reduced ocular perfusion due to intraoperative systemic hypotension may be a contributing risk factor in some eyes.

▶ Postoperative optic neuropathy with significant visual loss after either ophthalmic or nonophthalmic surgery is one of the most devastating developments following otherwise successful surgery. Although limited by the usual caveats of a retrospective study, this analysis suggests the possibility of intraoperative systemic hypotension as a contributing risk factor.

R. C. Sergott, MD

Optic Disk Pit Morphology and Retinal Detachment: Optical Coherence Tomography with Intraoperative Correlation

Gregory-Roberts EM, Mateo C, Corcòstegui B, et al (Columbia Univ Med Ctr, NY; Instituto de Microcirugia Ocular de Barcelona, Spain; et al)
Retina 33:363-370, 2013

Background.—The pathogenesis of optic nerve head pits and associated retinal detachment, and the most effective surgical intervention when visual loss develops, remains unclear.

Methods.—The morphology of the optic disk in patients with pits was investigated with optical coherence tomography. For those who underwent surgical treatment for pit-associated retinal detachment, the efficacy of treatment by vitrectomy and separation of the posterior hyaloid, with and without additional peeling of peripapillary tissue, was assessed.

Results.—On optical coherence tomography imaging, 14 of 18 pits (78%) demonstrated a localized pit-like invagination, whereas 3 (17%) had disks with a generally excavated structure. For 16 of 18 pits (89%), there was evidence of condensed vitreous or glial tissue seen extending from the pit or inside the optic disk. Nine eyes with retinal detachment underwent vitrectomy, posterior hyaloid separation, and endolaser. The retinal detachment completely resolved in 6 of 6 cases where the surgeon additionally peeled the fibrous tissue from the pit and 2 of 3 cases where this was not performed.

Conclusion.—Spectral domain optical coherence tomography demonstrates the varying morphology of optic pit anatomy. Condensed vitreous strands or glial tissue in the optic nerve pit may also contribute to retinal detachment development.

▶ Once again, high-resolution spectral domain optical coherence tomography shows the beautiful pathologic anatomy of this rare condition. However, from these cases, we learn how the optic nerve and macular area may interact. The unexpected finding was the discovery of vitreous strands/glial tissue in the optic nerve area, raising the possibility of a component of vitreous peripapillary/optic disc traction in the pathogenesis of this disorder. If traction does exist, then clinicians need to consider lysis of the vitreous traction enzymatically with ocriplasmin before proceeding with vitrectomy.

R. C. Sergott, MD

Ability and Reproducibility of Fourier-Domain Optical Coherence Tomography to Detect Retinal Nerve Fiber Layer Atrophy in Parkinson's Disease

Garcia-Martin E, Satue M, Fuertes I, et al (Miguel Servet Univ Hosp, Zaragoza, Spain)
Ophthalmology 119:2161-2167, 2012

Purpose.—To evaluate and compare the ability of 3 protocols of Fourier-domain optical coherence tomography (OCT) to detect retinal thinning and retinal nerve fiber layer (RNFL) atrophy in patients with Parkinson's disease (PD) compared with healthy subjects. To test the intrasession reproducibility of RNFL thickness measurements in patients with PD and healthy subjects using the Cirrus (Carl Zeiss Meditec Inc., Dublin, CA) and Spectralis (Heidelberg Engineering, Inc., Heidelberg, Germany) OCT devices.

Design.—Observational, cross-sectional study.

Participants.—Patients with PD (n = 75) and age-matched healthy subjects (n = 75) were enrolled.

Methods.—All subjects underwent three 360-degree circular scans centered on the optic disc by the same experienced examiner using the Cirrus OCT instrument, the classic glaucoma application, and the new Nsite Axonal Analytics of the Spectralis OCT instrument.

Main Outcome Measures.—Differences between the eyes of healthy subjects and the eyes of patients with PD were compared using the 3 protocols. The relationship between measurements provided by each OCT protocol was evaluated. Repeatability was studied by intraclass correlation coefficients and coefficients of variation.

Results.—Retinal nerve fiber layer atrophy was detected in eyes of patients with PD ($P = 0.025$, $P = 0.042$, and $P < 0.001$) with the 3 protocols used, but the Nsite Axonal Analytics of the Spectralis OCT device was the most sensitive for detecting subclinical defects. In eyes of patients with PD, RNFL thickness measurements determined by the OCT devices were correlated, but they were significantly different between the Cirrus and Spectralis devices ($P = 0.038$). Reproducibility was good with all 3 protocols but better using the Glaucoma application of the Spectralis OCT device.

Conclusions.—Fourier-domain OCT can be considered a valid and reproducible device for detecting subclinical RNFL atrophy in patients with PD, especially the Nsite Axonal Analytics of the Spectralis device. Retinal nerve fiber layer thickness measurements differed significantly between the Cirrus and Spectralis devices despite a high correlation of the measurements between the 2 instruments.

▶ New measurements of retinal and optic nerve structure and function promise to unlock secrets of primary ophthalmic diseases but also of neurodegenerative diseases. This study provides excellent data about retinal nerve fiber layer changes in Parkinson disease. Ophthalmologists must be aware of these changes in Parkinson disease and not overdiagnose glaucoma in these patients.

As segmentation of the outer and midretinal layers becomes standardized, we anticipate seeing changes in these cellular locations in neurodegenerative syndromes. More anatomically localized physiologic measurements, such as multifocal electroretinography and multifocal visually evoked potentials, will also have great value in diagnosing and following up with patients who have neurodegenerative diseases.

In the future, the applications of OCT for neurodegenerative disease may surpass those for ophthalmology.

R. C. Sergott, MD

Sex-specific differences in retinal nerve fiber layer thinning after acute optic neuritis

Costello F, Hodge W, Pan YI, et al (Univ of Calgary, Ontario, Canada; Univ of Western Ontario, London, Canada; et al)
Neurology 79:1866-1872, 2012

Objective.—The primary objective of this study was to explore the potential influence of gender on recovery from optic neuritis (ON) by determining whether differences in retinal nerve fiber layer (RNFL) thickness can be detected between men and women 6 months after an ON event.

Methods.—In this prospective cohort study, 39 men and 105 women with acute ON underwent repeat visual and optical coherence tomography (OCT) testing. The main outcome measures were change in RNFL measurements for male and female patients 6 months after ON.

Results.—Men were older (mean age = 39 years) than women (35 years) ($p = 0.05$) in this study, and more men (62%) than women (41%) had a diagnosis of relapsing-remitting multiple sclerosis (MS) ($p = 0.02$). Because age and MS subtype were 2 significant covariates, both variables were controlled for in multiple regression analyses. Other covariates controlled for in the multivariate regression included disease duration (years), use of disease-modifying therapy (yes/no), and use of high-dose corticosteroids for acute ON (yes/no). After 6 months, mean RNFL values were lower in men (74 μm) than women (91 μm) ($p < 0.001$). Men showed more apparent change in RNFL thickness in their ON eyes from baseline to 6 months after ON than women ($p = 0.003$).

Conclusions.—There may be differences in recovery between men and women after ON, which can be difficult to detect with conventional visual testing. Our findings raise interesting questions about the potential influence of gender in MS, which may be explored in future studies.

▶ This study reports an interesting observation about the potential for a gender-related difference in the susceptibility of the retinal nerve fiber layer to injury after optic neuritis. The authors controlled for differences in the study populations with age and the diagnosis of remitting relapsing multiple sclerosis. However, issues arise about using time domain optical coherence tomography (OCT) to draw significant conclusions. Despite experienced technicians, these measurements can be quite variable, especially for serial, longitudinal analysis. These observations will need to be validated with spectral domain OCT using devices with the lowest coefficient of variability for serial measurements.

R. C. Sergott, MD

Peripheral Nonperfusion and Tractional Retinal Detachment Associated with Congenital Optic Nerve Anomalies

Shapiro MJ, Chow CC, Blair MP, et al (Univ of Illinois at Chicago; et al)
Ophthalmology 120:607-615, 2013

Purpose.—To report an association of congenital optic nerve anomalies with peripheral retina nonperfusion and to describe the clinical manifestations and treatment.

Design.—Retrospective, observational case series.

Participants.—Fifteen patients with congenital optic nerve anomalies referred for pediatric retina consultation were studied. Sixteen eyes of 9 patients with optic nerve hypoplasia and 8 eyes of 6 patients with other congenital optic nerve anomalies, including optic nerve coloboma, morning glory disc, and peripapillary staphyloma, were included.

Methods.—All patients underwent examinations under anesthesia. Wide-angle retina photographs and fluorescein angiograms were reviewed. The severity of nonperfusion was graded. The presence of fibrovascular proliferation (FP), vitreous hemorrhage (VH), and tractional retinal detachment (TRD) were documented. Anatomic outcome after treatment was recorded.

Main Outcome Measures.—Severity of nonperfusion, occurrence of secondary complications, and the anatomic outcome of patients who underwent laser treatment.

Results.—In patients with optic nerve hypoplasia, 12 of 16 eyes (75%) had severe peripheral nonperfusion, 12 of 16 eyes (75%) had FP, 3 of 16 eyes (19%) had VH, and 10 of 16 eyes (63%) had TRD. Six of these eyes with severe nonperfusion received laser photocoagulation to the nonperfused retina; laser-treated retinas remained attached in all 6 eyes. In patients with the other optic nerve anomalies, 7 of 8 eyes (88%) had mild to moderate nonperfusion, 2 of 8 eyes (25%) had FP, 1 of 8 eyes (12%) had VH, and 2 of 8 eyes (25%) had TRD. Six of 9 patients (67%) with optic nerve hypoplasia and 1 of 6 patients (17%) with other anomalies had a coexisting congenital brain disease.

Conclusions.—Congenital optic nerve anomalies may be associated with peripheral retina nonperfusion and the secondary complications of FP, VH, and TRD. In this select group of patients, the nonperfusion associated with optic nerve hypoplasia seemed to be more severe and associated more frequently with secondary complications. Peripheral retina examination in eyes with optic nerve anomalies may identify nonperfusion or FP. Laser treatment of the avascular retina may have helped prevent complications from proliferative retinopathy in eyes clinically observed to have progressed or considered at risk for progression to proliferative retinopathy.

▶ A very surprising association was discovered by the authors—congenital optic nerve abnormalities and peripheral retinal nonperfusion. Relative optic nerve hypoplasia is not an uncommon disorder, so this report has importance for all ophthalmologists. The other associated optic nerve abnormalities—of optic nerve coloboma, morning glory syndrome, and peripapillary staphyloma—are much less common. Therefore, optic nerve abnormalities are no longer a simple fundoscopic curiosity but maybe the harbinger of serious peripheral retinal fibrovascular proliferation that can lead to vitreous hemorrhage and tractional retinal detachment. The pathophysiology of this association remains unknown.

R. C. Sergott, MD

Intravitreal bevacizumab for the treatment of nonarteritic anterior ischemic optic neuropathy: A prospective trial
Rootman DB, Gill HS, Margolin EA (Univ of Toronto, Ontario, Canada)
Eye 27:538-544, 2013

Purpose. There is currently no accepted treatment for Nonarteritic Anterior Ischemic Optic Neuropathy (NAION). One new therapeutic approach involves decreasing optic nerve edema with intravitreal bevacizumab in order to resolve a proposed compartment syndrome.

Methods.—In this non-randomized controlled clinical trial, 1.25 mg intravitreal bevacizumab was compared with natural history. Patients were examined at baseline, 1, 3, and 6 months with a full neuro-ophthalmic exam, automated perimetry, and optic nerve optical coherence tomography (OCT) measurements. The primary outcome measure was change in mean deviation on Humphrey visual field testing. Secondary outcome measures were change in visual acuity and optic nerve OCT thickness. Incidence and type of complications were also recorded.

Results.—Twenty-five patients were enrolled (17 treatment and 8 control). There was no significant effect of treatment on the primary outcome measure of mean deviation score ($P = 0.4$). There was similarly no effect of group assignment on the secondary outcome measures of change in mean Early Treatment Diabetic Retinopathy Study letters ($P = 0.33$) or nerve fiber layer thickness on OCT ($P = 0.11$). In the bevacizumab group, there was one case of a corneal abrasion and two cases of recurrent NAION. No other complications were noted.

Conclusions.—We found no difference between bevacizumab and natural history for change in visual field, visual acuity, or optic nerve OCT thickness. Based on the current evidence we would not recommend the use of intravitreal bevacizumab to treat patients with the new onset of NAION.

▶ This study reports yet another unsuccessful treatment for nonarteritic ischemic optic neuropathy, the most common optic nerve condition without any therapeutic options. The authors found no treatment effect not only for functional metrics such as visual field and visual acuity but also for structural change with optical coherence tomography. Currently, the only option available for clinicians is to indicate to the patient that no treatment is available for the acutely involved eye and that all efforts need to be directed to reducing vasculopathic risk factors in the hopes of reducing the chances of second eye involvement.

R. C. Sergott, MD

Postoperative increase in grey matter volume in visual cortex after unilateral cataract surgery

Lou AR, Madsen KH, Julian HO, et al (Glostrup Hosp, Copenhagen, Denmark; Copenhagen Univ Hosp Hvidovre, Denmark; et al)
Acta Ophthalmol 91:58-65, 2013

Purpose.—The developing visual cortex has a strong potential to undergo plastic changes. Little is known about the potential of the ageing visual cortex to express plasticity. A pertinent question is whether therapeutic interventions can trigger plastic changes in the ageing visual cortex by restoring vision.

Methods.—Twelve patients aged 50–85 years underwent structural high-resolution T1-weighted MRI of the whole brain 2 days and 6 weeks after unilateral cataract surgery. Voxel-based morphometry (VBM) based on T1-weighted magnetic resonance imaging (MRI) was employed to test whether cataract surgery induces a regional increase in grey matter in areas V1 and V2 of the visual cortex.

Results.—In all patients, cataract surgery immediately improved visual acuity, contrast sensitivity and mean sensitivity in the visual field of the operated eye. The improvement in vision was stable throughout the 6 weeks after operation. VBM revealed a regional expansion of grey matter volume in area V2 contralateral to the operated eye during the 6-week period after surgery. Individual increases in grey matter were predicted by the symmetry in visual acuity between the operated eye and nonoperated eye. The more symmetrical visual acuity became after unilateral cataract surgery, the more pronounced was the grey matter increase in visual cortex.

Conclusion.—The data suggest that cataract surgery triggered a use-dependent structural plasticity in V2 presumably through improved

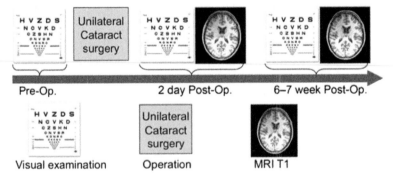

FIGURE 1.—Timeline of the experimental procedures. In the week before unilateral cataract surgery, patients with senile cataract underwent a standardized visual examination of both eyes. The examination schedule comprised biomicroscopy examination, assessment of visual acuity using the ETDRS chart, assessment of contrast sensitivity using the Pelli-Robson chart, and autoperimetry of the visual field. The same examination was repeated two times postoperatively, at day 2 and 6–7 week after surgery. The postoperative visual examination program was followed by an MRI scan. The MRI protocol consisted of a high-resolution structural T1 image of the whole brain. (Reprinted from Lou AR, Madsen KH, Julian HO, et al. Postoperative increase in grey matter volume in visual cortex after unilateral cataract surgery. *Acta Ophthalmol.* 2013;91:58-65, Copyright 2013, Acta Ophthalmologica Scandinavica Foundation.)

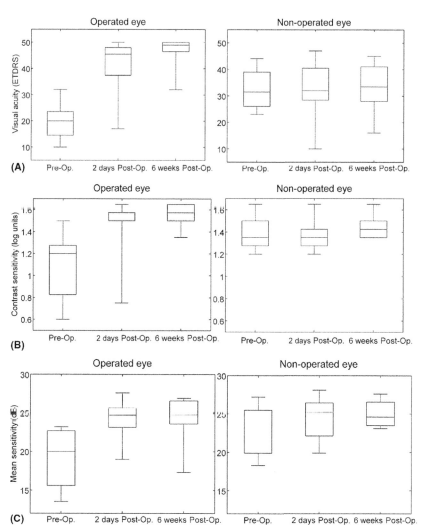

FIGURE 2.—Changes in vision after unilateral cataract surgery. The group data are presented as whisker plots. Each plot gives the results of the preoperative and the two postoperative measurements of visual acuity (**A**), contrast sensitivity (**B**) and mean sensitivity in the visual field (**C**). The red line indicates the group median. The upper and lower blue lines represent the 75 and 25 percentile, respectively. The black lines give the whole range. Visual acuity, contrast sensitivity and mean sensitivity in the visual field was increased in the operated eye 2 days after surgery, whereas there was no significant change in the postoperative period between day 2 and week 6. There was no consistent change in vision in the non-operated eye. For interpretation of the references to color in this figure legend, the reader is referred to web version of this article. (Reprinted from Lou AR, Madsen KH, Julian HO, et al. Postoperative increase in grey matter volume in visual cortex after unilateral cataract surgery. *Acta Ophthalmol.* 2013;91:58-65, Copyright 2013, Acta Ophthalmologica Scandinavica Foundation.)

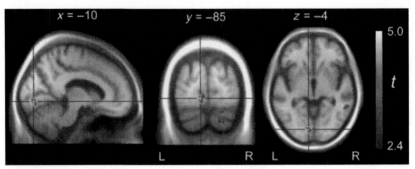

FIGURE 3.—Structural grey matter change in the visual cortex after cataract surgery. The statistical parametric map indicates relative increases in regional grey matter volume during the postoperative observation period (i.e., from day 2 to week 6–7 after s surgery). The operated side corresponds to the right. The red cross indicates the voxel at stereotactic coordinate $x, y, z = -11, -85, -6$ where VBM analysis identified peak increase in grey matter volume in the V2 contralateral to the operated eye. The coloured bar indicates the scaling of the T-score map. For interpretation of the references to color in this figure legend, the reader is referred to web version of this article. (Reprinted from Lou AR, Madsen KH, Julian HO, et al. Postoperative increase in grey matter volume in visual cortex after unilateral cataract surgery. *Acta Ophthalmol.* 2013;91:58-65, Copyright 2013, Acta Ophthalmologica Scandinavica Foundation.)

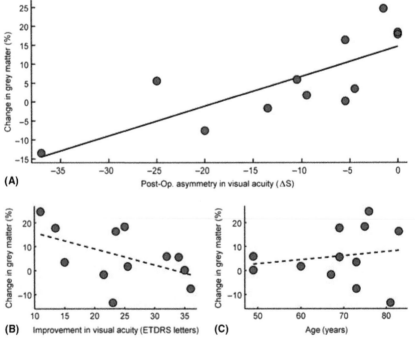

FIGURE 4.—Factors determining post-operative change in grey matter in V2. Three scatter plots showing the linear relationship between the change of regional grey matter in V2 with (**A**) the post-operative symmetry in visual acuity (**B**) the improvement in visual acuity (measured by the improvement in visual acuity between the pre-operative examination and the mean of the two post-operative examinations), and age of the patients (**C**). Only the post-operative improvement in symmetry in visual acuity of the operated and non-operated eye showed a statistical significant relationship ($p = 0.00288$) to change in grey matter volume in V2 (positive linear relationship, V2 ($R2 = 0.6055$). (Reprinted from Lou AR, Madsen KH, Julian HO, et al. Postoperative increase in grey matter volume in visual cortex after unilateral cataract surgery. *Acta Ophthalmol.* 2013;91:58-65, Copyright 2013, Acta Ophthalmologica Scandinavica Foundation.)

binocular integration of visual input from both eyes. We conclude that activity-dependent cortical plasticity is preserved in the ageing visual cortex and may be triggered by restoring impaired vision (Figs 1-4).

▶ This is an absolutely fascinating study using advanced regional brain volume measurements showing the effect of unilateral cataract surgery on the occipital cortex. Who would have ever dreamed that the aging brain was capable of undergoing structural improvement after anterior segment surgery. The more symmetric the visual acuity became between the operated and unoperated eye, the more striking was the gray matter increase. This well-done, innovative study has major implications for all forms of visual loss, not only in elderly patients with cataracts but also in all age groups with any type of visual loss. Because the occipital lobe is not an isolated region of brain but has many connections to other areas, one has to wonder if those other connected areas demonstrate similar changes.

R. C. Sergott, MD

Optic Neuropathy in McCune-Albright Syndrome: Effects of Early Diagnosis and Treatment of Growth Hormone Excess

Boyce AM, Glover M, Kelly MH, et al (Natl Insts of Health (NIH), Bethesda, MD; et al)
J Clin Endocrinol Metab 98:E126-E134, 2013

Context.—Growth Harmone Excess (GH excess) is a serious complication of McCune-Albright syndrome (MAS) and has been associated with craniofacial morbidity.

Objective.—The aim of the study was to determine whether early diagnosis and treatment of MAS-associated GH excess prevents optic neuropathy and hearing impairment, the major morbidities associated with GH excess.

Design and Setting.—A retrospective cross-sectional analysis was conducted at a clinical research center.

Patients.—Twenty-two subjects with MAS-associated GH excess and 21 control MAS subjects without GH excess were included in the study.

Intervention.—Biochemical testing included random GH, nadir GH after glucose load, nadir GH on frequent sampling, and IGF-I Z-score. Subjects underwent imaging, ophthalmological, audiological, and otolaryngological assessment. Treatment included octreotide, pegvisomant, transphenoidal surgery, and/or radiotherapy as indicated.

Main Outcome Measure.—Association of optic neuropathy and hearing impairment to age at GH excess diagnosis/treatment was measured.

Results.—Of 129 MAS subjects, 26 (20%) were diagnosed with GH excess based on elevation of two measures of GH function. Of these, 22 subjects were candidates for pharmacological intervention. Optic neuropathy was significantly correlated with intervention status, with no cases in the early intervention group (diagnosed/treated before age 18) or the control group, and four of seven (57%) in the late intervention group (diagnosed/treated after age 18) (Fisher's exact test; odds ratio, 0.027; $P = 0.0058$).

Early diagnosis/intervention was not associated with reduction in hearing deficits (odds ratio, 1.25; $P = 1.00$). Mean head circumference SD score was significantly higher in the late (6.08; range, 2.70 to 22.56) than the early intervention (2.67; range, -0.65 to 6.72) or control groups (2.13; range, -2.06 to 7.79) ($P = 0.003$).

Conclusions.—Early diagnosis/treatment of GH excess in MAS is important to prevent optic neuropathy and craniofacial expansion. The relationship between hearing deficits and GH excess remains less clear and requires further study.

▶ Although the McCune-Albright syndrome is a rare entity, this study is important for both comprehensive ophthalmologists and subspecialty neuro-ophthalmologists, because early diagnosis and treatment can prevent optic nerve dysfunction. The study clearly shows that early intervention was associated with better optic nerve function. Therapy directed against growth hormone excess before age 18 was associated with smaller head circumference and better optic nerve function.

R. C. Sergott, MD

Adult-Onset Opsoclonus-Myoclonus Syndrome
Klaas JP, Ahlskog JE, Pittock SJ, et al (Mayo Clinic College of Medicine, Rochester, MN; et al)
Arch Neurol 69:1598-1607, 2012

Background.—Little is known about adult-onset opsoclonus-myoclonus syndrome (OMS) outside of individual case reports.
Objective.—To describe adult-onset OMS.
Design.—Review of medical records (January 1, 1990, through December 31, 2011), prospective telephone surveillance, and literature review (January 1, 1967, through December 31, 2011).
Setting.—Department of Neurology, Mayo Clinic, Rochester, Minnesota.
Patients.—Twenty-one Mayo Clinic patients and 116 previously reported patients with adult-onset OMS.
Main Outcome Measures.—Clinical course and longitudinal outcomes.
Results.—The median age at onset of the 21 OMS patients at the Mayo Clinic was 47 years (range, 27-78 years); 11 were women. Symptoms reported at the first visit included dizziness, 14 patients; balance difficulties, 14; nausea and/or vomiting, 10; vision abnormalities, 6; tremor/tremulousness, 4; and altered speech, 2. Myoclonus distribution was extremities, 15 patients; craniocervical, 8; and trunk, 4. Cancer was detected in 3 patients (breast adenocarcinoma, 2; and small cell lung carcinoma, 1); a parainfectious cause was assumed in the remainder of the patients. Follow-up of 1 month or more was available for 19 patients (median, 43 months; range, 1-187 months). Treatment (median, 6 weeks) consisted of immunotherapy and symptomatic therapy in 16 patients, immunotherapy alone for 2, and clonazepam alone for 1. Of these 19 patients, OMS remitted in

13 and improved in 3; 3 patients died (neurologic decline, 1; cancer, 1; and myocardial infarction, 1). The cause of death was of paraneoplastic origin in 60 of 116 literature review patients, with the most common carcinomas being lung (33 patients) and breast (7); the most common antibody was anti-neuronal nuclear antibody type 2 (anti-Ri, 15). Other causes were idiopathic in origin, 38 patients; parainfectious, 15 (human immunodeficiency virus, 7); toxic/metabolic, 2; and other autoimmune, 1. Both patients with N-methyl-D-aspartate receptor antibody had encephalopathy. Improvements were attributed to immunotherapy alone in 22 of 28 treated patients.

Conclusions.—Adult-onset OMS is rare. Paraneoplastic and parainfectious causes (particularly human immunodeficiency virus) should be considered. Complete remission achieved with immunotherapy is the most common outcome.

▶ Although opsoclonus-myoclonus is a rare condition, these patients naturally always seek neurologic and ophthalmologic attention. This review provides the largest series of patients with this disorder with complete and clear clinical facts and treatment outcomes. The most common causes are paraneoplastic and parainfectious syndromes, especially human immunodeficiency virus.

R. C. Sergott, MD

Acquired bilateral myelinated retinal nerve fibers after unilateral optic nerve sheath fenestration in a child with idiopathic intracranial hypertension

Prakalapakorn SG, Buckley EG (Duke Eye Ctr, Durham, NC)
J AAPOS 16:534-538, 2012

Purpose.—To report the unusual development of bilateral myelinated retinal nerve fibers (MRNF) adjacent to the optic nerve in a child after treatment of idiopathic intracranial hypertension (IIH) with unilateral optic nerve sheath fenestration (ONSF) and to discuss the etiology of acquired MRNF.

Methods.—The patient's clinical history, including visual acuity, refractive error, ocular alignment, fundus examination, and optic nerve photographs, was retrospectively reviewed. A literature review was performed for acquired MRNF in children using PubMed. The results of the demographic and clinical findings of our patient were compared with those of previously reported cases.

Results.—The child developed bilateral MRNF adjacent to the optic nerve 5 months after unilateral ONSF. In reviewing the literature, 8 of 10 cases of acquired MRNF in children had previous abnormalities of the optic nerve, 4 of 10 had associated bilateral optic nerve head drusen, 3 of 10 had associated optic nerve glioma, and 3 of 10 had a history of significant increased intracranial pressure requiring surgical intervention.

Conclusions.—Although the etiology of acquired MRNF is uncertain, this case plus a review of the literature suggest that it may be related to

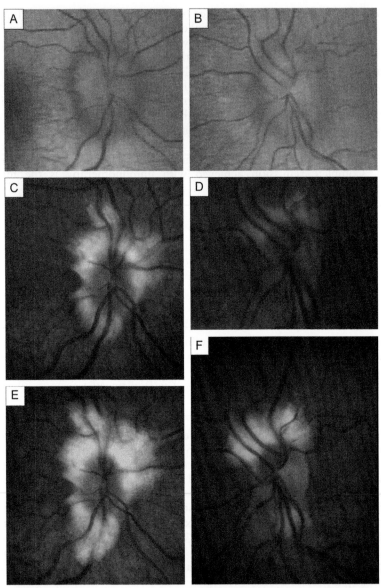

FIGURE.—Optic nerve photographs of the right eye (A, C, E) and left eye (B, D, F) of a 17-month-old girl showing bilateral disk edema at presentation (A-B) and the presence and expansion of myelinated retinal nerve fibers at 9 (C-D), and at 33 months (E-F) after optic nerve sheath fenestration in the right eye. (Reprinted from Journal of AAPOS. Prakalapakorn SG, Buckley EG. Acquired bilateral myelinated retinal nerve fibers after unilateral optic nerve sheath fenestration in a child with idiopathic intracranial hypertension. *J AAPOS*. 2012;16:534-538, Copyright 2012, with permission from American Association for Pediatric Ophthalmology and Strabismus.)

changes in the lamina cribosa combined with possible optic nerve injury caused by optic nerve head drusen, optic nerve glioma, or increased intracranial pressure and that it can occur months to years after intervention (Fig).

▶ The authors of this article present a fascinating case report of bilateral myelinated peripapillary retinal nerve fibers developing after unilateral optic nerve sheath fenestration (ONSF). The ONSF was performed for idiopathic intracranial hypertension. Similar cases of acquired myelinated retinal nerve fibers have been reported after the development of an optic neuropathy with optic disc drusen, optic nerve glioma, and increased intracranial pressure. The stimulation of myelination is a topic of critical importance to neurobiology. The observations in these cases clearly show that oligodendrocytes within the optic nerve can respond to various pathologic processes by producing myelin. If the stimulus for this response can be identified, then a pharmacologic means may be developed.

R. C. Sergott, MD

Axonal loss in non—optic neuritis eyes of patients with multiple sclerosis linked to delayed visual evoked potential
Klistorner A, Garrick R, Barnett MH, et al (Univ of Sydney, Australia; St Vincent Hosp, Sydney, Australia; Univ of Sydney, Australia; et al)
Neurology 80:242-245, 2013

Objective.—Recent studies demonstrate significant thinning of the retinal nerve fiber layer (RNFL) in multiple sclerosis (MS) non—optic neuritis (MS-NON) eyes. However, the pathologic basis of this reduction is not clear. The aim of the current study was to investigate the relationship of the RNFL thickness in MS-NON eyes with latency delay of the multifocal visual evoked potential (mfVEP), a surrogate marker of the visual pathway demyelination.

Methods.—Total and temporal RNFL thickness and latency of the mfVEP in 45 MS-NON eyes of 45 patients with relapsing-remitting MS and 25 eyes of age- and gender-matched controls were measured and analyzed.

Results.—There was significant reduction of total and temporal RNFL thickness ($p = 0.015$ and $p = 0.006$, respectively) and significant latency delay ($p < 0.0001$) in MS-NON eyes. Both total and temporal RNFL thickness were associated with latency of the mfVEP ($r^2 = 0.43$, $p < 0.0001$ and $r^2 = 0.36$, $p = 0.001$, respectively). MS-NON eyes with normal latency (n = 26) showed no significant reduction of RNFL thickness compared with controls ($p = 0.44$ and $p = 0.1$ for total and temporal RNFL, respectively), whereas eyes with delayed latency (n = 19) demonstrated significantly thinner RNFL ($p = 0.001$ and $p = 0.0005$). MS-NON eyes with delayed latency also had significantly thinner RNFL compared with those with normal latencies ($p = 0.013$ and $p = 0.02$). In patients with no previous optic neuritis in either eye, delayed latency and reduced RNFL were bilateral whenever present.

Conclusions.—The study demonstrated significant association between RNFL loss and a latency delay of the mfVEP in MS-NON eyes.

▶ The authors of this article have performed a potentially very important study, linking structural findings with spectral domain optical coherence tomography and multifocal visual evoked potential in patients with multiple sclerosis who have not had a clinical event of optic neuritis. The total and temporal quadrant retinal nerve fiber layer thickness correlated with the latency delay in both eyes. These observations may provide the basis for merging structural and functional metrics in clinical trials designed to investigate pharmaceutical compounds for neuroprotective properties.

R. C. Sergott, MD

A Novel Rodent Model of Posterior Ischemic Optic Neuropathy
Wang Y, Brown DP Jr, Duan Y, et al (Fudan Univ, Shanghai, China; Univ of Miami Miller School of Medicine, FL)
JAMA Ophthalmol 131:194-204, 2013

Objectives.—To develop a reliable, reproducible rat model of posterior ischemic optic neuropathy (PION) and study the cellular responses in the optic nerve and retina.

Methods.—Posterior ischemic optic neuropathy was induced in adult rats by photochemically induced ischemia. Retinal and optic nerve vasculature was examined by fluorescein isothiocyanate–dextran extravasation. Tissue sectioning and immunohistochemistry were used to investigate the pathologic changes. Retinal ganglion cell survival at different times after PION induction, with or without neurotrophic application, was quantified by fluorogold retrograde labeling.

Results.—Optic nerve injury was confirmed after PION induction, including local vascular leakage, optic nerve edema, and cavernous degeneration. Immunostaining data revealed microglial activation and focal loss of astrocytes, with adjacent astrocytic hypertrophy. Up to 23%, 50%, and 70% retinal ganglion cell loss was observed at 1 week, 2 weeks, and 3 weeks, respectively, after injury compared with a sham control group. Experimental treatment by brain-derived neurotrophic factor and ciliary neurotrophic factor remarkably prevented retinal ganglion cell loss in PION rats. At 3 weeks after injury, more than 40% of retinal ganglion cells were saved by the application of neurotrophic factors.

Conclusions.—Rat PION created by photochemically induced ischemia is a reproducible and reliable animal model for mimicking the key features of human PION.

Clinical Relevance.—The correspondence between the features of this rat PION model to those of human PION makes it an ideal model to study the pathophysiologic course of the disease, most of which remains to be elucidated. Furthermore, it provides an optimal model for testing therapeutic approaches for optic neuropathies.

▶ The development of rational therapies for ischemic optic neuropathy has been severely limited by a lack of acceptable animal models. This work may solve this unmet medical need. The authors followed the loss of retinal ganglion cells at 1, 2, and 3 weeks after the injury. Interestingly, treatment with brain-derived neurotrophic factor and ciliary neurotrophic factor prevented ganglion cell loss, an observation that may enable treatment of other neuropathies in which retinal ganglion cell loss is a final common pathway.

R. C. Sergott, MD

9 Imaging

Contrasting disease patterns in seropositive and seronegative neuromyelitis optica: A multicentre study of 175 patients
Jarius S, Ruprecht K, Wildemann B, et al (Univ of Heidelberg, Germany; Charité -
Univ Medicine Berlin, Germany; et al)
J Neuroinflammation 9:14, 2012

Background.—The diagnostic and pathophysiological relevance of antibodies to aquaporin-4 (AQP4-Ab) in patients with neuromyelitis optica spectrum disorders (NMOSD) has been intensively studied. However, little is known so far about the clinical impact of AQP4-Ab seropositivity.

Objective.—To analyse systematically the clinical and paraclinical features associated with NMO spectrum disorders in Caucasians in a stratified fashion according to the patients' AQP4-Ab serostatus.

Methods.—Retrospective study of 175 Caucasian patients (AQP4-Ab positive in 78.3%).

Results.—Seropositive patients were found to be predominantly female ($p < 0.0003$), to more often have signs of co-existing autoimmunity ($p < 0.00001$), and to experience more severe clinical attacks. A visual acuity of <0.1 during acute optic neuritis (ON) attacks was more frequent among seropositives ($p < 0.002$). Similarly, motor symptoms were more common in seropositive patients, the median Medical Research Council scale (MRC) grade worse, and MRC grades ≤ 2 more frequent, in particular if patients met the 2006 revised criteria ($p < 0.005$, $p < 0.006$ and $p < 0.01$, respectively), the total spinal cord lesion load was higher ($p < 0.006$), and lesions ≥ 6 vertebral segments as well as entire spinal cord involvement more frequent ($p < 0.003$ and $p < 0.043$). By contrast, bilateral ON at onset was more common in seronegatives ($p < 0.007$), as was simultaneous ON and myelitis ($p < 0.001$); accordingly, the time to diagnosis of NMO was shorter in the seronegative group ($p < 0.029$). The course of disease was more often monophasic in seronegatives ($p < 0.008$). Seropositives and seronegatives did not differ significantly with regard to age at onset, time to relapse, annualized relapse rates, outcome from relapse (complete, partial, no recovery), annualized EDSS increase, mortality rate, supratentorial brain lesions, brainstem lesions, history of carcinoma, frequency of preceding infections, oligoclonal bands, or CSF pleocytosis. Both the time to relapse and the time to diagnosis was longer if the disease started with ON ($p < 0.002$ and $p < 0.013$). Motor symptoms or tetraparesis at first myelitis and >1 myelitis attacks in the first year were identified as possible predictors of a worse outcome.

Conclusion.—This study provides an overview of the clinical and paraclinical features of NMOSD in Caucasians and demonstrates a number of distinct disease characteristics in seropositive and seronegative patients.

▶ Neuromyelitis optica (NMO), also known as Devic disease or Devic syndrome, is a severe inflammatory demyelination that has predilection for the optic nerves and the spinal cord. NMO, initially thought to be a variant of multiple sclerosis, is now considered a distinct disease process with several different clinical, laboratory, and imaging characteristics when compared with multiple sclerosis. An important difference is the presence of serum antibodies to aquaporin-4, a water channel in the central nervous system. The role of aquaporin-4 antibody testing in the diagnosis of NMO is now well established. Magnetic resonance imaging of the spinal cord and brain form an important aspect of the diagnostic workup. This retrospective study of 175 patients investigates the clinical and paraclinical features of NMO spectrum disorders according to the patient's aquaporin-4 antibody serostatus. The authors report several clinical and radiologic differences between these 2 subgroups. From an imaging perspective, a long spinal cord lesion (spanning over 3 vertebral segments) and a negative brain study help differentiate NMO from multiple sclerosis; the investigators in this study have observed that this is especially important in the seronegative subgroup.

A. Flanders, MD

Concurrent Acute Brain Infarcts in Patients with Monocular Visual Loss
Helenius J, Arsava EM, Goldstein JN, et al (Massachusetts General Hosp, Boston; et al)
Ann Neurol 72:286-293, 2012

Objective.—Embolism from a proximal source to the retinal circulation could be a sign of embolism from the same source to the hemispheric circulation. We sought to determine the frequency of acute brain infarcts on diffusion-weighted imaging (DWI) in patients with monocular visual loss of presumed ischemic origin (MVL).

Methods.—We retrospectively studied 129 consecutive patients with MVL secondary to retinal ischemia. All patients underwent DWI, comprehensive ophthalmologic and neurologic examination, and diagnostic evaluations for the underlying etiology. Statistical analyses explored univariate and multivariate predictors of DWI evidence of acute brain infarcts.

Results.—DWI revealed concurrent acute brain infarct(s) in 31 of the 129 patients (24%). The probability of positive DWI was higher in embolic versus nonembolic MVL (28 vs 8%, $p = 0.04$), in MVL characterized by permanent visual loss versus transient symptoms (33 vs 18%, $p = 0.04$), and in MVL associated with concurrent hemispheric symptoms versus isolated MVL (53 vs 20%, $p < 0.01$). Patients with positive DWI were more likely to harbor a major underlying etiology as compared to those with normal DWI (odds ratio, 3.7; 95% confidence interval, 1.5−9.4).

Interpretation.—This study demonstrates that MVL does not always represent an isolated disease of the retina; approximately 1 of every 4 patients with MVL demonstrates acute brain infarcts on DWI. Because patients with concurrent brain infarcts are more likely to exhibit a cardiac or vascular source of embolism, imaging evidence of brain injury in patients with MVL may be a useful marker to guide the timing and extent of diagnostic examinations.

▶ Magnetic resonance imaging (MRI) has been shown in clinical studies to be an important tool in the work-up of patients with transient ischemic attack (TIA). The 2009 American Heart Association/American Stroke Association Scientific Statement on TIA[1] also recommends neuroimaging, preferably with MRI, including diffusion-weighted imaging (DWI) among other recommendations, in a work-up of patients with neurological dysfunction, including retinal ischemia for risk stratification and management because of the risk of future stroke. This article investigates the occurrence of acute brain infarcts on DWI in patients with monocular visual loss of presumed ischemic origin (MVL). They report that approximately 1 in 4 patients with MVL has an acute infarct on DWI. They also suggest that presence of an embolic etiology (vs nonembolic), concurrent hemispheric symptoms, and permanent visual loss have a higher probability of positive DWI results.

A. Flanders, MD

Reference

1. Easton JD, Saver JL, Albers GW, et al. Definition and evaluation of transient ischemic attack: a scientific statement for healthcare professionals from the American Heart Association/American Stroke Association Stroke Council; Council on Cardiovascular Surgery and Anesthesia; Council on Cardiovascular Radiology and Intervention; Council on Cardiovascular Nursing; and the Interdisciplinary Council on Peripheral Vascular Disease. The American Academy of Neurology affirms the value of this statement as an educational tool for neurologists. *Stroke.* 2009;40:2276-2293.

10 Ocular Oncology

Clinical and Pathologic Characteristics of Biopsy-Proven Iris Melanoma: A Multicenter International Study

Khan S, Finger PT, Yu G-P, et al (New York Univ School of Medicine; et al)
Arch Ophthalmol 130:57-64, 2012

Objective.—To collaborate with multiple centers to identify representative epidemiological, clinical, and pathologic characteristics of melanoma of the iris. This international, multicenter, Internet-assisted study in ophthalmic oncology demonstrates the collaboration among eye cancer specialists to stage and describe the clinical and pathologic characteristics of biopsy-proven melanoma of the iris.

Methods.—A computer program was created to allow for Internet-assisted multicenter, privacy-protected, online data entry. Eight eye cancer centers in 6 countries performed retrospective chart reviews. Statistical analysis included patient and tumor characteristics, ocular and angle abnormalities, management, histopathology, and outcomes.

Results.—A total of 131 patients with iris melanoma (mean age, 64 years [range, 20-100 years]) were found to have blue-gray (62.2%), green-hazel (29.1%), or brown (8.7%) irides. Iris melanoma color was brown (65.6%), amelanotic (9.9%), and multicolored (6.9%). A mean of 2.5 clock hours of iris was visibly involved with melanoma, typically centered at the 6-o'clock meridian. Presentations included iritis, glaucoma, hyphema, and sector cataract. High-frequency ultrasonography revealed a largest mean tumor diameter of 4.9 mm, a mean maximum tumor thickness of 1.9 mm, angle blunting (52%), iris root disinsertion (9%), and posterior iris pigment epithelium displacement (9%). Using the American Joint Commission on Cancer–International Union Against Cancer classification, we identified 56% of tumors as T1, 34% of tumors as T2, 2% of tumors as T3, and 1% of tumors as T4. Histopathologic grades were G1-spindle (54%), G2-mixed (28%), G3-epithelioid (5%), and undetermined (13%) cell types. Primary treatment involved radiation (26%) and surgery (64%). Kaplan-Meier analysis found a 10.7% risk of metastatic melanoma at 5 years.

Conclusions.—Iris melanomas were most likely to be brown and found in the inferior quadrants of patients with light irides. Typically small and unifocal, melanomas are commonly associated with angle blunting and spindle cell histopathology. This multicenter, Internet-based, international

185

study successfully pooled data and extracted information on biopsy-proven melanoma of the iris.

▶ Iris melanoma is rare. There have been several single-center reports on the clinical features and outcomes in small cohorts of patients with iris melanoma. The largest single-center clinical cohort was from the Oncology Service at Wills Eye Institute in which 169 eyes with iris melanoma were evaluated for features predictive of outcomes of melanoma metastasis.[1] Metastasis was found in 3% at 5 years, 5% at 10 years, and 10% at 20 years. The authors noted that factors predictive of metastasis included older age, elevated intraocular pressure, extension of tumor into root of iris or angle, extraocular extension of tumor, and prior surgical biopsy. Another fairly large study, from a pathology laboratory, assessed 72 iris melanomas that were surgically removed.[2]

In this article, data from a collaboration of several ocular oncology centers in 6 countries in North America and Europe were compiled. A total of 131 patients with iris melanoma were identified. The tumors were classified according to the new 7th edition of the American Joint Committee on Cancer's (AJCC) *Cancer Staging Manuel* classification of iris melanoma. Using this classification, tumors are classified by T for tumor, N for node, and M for metastasis. A simplified understanding of the tumor classification includes:

T1 tumor limited to iris.

T2 tumor extending into ciliary body, choroid, or both.

T3 tumor extending into ciliary body, choroid, or both with scleral extension.

T4 tumor with extraocular extension.

Factored within each group are secondary glaucoma and other features. The gradual increase in features portends worse prognosis and is reflective of the prognostic factors previously published.[1]

In this analysis of 131 tumors, most were low grade at T1 (56%) or T2 (34%) and only 3% were higher grade T3 or T4. The tumors were managed by surgery (described as "resection") in 64% and radiation in 26%. It is unclear if enucleation was performed. Based on previous studies, enucleation is indeed necessary for iris melanoma management, particularly when there is secondary glaucoma or extrascleral extension.[1] The authors of this article found 11% metastasis at 5 years, somewhat higher than previous reports. Metastatic disease correlated with tumor classification. The 5-year metastatic rate for T1 was 0%, T2 was 10%, and T3 or T4 was 50%.

This study is important in that it incorporates the new AJCC 7th edition classification of iris melanoma into description and outcomes of iris melanoma. This collaborative effort of pooled data from several centers worldwide has provided relevant information on a rare tumor.

C. L. Shields, MD

References

1. Shields CL, Shields JA, Materin M, Gershenbaum E, Singh AD, Smith A. Iris melanoma: risk factors for metastasis in 169 consecutive patients. *Ophthalmology.* 2001;108:172-178.

2. Arentsen JJ, Green WR. Melanoma of the iris: report of 72 cases treated surgically. *Ophthalmic Surg.* 1975;6:23-37.

Minimal Exposure (One or Two Cycles) of Intra-arterial Chemotherapy in the Management of Retinoblastoma
Shields CL, Kaliki S, Shah SU, et al (Wills Eye Inst, Philadelphia, PA; et al)
Ophthalmology 119:188-192, 2012

Purpose.—To assess the efficacy of less than 3 cycles of intra-arterial chemotherapy (IAC) for retinoblastoma.
Design.—Retrospective, nonrandomized, interventional case series.
Participants.—Eight patients.
Intervention.—Intra-arterial chemotherapy.
Main Outcome Measures.—Tumor control and globe salvage.
Results.—Eight patients received fewer than 3 cycles of IAC for retinoblastoma because there was complete tumor control with no residual viable tumor (n = 7) or poor response (n = 1) with little hope that further therapy would benefit the patient. In 3 cases, additional vascular compromise precluded further IAC. The treatment was primary in 6 cases and secondary after failure of other treatment in 2 cases. The 8 eyes were classified (International Classification of Retinoblastoma) as group C (n = 2), group D (n = 3), group E (n = 1), and secondary treatment (n = 2). At initial examination, the main tumor showed a mean basal diameter of 16 mm, a thickness of 8.6 mm, vitreous seeds (n = 2), subretinal seeds (n = 6), and iris neovascularization (n = 1). Three patients were treated with a single cycle of IAC, and 5 patients were treated with 2 cycles of IAC. After IAC, complete tumor response was found in 7 eyes (88%) and partial response was found in 1 eye (13%). Over a mean of 13 months follow-up, there was intraretinal tumor recurrence (n = 1), subretinal seed recurrence (n = 1), and no case of vitreous seed recurrence. Globe salvage was achieved in 2 of 2 group C eyes (100%), 3 of 3 group D eyes (100%), 0 of 1 group E eye (0%), and 1 of 2 secondary treatment eyes (50%). Globe salvage was achieved in 6 of 8 eyes (75%), and 2 of 8 eyes (25%) required enucleation.
Conclusions.—One or 2 cycles of IAC can be sufficient for selected eyes with group C or D retinoblastoma, with remarkable tumor control.

▶ There is intense interest in the use of intra-arterial chemotherapy (IAC) for retinoblastoma. The main reason for this is because the technique is theoretically focused to provide chemotherapy to the eye via the ophthalmic artery with minimal escape of chemotherapy to the rest of the body. This is achieved by catheterization of the femoral artery, through the aorta, into the internal carotid artery and slipping into the ophthalmic artery with subsequent pulsatile chemotherapy flush. The good news is that it works. The bad news is that there are potential complications of vascular obstruction of the retinal or choroidal vessels leading to blindness, and, more seriously, there is a risk for spasm or obstruction of larger vessels in the brain leading to stroke or death. In our hands, there has been no case of stroke or death. Initially, retinal or choroidal reduction in flow was noted, but this feature has nearly disappeared now with better techniques. How do we avoid vascular toxicities? We do not enter the ophthalmic artery, as initially described. We just peek into the ostium of the artery, so there is no obstruction to flow and the chemotherapy is flushed to the eye admixed with blood.

In this article, the authors have shown that only 1 or 2 sessions of IAC are necessary for complete control of retinoblastoma in some instances. This is an important observation as most centers plan 3 sessions or more. However, with less advanced tumors that show minimal seeding, only 1 or 2 sessions are needed. This allows for reduction in complications.

Retinoblastoma is a dangerous, life-threatening malignancy of the eye, classically found in children. This cancer grows rapidly and can lead to metastasis and death of the child if it's not appropriately managed within a window of time. The use of IAC has allowed rapid control of this cancer with minimal systemic toxicity. Long-term data are not available regarding IAC, but hopefully the tumor control is lasting and the complications remain minimal.

C. L. Shields, MD

Success of Intra-arterial Chemotherapy (Chemosurgery) for Retinoblastoma: Effect of Orbitovascular Anatomy
Marr BP, Hung C, Gobin YP, et al (Memorial Sloan-Kettering Cancer Ctr, NY; Weill Cornell Med College, NY; et al)
Arch Ophthalmol 130:180-185, 2012

Objectives.—To review results of orbital angiography performed during intra-arterial chemotherapy (chemosurgery) for treatment of retinoblastoma to assess the association of angiographic variability in orbitovascular anatomy with tumor response and outcomes.

Methods.—Medical records and 64 orbital angiograms were reviewed for 56 pediatric patients with retinoblastoma undergoing chemosurgery using a combination of melphalan hydrochloride, topotecan hydrochloride, or carboplatin. The major orbital arteries and capillary blush patterns were graded, and tumor response and recurrence were compared using the log-rank and Fisher exact tests.

Results.—Statistically significant variables for tumor response were lacrimal artery prominence ($P = .001$), previous treatment ($P = .003$), and lacrimal blush ($P = .004$). The only statistically significant variable for vitreous seed response was ciliary body blush ($P = .03$). Statistically significant variables influencing time to recurrence and time to enucleation were choroidal blush absence ($P = .01$) and lacrimal artery presence ($P = .03$), respectively.

Conclusions.—The success of intra-arterial chemotherapy is dependent on delivery of drug to the target tumor within the eye via the ophthalmic artery. Because of the small volume of drug used (0.50-1.25 mL per treatment) and the selectivity of catheterization, variables affecting orbital blood flow greatly influence drug delivery and the success of chemosurgery.

▶ Intra-arterial chemotherapy (IAC) has become a somewhat accepted therapy for the management of retinoblastoma.[1] The success depends on many factors, including extent of tumor seeding, tumor classification, and whether the treatment is primary or secondary. Eyes classified as group C or D show nearly 100% control, whereas group E shows approximately 33% control.[2] Primary treatment shows up to 90% success, whereas secondary treatment displays about 50% to 60% success.[3] One factor that could contribute to success is the vascular anatomy of the orbit, a feature that determines blood flow and delivery of potent chemotherapy to the ocular malignancy.

Orbital vascular flow has been studied previously in cadaver eyes, and noted differences were found to be relatively common. In most cases, the ophthalmic artery supplies the orbital tissue from the internal carotid artery. However, in some instances, the main flow to the eye comes from the middle meningeal and not the ophthalmic artery. Furthermore, in approximately 5% of orbits, the ophthalmic artery emanates from the middle meningeal and not the internal carotid artery.

In this report, these authors reviewed 64 orbital angiograms of 56 children. They noted that prominence of the lacrimal artery was an important factor in tumor response, perhaps related to steal of flow and reduction of chemotherapy to target tissue. This important observation should be considered by interventional neuroradiologists and endovascular neurosurgeons who participate in catheterization of the ophthalmic artery for IAC.

C. L. Shields, MD

References

1. Shields CL, Shields JA. Intra-arterial chemotherapy for retinoblastoma: the beginning of a long journey [editorial]. *Clin Experiment Ophthalmol.* 2010;38:638-643.
2. Shields CL, Bianciotto CG, Jabbour P, et al. Intra-arterial chemotherapy for retinoblastoma: report No. 1, control of retinal tumors, subretinal seeds, and vitreous seeds. *Arch Ophthalmol.* 2011;129:1399-1406.
3. Abramson DH. Super selective ophthalmic artery delivery of chemotherapy for intraocular retinoblastoma: 'Chemosurgery' the first Stallard lecture. *Br J Ophthalmol.* 2010;94:396-399.

Topical Interferon Alfa-2b for Management of Ocular Surface Squamous Neoplasia in 23 Cases: Outcomes Based on American Joint Committee on Cancer Classification

Shah SU, Kaliki S, Kim HJ, et al (Thomas Jefferson Univ, Philadelphia, PA)
Arch Ophthalmol 130:159-164, 2012

Objective.—To evaluate the efficacy of topical interferonalfa-2b in the management of ocular surface squamous neoplasia (OSSN).

Methods.—Clinically visible OSSN in 20 patients (23 tumors) was managed with topical interferon alfa-2b, 1 million IU/mL, 4 times daily. Tumor control and complications were evaluated according to American Joint Committee on Cancer classification.

Results.—Complete tumor resolution was achieved in 19 tumors (83%) following topical interferon alfa-2b treatment for a median period of 6 months (mean, 7 months; range, 1-12 months) and maintained for up to 24 months of follow-up. Of the 4 tumors with partial resolution (17%), tumor surface area was reduced 44% (median) during 4 months (median) without further response and alternative therapy was used. Based on American Joint Committee on Cancer classification, complete control was achieved in 2 of 3 Tis (67%), 17 of 20 T3 (85%), 19 of 23 N0 (83%), and 19 of 23 M0 (83%) category tumors. Tumors involving the cornea responded earlier compared with those without corneal involvement ($P = .01$). Initial tumor size did not correlate with time to response ($P = .27$). Recurrence was noted in 1 case (Tis, 4%) at 3 months. Adverse effects included conjunctival hyperemia (2 [10%]), follicular hypertrophy (2 [10%]), giant papillary conjunctivitis (1 [5%]), irritation (1 [5%]), corneal epithelial defect (1 [5%]), and flu like symptoms (1 [5%]); all resolved within 1 month of medication discontinuation.

Conclusion.—According to American Joint Committee on Cancer classification, complete control with topical interferonalfa-2b can be achieved in 67% of Tis, 85% ofT3, and 83% of all OSSN.

▶ Ocular surface squamous neoplasia (OSSN) is a spectrum of epithelial neoplastic infiltration on the surface of the eye ranging from in situ to invasive disease. Management of this condition involves surgical or medical strategies. Surgically, complete microscopic dissection using no touch technique is advised. Medically, application of topical chemotherapeutics like mitomycin C (MMC) or 5 fluorouracil (5FU) are effective. Another medical alternative is topical or injection immunotherapy with interferon (IFN) α2b.

In this report, Shah et al evaluated 23 patients treated with topical IFN and note that 83% achieved complete resolution and 17% showed partial resolution. Those with partial response showed definite reduction in tumor volume and were treated with other therapies to achieve complete control. Tumors on the corneal surface showed faster response than those on the bulbar, forniceal, or tarsal surface.

IFN works by binding to cell receptors and triggering synthesis of proteins to inhibit viruses, activate immunocompetent cells, and regulate oncogenes. A study by Poothullil and Colby[1] found in situ OSSN regression to be similar for both chemotherapy (MMC, 5FU) and immunotherapy (IFN) medications. It should be noted that cost is a factor, as IFN, at a cost of $300 per treatment, is more expensive than the others that cost $100 to $150 per treatment. However, the superior safety profile with few complications from IFN compared with MMC or 5FU outweighs the cost issue.

The preference in our practice of ocular oncology is for resection of small or limited cases of OSSN and treatment with topical or injection IFN for more extensive OSSN or those in nonsurgical candidates. We prefer this therapy over topical chemotherapy because of the gentle control and few side effects offered by this method.

C. L. Shields, MD

Reference

1. Poothullil AM, Colby KA. Topical medical therapies for ocular surface tumors. *Semin Ophthalmol.* 2006;21:161-169.

Choroidal Abnormalities Detected by Near-Infrared Reflectance Imaging as a New Diagnostic Criterion for Neurofibromatosis 1
Viola F, Villani E, Natacci F, et al (Università degli Studi di Milano, Italy)
Ophthalmology 119:369 376, 2012

Objective.—To investigate in a large sample of consecutive patients with neurofibromatosis type 1 (NF1) the possibility of including the presence of choroidal abnormalities detected by near-infrared reflectance (NIR) as a new diagnostic criterion for NF1.

Design.—Cross-sectional evaluation of a diagnostic test.

Participants and Controls.—Ninety-five consecutive adult and pediatric patients (190 eyes) with NF1, diagnosed based on the National Institutes of Health (NIH) criteria. Controls included 100 healthy age- and gender-matched control subjects.

Methods.—Confocal scanning laser ophthalmoscopy was performed for each subject, investigating the presence and the number of choroidal abnormalities.

Main Outcome Measures.—Sensitivity, specificity, and diagnostic accuracy for the different cutoff values of the criterion choroidal nodules detected by NIR compared with the NIH criteria.

Results.—Choroidal nodules detected by NIR imaging were present in 79 (82%) of 95 of the NF1 patients, including 15 (71%) of the 21 NF1 pediatric patients. Similar abnormalities were present in 7 (7%) of 100 healthy subjects, including 2 (8%) of the 25 healthy pediatric subjects. The highest accuracy was obtained at the cutoff value of 1.5 choroidal nodules detected by NIR imagery. Sensitivity and specificity of the examination at the optimal cutoff point were 83% and 96%, respectively. Diagnostic accuracy was 90% in the overall population and 83% in the pediatric population. Both of these values were in line with the most common NIH diagnostic criteria.

Conclusions.—Choroidal abnormalities appearing as bright patchy nodules detected by NIR imaging frequently occurred in NF1 patients. The present study shows that NIR examination to detect choroidal involvement should be considered as a new diagnostic criterion for NF1.

▶ The diagnosis of neurofibromatosis type 1 (NF1) relies on 2 of the following characteristics: 6 or more cutaneous café au lait spots, freckling in the axilla or inguinal region, 2 or more cutaneous neurofibromas, one plexiform neurofibroma, osseous lesions like pseudarthrosis or sphenoid wing hypoplasia, optic nerve glioma, multifocal iris Lisch nodules, and a first-degree relative with NF1. The eye has numerous features of NF1, including eyelid, conjunctival, and uveal (choroidal) neurofibroma; iris Lisch nodules; prominence of corneal nerves; choroidal freckling; congenital hypertrophy of the retinal pigment epithelium; retinal astrocytic hamartoma; optic nerve glioma; and choroidal or conjunctival melanoma.

Choroidal neurofibromatosis consists of Schwann cells enwrapping axons and forming ovoid bodies documented on histopathology. These findings are not visible on indirect ophthalmoscopy or fundus photography. In this report, the authors state that these findings can be imaged with near-infrared reflectance (NIR) photography without the need for invasive testing. NIR was measured at 815 nm using a special technique, and interpretation was performed blinded to patient vs control. The investigators found that in most cases, patients with NF1 showed no distinct features with fundus photography, autofluorescence (488 nm excitation, 500 nm filter), and red-free imaging (488 nm), but with NIR, the ovoid bodies were visible as bright choroidal focal defects. In fact, the controls showed the focal bright defects in 7% of cases compared with 82% of cases with NF1.

This feature on NIR photography was found more commonly than Lisch nodules, described in only 43% of NF1 patients. Most of the bright lesions were found in the posterior pole. Yasunari et al[1] and Nakakura et al[2] have previously identified this finding as a reliable marker for NF1, and Viola et al have confirmed their findings in a relatively large cohort. NIR is necessary to detect this NF1 marker, as it is not visible by fundus photography, fluorescein angiography, red-free imaging, or autofluorescence photography.

C. L. Shields, MD

References

1. Yasunari T, Shiraki K, Hattori H, Miki T. Frequency of choroidal abnormalities in neurofibromatosis type 1. *Lancet.* 2000;356:988-992.
2. Nakakura S, Shiraki K, Yasunari T, Hayashi Y, Ataka S, Kohno T. Quantification and anatomic distribution of choroidal abnormalities in patients with type I neurofibromatosis. *Graefes Arch Clin Exp Ophthalmol.* 2005;243:980-984.

Clinical Survey of 3680 Iris Tumors Based on Patient Age at Presentation
Shields CL, Kancherla S, Patel J, et al (Thomas Jefferson Univ, Philadelphia, PA)
Ophthalmology 119:407-414, 2012

Objective.—To report the spectrum of iris lesions based on patient age at presentation.
Design.—Retrospective, nonrandomized, single-center case series.
Participants.—We included 3680 iris tumors in 3451 patients.
Methods.—Chart review.
Main Outcome Measures.—Diagnostic category based on age.

TABLE 1.—Clinical Survey of 3680 Iris Tumors in 3451 Patients: Diagnostic Category

Diagnostic Category	Patients No. of Patients (n = 3451)	% of All Patients	Tumor No. of Tumors (n = 3680)	% of All Iris Tumors
Cystic	718	21	768	21
Solid	2733	79	2912	79
Melanocytic	2375	69	2510	68
Nonmelanocytic	358	10	402	11
Choristomatous	4	<1	4	<1
Vascular	53	2	57	2
Fibrous	2	<1	2	<1
Neural	2	<1	3	<1
Myogenic	2	<1	2	<1
Epithelial	35	1	35	1
Xanthomatous	8	<1	8	<1
Metastatic	65	2	67	2
Lymphoid	11	<1	12	<1
Leukemic	2	<1	2	<1
Secondary	12	<1	12	<1
Nonneoplastic simulating lesion	162	5	198	5

Results.—The mean age at presentation was 48 years and there were 449 (12%) tumors in children (≤20 years), 788 (21%) in young adults (21–40 years), 1308 (36%) in mid adults (41–60 years), and 1135 (31%) in senior adults (>60 years). Of 3680 tumors, the diagnostic category was cystic (n = 768; 21%) or solid (n = 2912; 79%). The cystic tumors originated from iris pigment epithelium (IPE; n = 672; 18%) or iris stroma (n = 96; 3%). The solid tumors included melanocytic (n = 2510; 68%) and nonmelanocytic (n = 402; 11%). The melanocytic tumors comprised nevus (n = 1503; 60%), melanocytoma (n = 68; 3%), melanoma (n = 645; 26%), and melanocytosis (n = 64; 3%). Of 2510 melanocytic tumors, the first and second most common diagnoses by age (children, young adult, mid adult, senior adult) were nevus (53%, 57%, 63%, and 63%, respectively) and melanoma (17%, 27%, 26%, and 27%, respectively). The nonmelanocytic tumors included categories of choristomatous (n = 4; <1%), vascular (n = 57; 2%), fibrous (n = 2; <1%), neural (n = 3; <1%), myogenic (n = 2;, <1%), epithelial (n = 35; 1%), xanthomatous (n = 8; <1%), metastasis (n = 67; 2%), lymphoid (n = 12; <1%), leukemic (n = 2; <1%), secondary (n = 12; <1%), and nonneoplastic simulators (n = 198; 5%). The median age (in years) at diagnosis included cystic (39), melanocytic (52), choristomatous (0.7), vascular (56), fibrous (53), neural (8), myogenic (42), epithelial (63), xanthomatous (1.9), metastasis (60), lymphoid (57), leukemic (25.5), secondary (59), and nonneoplastic simulators (49). Overall, the 3 most common specific diagnoses (children, young adult, mid adult, senior adult) were nevus (25%, 36%, 47%, and 47%, respectively), IPE cyst (28%, 30%, 15%, and 14%, respectively), and melanoma (8%, 16%, 20%, and 19%, respectively).

Conclusions.—In an ocular oncology practice, the spectrum of iris tumors includes cystic (21%) and solid (79%) tumors. The solid tumors were melanocytic (68%) or nonmelanocytic (11%). At all ages, the most common specific diagnoses were nevus (42%), IPE cyst (19%), and melanoma (17%) (Table 1).

▶ Iris tumors are uncommon, and there are just a few publications in the ophthalmic literature on the various types and frequencies of iris lesions. Some published series have emanated from pathology laboratories and rarely from clinical practice. These authors report the various diagnoses of iris tumors in a large clinical cohort of patients managed in an ocular oncology center and evaluated the tumors based on patient age at presentation.

The 3 most common diagnoses were nevus, iris pigment epithelial (IPE) cyst, and melanoma in all age groups. Overall, there were 21% cystic tumors and 79% solid tumors. The cystic tumors proved to be IPE cyst in 86%, iris stromal cyst in 11%, and epithelial ingrowth cyst in 2%. The solid tumors were melanocytic in 86% and nonmelanocytic in 14%. The solid tumor diagnoses included nevus, melanocytoma, melanoma, metastasis, adenoma, juvenile xanthogranuloma, and others. Based on age, the lesions (median age years) included cystic (39), melanocytic (52), choristomatous (0.7), vascular (56), fibrous (53), neural (8), myogenic (42), epithelial (63), xanthomatous (1.9), metastasis (60), lymphoid (57), leukemic (25.5), secondary (59), and nonneoplastic simulators (49).

Large series' like this one are important to allow the clinician the chance to evaluate and compare the features of various tumors. This series will serve as a basis for future comparative publications. Although there is inherent bias in this clinic-based ocular oncology series, there is value in its information.

C. L. Shields, MD

A Survey Study of Musculoskeletal Disorders Among Eye Care Physicians Compared With Family Medicine Physicians
Kitzmann AS, Fethke NB, Baratz KH, et al (Univ of Iowa Hosps and Clinics, Iowa City; Univ of Iowa, Iowa City; The Mayo Clinic, Rochester, MN; et al)
Ophthalmology 119:213-220, 2012

Purpose.—To evaluate the prevalence of musculoskeletal disorders among eye care physicians compared with family medicine physicians.

Design.—Case control study.

Participants and Controls.—Ophthalmologists and optometrists at the University of Iowa and Mayo Clinic (participants) and family medicine physicians at the University of Iowa and Mayo Clinic (controls).

Methods.—An electronic survey was e-mailed to all subjects.

Main Outcome Measures.—The prevalence of musculoskeletal symptoms between eye care providers and family medicine physicians (control group).

Results.—One hundred eight-six surveys were completed by 94 eye care physicians and 92 family medicine physicians with a response rate of 99% and 80%, respectively. There were no significant differences between the 2 groups with regard to mean age, gender, body mass index, years with

TABLE 2.—Participants Reporting Musculoskeletal Symptoms during the Previous 30 Days, by Body Region and Group

Body Region	Eye Care Physicians, n (%)	Family Medicine Physicians, n (%)	P-Value
Neck	(n = 93) 43 (46)	(n = 90) 19 (21)	<0.01
Shoulder	10 (11)	10 (11)	0.96
Elbow	1 (1)	(n = 91) 3 (3)	0.36*
Hand/wrist	(n = 93) 16 (17)	6 (7)	0.03
Upper back	(n = 93) 18 (19)	11 (12)	0.17
Lower back	(n = 93) 24 (26)	8 (9)	<0.01

Sample sizes are 94 eye care physicians and 92 family medicine physicians unless otherwise noted.
*Fisher's exact test used to compare groups.

current employer, or years in practice. Eye care providers, compared with their family medicine colleagues, reported a higher prevalence of neck (46% vs 21%; $P < 0.01$), hand/wrist pain (17% vs 7%; $P = 0.03$), and lower back pain (26% vs 9%; $P < 0.01$). A greater proportion of eye care physicians classified their job as a high-strain job (high demand, low control; 31% vs 20%) and a lower proportion classified their job as an active job (high demand, high control; 24% vs 47%; $P = 0.01$). Several job factors reported by eye care providers to contribute to musculoskeletal symptoms included performing the same task repeatedly, working in awkward/cramped positions, working in the same position for long periods, and bending/twisting the back (all $P < 0.01$).

Conclusions.—In this survey, the study group, composed of ophthalmologists and optometrists, had a higher prevalence of neck, hand/wrist, and lower back pain compared with family medicine physicians; repetitive tasks, prolonged or awkward/cramped positions, and bending/twisting were contributory factors. Given the ramifications of these findings, future efforts should concentrate on modifications to the eye care providers' work environment to prevent or alleviate musculoskeletal disorders and their personal and socioeconomic burden (Table 2).

▶ Musculoskeletal disorders (MSDs) are common. They can occur with any profession. For health care workers, MSDs have been reported with registered nurses, dental hygienists, and custodial workers. These employees encounter physical work, often in awkward positions and with repetitive tasks. Surgeons are also at risk for MSDs. In 1 study, 90% of surgeons reported some degree of MSD during surgery and 43% required rest to relieve pain during surgery.[1] Ophthalmologists are at particular risk for MSDs because of the unusual back twisting and neck torquing positions to perform fundus and slit lamp examination.

This article compares MSDs of 94 eye care physicians to 92 family medical physicians, both from practices at the University of Iowa or the Mayo Clinic. The comparison was based on a survey, and as expected, the compulsive eye care physicians showed 99% response compared with 80% response of family medical physicians (Table 2). Eye care physicians showed statistically higher prevalence of neck, hand, wrist, and lower back pain. The authors conclude that eye care workers need to improve working conditions by modification of the environment, musculoskeletal strain, and repetitive tasks.

Other studies on ophthalmologists have identified MSDs of the neck in 33% to nearly 70% and low back symptoms in 30% to 80%. This is a serious life-altering problem that ophthalmic care specialists need to consider on a daily basis. The factors related to MSDs included repetitive tasking, awkward cramped positions, and bending or twisting the back. Interestingly, the average number of patients per day and the amount of exercise per week were associated with neck symptoms. Similar to ophthalmologists, laparoscopic surgeons have reported a high frequency of MSDs. These 2 professions have similar bodily demands in positioning and long-standing procedures. Laparoscopic surgeons have incorporated methods to minimize MSDs, such as improved instrument design, video monitor placement, and surgeon body posture. Ophthalmologists should adapt the preventative philosophy at an early point in their careers to minimize MSDs. Techniques like sitting low and straight at the slit lamp and operating the microscope without bending the cervical spine, flexing at the knees rather than bending the neck for indirect ophthalmoscopy, frequent relaxation exercises, and stretching could all help to alleviate this potentially crippling profession-related disease.

C. L. Shields, MD

Reference

1. Soueid A, Oudit D, Thiagarajah S, Laitung G. The pain of surgery: pain experienced by surgeons while operating. *Int J Surg.* 2010;8:118-120.

A Five-Year Study of Slotted Eye Plaque Radiation Therapy for Choroidal Melanoma: Near, Touching, or Surrounding the Optic Nerve
Finger PT, Chin KJ, Tena LB (The New York Eye Cancer Ctr)
Ophthalmology 119:415-422, 2012

Objective.—To evaluate slotted eye plaque radiation therapy for choroidal melanomas near the optic disc.

Design.—A clinical case series.

Participants.—Twenty-four consecutive patients with uveal melanomas that were near, touching, or surrounding the optic disc.

Intervention.—Slotted eye plaque radiation therapy.

Main Outcome Measures.—Recorded characteristics were related to patient, clinical, and ophthalmic imaging. Data included change in visual acuity, tumor size, recurrence, eye retention, and metastasis.

Results.—From 2005 to 2010, 24 consecutive patients were treated with custom-sized plaques with 8-mm− wide, variable-depth slots. Radiation doses ranged from 69.3 to 163.8 Gy (mean, 85.0 Gy) based on delivering a minimum tumor dose of 85 Gy. All treatments were continuously delivered over 5 to 7 days. Mean patient age at presentation was 57 years. Tumors were within 1.5 mm of the optic nerve (n = 3, 13%), juxtapapillary (n = 6, 25%), touching ≥180 degrees (n = 7, 29%), or circumpapillary (n = 8, 33%). Ultrasound revealed dome-shaped tumors in 79% of patients, collar-button tumors in 17% of patients, irregular tumor in 1 patient (4%), and intraneural invasion in 2 patients. Mean initial largest basal dimension was 11.0 mm (standard deviation [SD] ± 3.5 mm; median, 11.4 mm; range, 5.9–16.4 mm). Mean initial tumor thickness was 3.5 mm (SD ± 1.7 mm; median, 3.0 mm; range, 1.4–6.9 mm). Initial visual acuities were a median 20/25 (range, 20/20 to hand motions) and decreased to a median 20/40 (range, 20/20 to no light perception). At a mean follow-up of 23 months, 12 patients required periodic intravitreal bevacizumab to suppress radiation optic neuropathy (RON) or maculopathy. To date, there has been a 100% local control rate. No patients have required secondary enucleation for recurrence or neovascular glaucoma. No patients have developed metastasis.

Conclusions.—Slotted plaque radiation therapy allows peripapillary, juxtapapilary, and circumpapillary choroidal melanomas (and a safety margin) to be included in the radiation targeted zone. Normalization of the plaque position beneath the tumor appears to increase RON and improve local control.

▶ Uveal melanoma near or touching the optic disc is termed juxtapapillary melanoma. This subset of tumors is the most difficult to treat with radiotherapy, as the procedure is performed on the back wall of the eye with extreme globe rotation and in a region that is barely visualized. Much of the procedure is done by indirect ophthalmoscopic localization and understanding of the posterior anatomy of the globe. The optic disc within the eye has a mean diameter of 1.8 mm, whereas the optic nerve with its sheath immediately outside the eye has a mean diameter of 4.5 to 6 mm. These measurements are important for plaque radiotherapy design.

From a practical perspective, any tumor that is within 2 mm of the optic disc is treated with a posteriorly notched plaque. This allows radioactive seeds to be placed in the side legs of the plaque to adequately cover the juxtapapillary portion. If a tumor touches the disc for 3 clock hours or more, then a deeply notched plaque is applied with deeper indentation of the posterior margin and longer legs.

In this report, Finger et al look at their design of posterior notching that they term *slotted* plaque. They studied 24 patients who had tumors near or touching the optic disc, most of which had small melanoma, as the median tumor thickness was 3.0 mm. There were 12 (50%) to receive intravitreal bevacizumab. The local control rate at median follow-up of 22 months was 100%. It should be noted that they included patients with only one follow-up examination at 4 months, which is far too short to find radiation complications (occur at median of 18 months) and tumor recurrence (occur at median of 48 months). This report would benefit by longer follow-up and inclusion of only those patients with follow-up of perhaps 1 year or longer, as short follow-up skews the data in this small cohort toward better results.

In comparison with this study on 24 eyes, Sagoo et al[1-3] evaluated a larger, more robust cohort of 650 patients with juxtapapillary melanoma treated with plaque radiotherapy over a 30-year period. They used Kaplan-Meier analysis and included only those with specific lengths of follow-up at 1 year, 2 years, 5 years, and 10 years. They found that patients treated with round (not notched) plaques had higher recurrence than those treated with notched plaques. They recognized treatment complications and some tumor recurrences in those with longer follow-up. Melanoma-related death at 1 year was 0%, 2 years was 1%, 5 years was 4%, and 10 years was 9%, further emphasizing the need for long-term accurate reporting of data. This is particularly important with uveal melanoma results, as disease recurrence or metastasis can take years or decades to be recognized.

C. L. Shields, MD

References

1. Sagoo MS, Shields CL, Mashayekhi A, et al. Plaque radiotherapy for choroidal melanoma encircling the optic disc (circumpapillary choroidal melanoma). *Arch Ophthalmol.* 2007;125:1202-1209.
2. Sagoo MS, Shields CL, Mashayekhi A, et al. Plaque radiotherapy for juxtapapillary choroidal melanoma overhanging the optic disc in 141 consecutive patients. *Arch Ophthalmol.* 2008;126:1515-1522.
3. Sagoo MS, Shields CL, Mashayekhi A, et al. Plaque radiotherapy for juxtapapillary choroidal melanoma: tumor control in 650 consecutive cases. *Ophthalmology.* 2011; 118:402-407.

Clinicopathologic and Immunohistochemical Features of Pigmented Basal Cell Carcinomas of the Eyelids
Kirzhner M, Jakobiec FA (Massachusetts Eye and Ear Infirmary and Harvard Med School, Boston)
Am J Ophthalmol 153:242-252, 2012

• *Purpose.*—To describe the clinical and microscopic features of pigmented basal cell carcinomas (pBCC) of the eyelid.

• *Design.*—Retrospective observational case series collected at one institution.

• *Methods.*—An analysis of clinical records, photographs, and histopathologic characteristics of 257 BCCs with a review of the literature. The frequencies of clinically pigmented, and of microscopically pigmented but clinically nonpigmented, BCCs were determined. Cytochemical stains (Fontana-Masson, Prussian blue) and immunohistochemical probes (S-100, microphthalmia-associated transcription factor [MiTF], HMB-45, MART-1, CK20, synaptophysin, chromogranin, CD1a, Ki-67) were then employed and the findings correlated with the degree of clinical pigmentation.

• *Results.*—Histopathologically, 13 of 257 cases (5.06%) were found to have pigment; of these 13, 6 (all white patients) had clinically apparent pigmentation (2.33%), either focal or diffuse. Eight of 13 lesions developed on the lower eyelids. All stained positively for melanin but negatively for iron. MiTF highlighted numerous melanocytic nuclei in the tumor lobules, while MART-1 and HMB-45 revealed the dendritic shapes of the entrapped melanocytes. There was a subtotal blockage of melanin transfer to the surrounding basaloid cells. Intralobular S-100-positive cells included CD1a-positive Langerhans cells, while CK20 did not identify any Merkel cells.

• *Conclusions.*—Only 1 of 6 lesions was uniformly clinically pigmented, whereas the other 5 were only focally brown-black. The clinical pigmentation was imparted by varying densities and distributions of melanocytes with arborizing dendrites, which were present in all BCCs. Melanophages within the stroma and basaloid cell melanization also contributed to pigmentation. No behavioral or biologic differences in pBCC were documented compared with clinically nonpigmented lesions.

▶ Basal cell carcinoma is the most common eyelid malignancy in the Western world. Basal cell carcinoma is classically found on the lower eyelid or medial canthus as a pink, slightly vascular mass with loss of cilia and often central erosion. Pigmentation can be found within basal cell carcinoma, causing confusion with cutaneous nevus and melanoma. The pigmentation is usually partial and not complete.

In this article the authors reviewed 257 cases of eyelid basal cell carcinoma from a pathology laboratory and found 13 (5%) with pigment, mostly focal and not diffuse pigment. This finding is similar to clinical series in which it was found that 9% of basal cell carcinomas were pigmented.[1] Most clinicians indicate that this variant is found in dark-skinned individuals. These authors found that the pigmentation was attributed to extra melanocytes, melanophages infiltrating the tumor, or dendritic cells filled with melanin. Pigmentation within tumors is not limited to cutaneous tumors because pigmentation within conjunctival squamous cell carcinoma can also be found, mostly in dark-skinned individuals.[2]

The authors conclude that this rare variant of basal cell carcinoma was no different in behavior than the nonpigmented counterparts. The wide spectrum of basal cell carcinoma includes many different clinical types, such as nodular, micronodular, superficial, adenoidal, cystic, morpheaform, and rare types like fibroepitheliomatous, ductular, neuroendocrine, and amyloid-producing malignancies. We can now add pigmented basal carcinoma to this special list.

C. L. Shields, MD

References

1. Hornblass A, Stefano JA. Pigmented basal cell carcinoma of the eyelids. *Am J Ophthalmol.* 1981;92:193-197.
2. Shields CL, Manchandia A, Subbiah R, Eagle RC Jr, Shields JA. Pigmented squamous cell carcinoma in situ of the conjunctiva in 5 cases. *Ophthalmology.* 2008;115: 1673-1678.

Uveal Melanoma: Molecular Pattern, Clinical Features, and Radiation Response
Chappell MC, Char DH, Cole TB, et al (California Pacific Med Ctr (CPMC), San Francisco; The Tumori Foundation, San Francisco, CA; et al)
Am J Ophthalmol 154:227-232.e2, 2012

Purpose.—To characterize the clinical spectrum of class 1 and class 2 uveal melanomas and their relationship with intraocular proton radiation response.

Design.—Masked retrospective case series of uveal melanoma patients with fine needle biopsy based molecular profiles.

Methods.—197 uveal melanoma patients from a single institution were analyzed for pathology, clinical characteristics, and response to radiation therapy.

Results.—126 patients (64%) had class 1 tumors and 71 (36%) had class 2 tumors. Patients with class 2 tumors had more advanced age (means: 64 years vs. 57 years; $p = 0.001$), thicker initial mean ultrasound measurements (7.4 mm vs. 5.9 mm; $p = 0.0007$), and were more likely to have epithelioid or mixed cells on cytopathology (66% vs. 38%; $p = 0.0004$). Although mean pre-treatment and post-treatment ultrasound thickness were significantly different between class 1 and class 2 tumors, there was no difference in the mean change in thickness 24 months after radiation therapy (mean difference: class $1 = -1.64$ mm, class $2 = -1.47$; $p = 0.47$), or in the overall rate of thickness change (slope: $p = 0.64$). Class 2 tumors were more likely to metastasize and cause death than class 1 tumors (DSS: $p < 0.0001$).

Conclusions.—At the time of radiation therapy, thicker tumors, epithelioid pathology, and older patient age are significantly related to class 2 tumors, and class 2 tumors result in higher tumor-related mortality. We found no definitive clinical marker for differentiating class 1 and class 2 tumors.

▶ Uveal melanoma is a deadly tumor. Based on long-term follow-up of nearly 40 years, more than 50% of affected patients die from this malignancy, and the greater the thickness, the more guaranteed the metastatic doom.[1] Investigators worldwide are searching for genetic and molecular pathways leading to uveal melanoma development and metastatic spread. Teams have focused on delineating alterations in melanoma DNA, RNA, or more clinically applicable biologic signaling pathways. Others have looked at techniques for harvesting adequate microscopic tissue for evaluation using needle biopsy without the need for enucleation.

Chappell et al performed gene expression profiling (RNA analysis) on 126 patients with uveal melanoma using tissue harvested by needle biopsy. They identified 64% class 1 (good prognosis) and 36% class 2 (poor prognosis) melanomas. Thicker tumors, epithelioid cell type, and older age correlated with the more ominous class 2 tumors. Unlike previous similar publications, these authors found that tumor class did not predict rate of tumor regression after radiotherapy.

These findings are distinctly contrary to previous reports on this topic. Previous studies from Philadelphia,[2,3] Boston,[4] Jerusalem,[5] and Los Angeles[6] have indicated that high-grade melanoma at greater risk for metastasis (epithelioid cell type, monosomy 3) show more rapid regression after radiotherapy. In this study, class 2 melanomas, designated as high-grade tumors, did not show more rapid regression. This finding, which the authors describe as "surprising" to them, is contradictory to that of previous publications. The authors did not specify why this occurred. We speculate that the disparity could represent an inadequate cohort size for reliable analysis, and we doubt that these experienced clinicians had inaccuracies in treatment parameters or genetic analyses. Despite these findings, this does not detract from the importance of genetic evaluation.

Now is an exciting time for uveal melanoma investigators. Major strides in understanding the development of melanoma emanate from teams around the world, and we anticipate further work will expose the "uveal melanoma code."

C. L. Shields, MD

References

1. Shields CL, Furuta M, Thangappan A, et al. Metastasis of uveal melanoma millimeter-by-millimeter in 8033 consecutive eyes. *Arch Ophthalmol.* 2009;127: 989-998.
2. Augsburger JJ, Gamel JW, Shields JA, Markoe AM, Brady LW. Post-irradiation regression of choroidal melanomas as a risk factor for death from metastatic disease. *Ophthalmology.* 1987;94:1173-1177.
3. Shields CL, Bianciotto C, Rudich D, Materin MA, Ganguly A, Shields JA. Regression of uveal melanoma after plaque radiotherapy and thermotherapy based on chromosome 3 status. *Retina.* 2008;28:1289-1295.
4. Glynn RJ, Seddon JM, Gragoudas ES, Egan KM, Hart LJ. Evaluation of tumor regression and other prognostic factors for early and late metastasis after proton irradiation of uveal melanoma. *Ophthalmology.* 1989;96:1566-1573.
5. Kaiserman I, Anteby I, Chowers I, Blumenthal EZ, Kliers I, Pe'er J. Post-brachytherapy initial tumor regression rate correlates with metastatic spread in posterior uveal melanoma. *Br J Ophthalmol.* 2004;88:892-895.
6. Marathe OS, Wu J, Lee SP, et al. Ocular response of choroidal melanoma with monosomy 3 versus disomy 3 after iodine-125 brachytherapy. *Int J Radiat Oncol Biol Phys.* 2011;81:1046-1048.

11 Pathology

Recommendations for Genetic Testing of Inherited Eye Diseases: Report of
the American Academy of Ophthalmology Task Force on Genetic Testing
Stone EM, Aldave AJ, Drack AV, et al (Foundation of the American Academy of
Ophthalmology, San Francisco, CA)
Ophthalmology 119:2408-2410, 2012

Genetic testing can make a very positive impact on individuals and families affected with inherited eye disease in a number of ways. When properly
performed, interpreted, and acted on, genetic tests can improve the accuracy
of diagnoses and prognoses, can improve the accuracy of genetic counseling,
can reduce the risk of disease occurrence or recurrence in families at risk, and
can facilitate the development and delivery of mechanism-specific care.
However, like all medical interventions, genetic testing has some specific
risks that vary from patient to patient. For example, the results of a genetic
test can affect a patient's plans to have children, can create a sense of anxiety
or guilt, and can even perturb a patient's relationships with other family
members. For these reasons, skilled counseling should be provided to all
individuals who undergo genetic testing to maximize the benefits and minimize the risks associated with each test.

▶ Genetic analysis is becoming an integral part of pathology and clinical practice.
In this report by the American Academy of Ophthalmology Task Force on Genetic
Testing, the leaders in the field, provide general and specific recommendations for
ophthalmologists regarding genetic testing of inherited eye diseases. The role of
presymptomatic testing, parallel testing of numerous genetic loci, and genetic
testing for complex diseases is discussed. The authors recommend offering
genetic tests primarily to patients with Mendelian disorders whose causative
genes have been identified and ensure that the patient receives a copy of a genetic
test report and counseling from a physician with expertise in an inherited disease.
In addition, the article provides guidelines to locating the laboratories and specialists with expertise in genetic testing. The experts caution against direct-to-
consumer genetic testing, unnecessary testing of numerous genetic loci or
complex diseases, and testing of asymptomatic minors for untreatable disorders,
except in extraordinary circumstances.

T. Milman, MD

Diffuse Large B-Cell Lymphoma of the Orbit: Clinicopathologic, Immunohistochemical, and Prognostic Features of 20 Cases
Stacy RC, Jakobiec FA, Herwig MC, et al (Harvard Med School, Boston, MA; Emory Univ School of Medicine, Atlanta, GA; et al)
Am J Ophthalmol 154:87-98, 2012

Purpose.—To evaluate a series of orbital diffuse large B-cell lymphomas (DLBCL) for prognostic features and therapeutic outcomes.

Design.—Retrospective multicenter case study of clinical and immunohistochemical features of 20 patients.

Methods.—Clinical, histopathologic, and immunohistochemical features were correlated with outcomes. Immunohistochemistry for biomarkers including Bcl-6, CD5, CD10, CD20, FOXP1, GCET1, and MUM1 was performed to differentiate between 2 major genetic subtypes of DLBCL: activated B-cell-like (ABC) and germinal center B-cell-like (GCB).

Results.—Sixteen patients presented with unilateral and 4 with bilateral tumors. Three had bony erosion of the orbit on imaging studies. Of 14 patients with detailed follow-ups, 3 had a prior or concurrent lymphomatous disease; 8 had stage I disease (limited to the orbit) at presentation; and 3 were newly diagnosed with systemic (stage IV) DLBCL. Localized disease was treated with combined systemic chemotherapy, including rituximab and radiation with no deaths to date; there was 1 death related to systemic DLBCL. Clinical staging was the best predictive method and no immunohistochemical feature or subcategory (ABC vs GCB) correlated with outcome.

Conclusions.—Primary orbital DLBCL has a more favorable prognosis than systemic DLBCL and may arise from a preexistent hematolymphomatous neoplasm (4 out of 20 cases). In our series, orbital DLBCL had a 57% likelihood of being restricted to the ocular adnexa. Clinical staging was more helpful in predicting outcome than any single immunohistopathologic feature or combination of biomarkers. Orbital radiation of 30 gray in conjunction with systemic chemotherapy with rituximab can achieve disease-specific survival approaching 100% in purely localized cases (Figs 1-3).

▶ Although diffuse large B-cell lymphoma (DLBCL) is the most common nonocular lymphoma, it is rare in the orbit, where extranodal marginal B-cell lymphoma of mucosa-associated tissue type predominates. Nonocular DLBCL is an aggressive disease with an approximately 50% 5-year mortality rate. It has been shown that DLBCL is not a single disease entity but rather a group of histologically similar lymphomas with distinct immunohistochemical, cytogenetic, and molecular genetic profiles. Recent evidence suggests that subtyping of DLBCL in accordance with these parameters is useful in predicting survival.

In this retrospective multicenter study, Stacy and colleagues evaluate the clinical, histopathologic, and immunohistochemical characteristics of ocular adnexal DLBCL from 20 patients and correlate these data with prognosis (Figs 1-3). The outcomes are concordant with previously published data, which show that ocular adnexal DLBCL has high association with diffuse systemic disease (~50%) and,

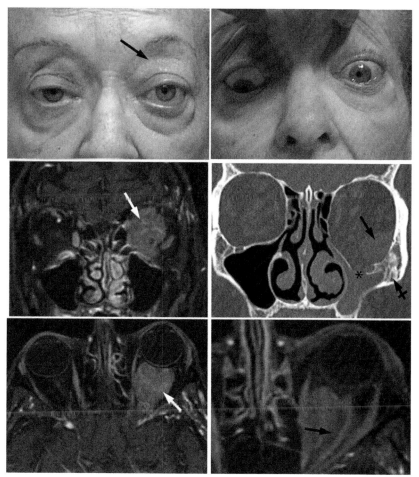

FIGURE 1.—Clinical and radiographic features of diffuse large B-cell lymphoma of the orbit. (Top left) Patient with mass in the left upper orbit (arrow) producing mild, noncongestive proptosis. (Top right) The lesion's mass effect resulted in limited eye movements, including infraduction of the left globe. (Middle left) Typical location of an orbital lymphoid tumor (arrow) in the superior and superonasal regions of the orbit. There is no bone erosion. (Middle right) An unusual inferotemporal tumor (arrow) has created adjacent bone changes (crossed arrow). An old inferior, post-traumatic orbital floor fracture (*) explains the absence of clinical proptosis. (Bottom left) An intraconal, retrobulbar mass (arrow) is accompanied by moderate proptosis (3—4 mm). (Bottom right) In the same patient portrayed in Bottom left, an axial computed tomography image at the level of the optic nerve reveals that the tumor encases it (arrow) asymmetrically, with a more prominent component found nasally. The patient had a decline in visual acuity and an afferent pupillary defect. (Reprinted from American Journal of Ophthalmology. Stacy RC, Jakobiec FA, Herwig MC, et al. Diffuse large B-cell lymphoma of the orbit: clinicopathologic, immunohistochemical, and prognostic features of 20 cases. *Am J Ophthalmol.* 2012;154:87-98, Copyright 2012, with permission from Elsevier.)

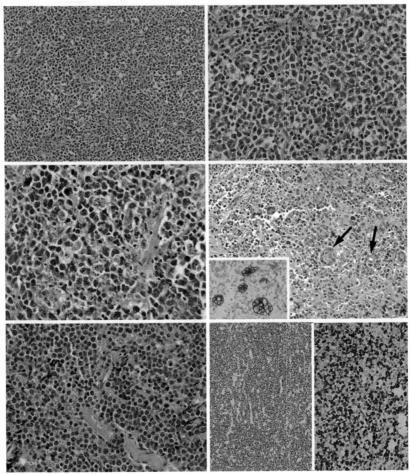

FIGURE 2.—Histopathologic and immunohistochemical features of orbital diffuse large B-cell lymphoma. (Top left) Low-power photomicrograph demonstrates uniform arrangement of the lymphoma cells without a follicular pattern. (Top right) Higher power displays viable cells with irregular nuclei with prominent nucleoli, usually in multiples and arranged peripherally at the nuclear membrane. (Middle left) Karyorrhexis, apoptosis, and cellular debris are prominent. (Middle right) The lacrimal gland is mostly necrotic and invaded by hyperchromatic lymphoma cells. Some remaining acini (arrows) simulating giant cells are highlighted by pancytokeratin staining (inset). (Bottom left) Lymphoplasmacytic lymphoma from the neck of a patient who later developed orbital DLBCL. This original lesion displays smaller cells with more abundant, amphophilic cytoplasm and more compact, rounder nuclei. (Bottom right) Cells staining positive for CD20 (left panel) were discovered in all lesions, and Ki-67 nuclear staining (right panel) was identified in >70% of cells. (All panels hematoxylin-eosin, except for inset from Middle right and 2 panels in Bottom right, which were immunoperoxidase reaction, diaminobenzidine chromogen; original magnifications: 200×, 400×, 400×, 200×, 400×, 200×.) (Reprinted from American Journal of Ophthalmology. Stacy RC, Jakobiec FA, Herwig MC, et al. Diffuse large B-cell lymphoma of the orbit: clinicopathologic, immunohistochemical, and prognostic features of 20 cases. *Am J Ophthalmol.* 2012;154:87-98, Copyright 2012, with permission from Elsevier.)

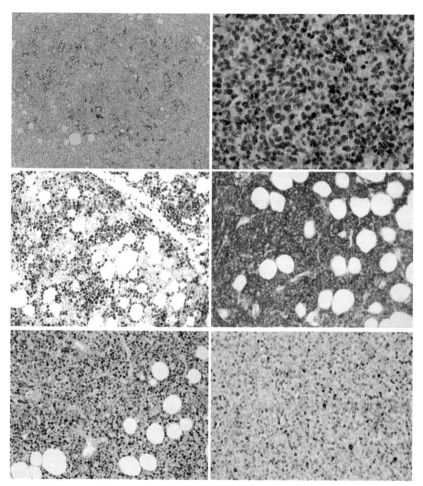

FIGURE 3.—Immunohistochemical features of orbital diffuse large B-cell lymphoma. (Top left) CD21 staining discloses a cluster of widely separated dendritic cells of an orbital DLBCL, suggesting that the tumor arose either from a preexisting extranodal marginal zone or follicular lymphoma. (Top right) FOXP1 staining is positive in >80% of cells. (Middle left) Bcl-6 stains the nuclei of >30% of cells. (Middle right) CD10 stains the cell membranes of the majority of cells in this specimen. Infiltration of the orbital fat is apparent. (Bottom left) MUM1 nuclear positivity is demonstrated at greater than 80% of cells. (Bottom right) MUM1 positivity in this lesion is identified in fewer than 80% of cells. (All panels immunoperoxidase reaction, diaminobenzidine chromogen; original magnifications: 200×, except for upper right: 400×.) (Reprinted from American Journal of Ophthalmology. Stacy RC, Jakobiec FA, Herwig MC, et al. Diffuse large B-cell lymphoma of the orbit: clinicopathologic, immunohistochemical, and prognostic features of 20 cases. *Am J Ophthalmol.* 2012;154:87-98, Copyright 2012, with permission from Elsevier.)

when disseminated, with high mortality. Localized orbital DLBCL, in contrast, has survival rates approaching 100% with appropriate therapy. The authors found no prognostic benefit from immunohistochemical subtyping of DLBCL, but a larger sample size and molecular genetic studies may be required to validate this conclusion.

For enhanced understanding of how aberrations in normal germinal center physiology can give rise to lymphomas, including DLBCL, please read an excellent article by Klein and Dalla-Favera.[1]

T. Milman, MD

Reference

1. Klein U, Dalla-Favera R. Germinal centres: role in B-cell physiology and malignancy. *Nat Rev Immunol.* 2008;8:22-33. www.nature.com/reviews/immunol.

Shrinkage Revisited: How Long Is Long Enough?
Murchison AP, Bilyk JR, Eagle RC Jr, et al (Wills Eye Inst, Philadelphia, PA; et al)
Ophthal Plast Reconstr Surg 28:261-263, 2012

Purpose.—Temporal artery biopsy (TAB) is considered the gold standard in the diagnosis of suspected giant cell arteritis. The most commonly accepted length for an adequate postfixation TAB specimen is 20 mm. There is a reported 2.4-mm mean shrinkage with the fixation process, but to date, there is no data correlating shrinkage after specimen fixation with the biopsy results.

Methods.—A prospective, Institutional Review Board—approved study of all patients undergoing TAB over 1 year was performed. The pre- and postfixation measurements were recorded. Comparison of the pre- and postfixation lengths was performed, and potential correlation was sought with biopsy results and patient gender, age, and race/ethnicity.

Results.—Sixty-two TABs were performed over a 1 year period with 53 (85.5%) negative for giant cell arteritis. The mean shrinkage length was 4.61 mm ± 2.97 overall, and the amount of shrinkage between positive and negative TAB specimens was not significant ($p = 0.43$). Linear regression analysis did not show any correlation between the amount of shrinkage and the length of the specimen or duration in fixative. There was no significant difference between the amount of shrinkage by surgeon ($p = 0.82$), patient gender ($p = 1.00$), or race/ethnicity ($p = 0.695$).

Conclusions.—Surgeons should be aware of the amount of shrinkage of TAB specimens to meet the commonly accepted goal of 20 mm postfixation length. Based on the 4.61-mm mean shrinkage with 2.97-mm standard deviation, a 27.58-mm specimen would have to be obtained to reach the 20-mm goal. Surgeon, patient age, gender, race/ethnicity, and biopsy results did not have a significant impact on the amount of TAB specimen shrinkage (Fig).

▶ Histopathologic evaluation of superficial temporal artery biopsy (TAB) plays an important role in confirming clinically suspected diagnosis of giant cell arteritis (GCA). Adequate sampling of the TAB is essential for accurate histopathologic diagnosis, because GCA is known for its discontinuous involvement of the vessel

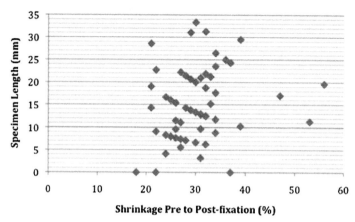

FIGURE.—Scatter plot of specimen length in millimeters (x axis) versus percentage shrinkage of specimen pre- to postfixation (y axis). (Reprinted from Murchison AP, Bilyk JR, Eagle RC Jr, et al. Shrinkage revisited: how long is long enough? *Ophthal Plast Reconstr Surg.* 2012;28:261-263, with permission from The American Society of Ophthalmic Plastic and Reconstructive Surgery, Inc.)

wall, or skip lesions. The optimal recommended TAB length for maximal diagnostic yield varies from study to study, generally ranging from 10 mm to 35 mm. Most ophthalmologists are aware of 2 cm as the recommended cutoff for minimal TAB length. However, not many are aware that this is a postfixation length measurement, and that prefixation biopsy length has to be adjusted to take into account postfixation shrinkage of tissue.

In this prospective masked study, Murchison and colleagues investigated the amount of shrinkage TAB specimens undergo with fixation and if the degree of shrinkage correlates with biopsy results. The study was performed by 2 oculoplastic surgeons using the same surgical technique and by one pathologist masked to the clinical diagnosis; thus, there was uniformity in the measurements obtained. The authors did not find a significant difference in postfixation shrinkage between the positive and negative temporal biopsies. The average shrinkage length was approximately 4.61 mm with approximately 3 mm of standard deviation. This value was not dependent on the surgeon, specimen length, fixation time, patient gender, or ethnicity (Fig). The authors' study showed a greater amount of postfixation shrinkage than previously reported, which is likely related to the measurement technique (the artery was gently straightened without being stretched postfixation) and, possibly, because of the larger sample size in this study (62 biopsies).

Although there is no clear or uniform data in the older literature regarding the exact measurement techniques used in assessing the optimal TAB length, this study provides clear and easily followed guidelines. The proposed rule for TABs: "excise 30 to get 20" will likely be quoted and followed.

T. Milman, MD

Validity of the American College of Rheumatology Criteria for the Diagnosis of Giant Cell Arteritis
Murchison AP, Gilbert ME, Bilyk JR, et al (Wills Eye Inst, Philadelphia, PA)
Am J Ophthalmol 154:722-729, 2012

Purpose.—To assess the clinical utility of the American College of Rheumatology criteria for the diagnosis of giant cell arteritis (GCA) in patients with positive and negative temporal artery biopsies.

Design.—Retrospective case series of all patients undergoing temporal artery biopsy.

Methods.—Retrospective chart review of all patients seen in the Neuro-ophthalmology Service of the Wills Eye Institute undergoing biopsy. One hundred twelve patients were identified between October 2001 and May 2006. Charts were reviewed for American College of Rheumatology criteria, biopsy results, and progression of visual loss after diagnosis.

Results.—Nine of 35 patients (25.7%) with positive biopsies would not have been diagnosed with GCA using American College of Rheumatology criteria alone. An additional 16 patients (45.7%) met only 2 criteria and required the positive biopsy to establish the American College of Rheumatology diagnosis of GCA. Eleven of 39 patients (28.2%) with negative biopsies met the criteria and would have been diagnosed with GCA. Diagnostic agreement between the American College of Rheumatology criteria without biopsy results and biopsy results alone was 51.4%; with the addition of biopsy results to the criteria, this increased to 73.0%.

Conclusions.—The current American College of Rheumatology criteria should not be used to diagnose GCA and all patients suspected of having GCA should undergo a temporal artery biopsy (Fig, Table 2).

▶ According to the American College of Rheumatology (ACR) diagnostic criteria, the diagnosis of giant cell arteritis (GCA) can be made if 3 of 5 criteria are satisfied: 1) age more than 50 years, 2) new onset of localized headache, 3) temporal artery tenderness or decreased temporal artery pulse, 4) erythrocyte sedimentation rate greater than or equal to 50 mm/hour, or 5) positive temporal artery biopsy. Thus, according to the ACR diagnostic criteria, temporal artery biopsy is not essential for diagnosis of GCA, and up to one third of physicians surveyed in one study would not recommend it.[1] It is not widely known that the ACR criteria were established initially for research purposes to distinguish between the different vasculitides in a patient with known vasculitis.[2] In this context, the ACR criteria have a reported sensitivity and specificity of 93.5% and 91.2%, respectively. These values are different if the ACR criteria are used to diagnose GCA in patients with previously undiagnosed vasculitis, especially those presenting to the ophthalmologist with purely ophthalmologic symptoms (approximately 20% of patients with GCA).

In this retrospective case series of patients undergoing temporal artery biopsy for suspected GCA, Murchison et al tried to determine if 1) ACR classification criteria are sufficient to accurately establish the diagnosis of GCA without temporal artery biopsy, and 2) the concordance between the ACR criteria vs

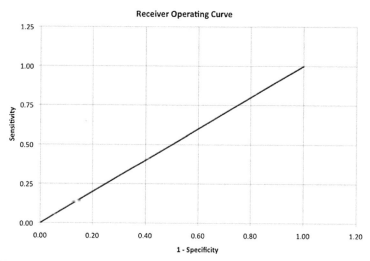

FIGURE.—Receiver operating curve (ROC) for model of comparing American College of Rheumatology criteria and temporal artery biopsy results as diagnostic methods. The area under the curve is 0.500. (Reprinted from American Journal of Ophthalmology. Murchison AP, Gilbert ME, Bilyk JR, et al. Validity of the American College of Rheumatology criteria for the diagnosis of giant cell arteritis. *Am J Ophthalmol.* 2012;154:722-729, Copyright 2012, with permission from Elsevier.)

TABLE 2.—Number of Patients With 1, 2, 3, or 4 American College of Rheumatology Criteria Present Prior to Temporal Artery Biopsy

Number of American College of Rheumatology Criteria Met Before Biopsy	Positive Temporal Artery Biopsy (n = 35)	Negative Temporal Artery Biopsy (n = 39)
1	9 (25.7%)	11 (28.2%)
2	16 (45.7%)	17 (43.9%)
3	8 (22.9%)	10 (25.6%)
4	2 (5.7%)	1 (2.6%)

temporal artery biopsy alone as diagnostic criteria for GCA. The authors found that one fourth of patients with positive biopsies would not have been diagnosed with GCA using the ACR criteria, whereas 28.2% of the patients with negative biopsies would have been diagnosed with GCA based on ACR criteria (Table 2). None of the patients with negative temporal artery biopsies developed GCA-related visual loss when corticosteroids were discontinued immediately after biopsy. The biopsy-positive group demonstrated significant further visual loss following diagnosis of GCA as compared with the biopsy negative group. Diagnostic agreement between the ACR criteria without biopsy results alone was 51.4% and increased to 73% with addition of biopsy results (Fig).

The authors make the following recommendations based on their observations:

1. The current criteria from the ACR should not be used to determine presence or absence of GCA.

2. All patients suspected of GCA should undergo temporal artery biopsy of at least 2 cm in length.
3. All patients with a positive temporal artery biopsy must be treated with systemic corticosteroids, even in the absence of other ACR criteria.
4. Education of all physicians who treat GCA should be undertaken to stress the importance of temporal artery biopsy in establishing the diagnosis of GCA.
5. The results of temporal artery biopsy, and not the ACR criteria, should be used as the only indicator of the presence or absence of disease in research regarding GCA.

Although it is difficult to argue with the first 4 recommendations, it is prudent to emphasize that the fifth statement is worded to guide GCA research, rather than clinical practice. In clinical practice, there is great variability in the surgical and pathologic sampling of temporal artery biopsies, contributing to the histopathologic diagnostic challenges. In addition, there is a subset of "healed" or "indeterminate" temporal artery biopsies, typically in patients on prolonged corticosteroid treatment, which need to be closely correlated with clinical findings.

T. Milman, MD

References

1. Danesh-Meyer HV. Temporal artery biopsy: skip it at your patient's peril. *Am J Ophthalmol.* 2012;154:617-619.
2. Zhou L, Luneau K, Weyand CM, Biousse V, Newman NJ, Grossniklaus HE. Clinicopathologic correlations in giant cell arteritis: a retrospective study of 107 cases. *Ophthalmology.* 2009;116:1574-1580.

BAP1 cancer syndrome: Malignant mesothelioma, uveal and cutaneous melanoma, and MBAITs
Carbone M, Ferris LK, Baumann F, et al (Univ of Hawai'i Cancer Ctr, Honolulu; Univ of Pittsburgh, PA; et al)
J Transl Med 10:179, 2012

Background.—BRCA1–associated protein 1 (*BAP1*) is a tumor suppressor gene located on chromosome 3p21. Germline *BAP1* mutations have been recently associated with an increased risk of malignant mesothelioma, atypical melanocytic tumors and other neoplasms. To answer the question if different germline *BAP1* mutations may predispose to a single syndrome with a wide phenotypic range or to distinct syndromes, we investigated the presence of melanocytic tumors in two unrelated families (L and W) with germline *BAP1* mutations and increased risk of malignant mesothelioma.

Methods.—Suspicious cutaneous lesions were clinically and pathologically characterized and compared to those present in other families carrying *BAP1* mutations. We then conducted a meta-analysis of all the studies reporting *BAP1*-mutated families to survey cancer risk related to the germline BAP1 mutation (means were compared using t-test and proportions were compared with Pearson χ^2 test or two-tailed Fisher's exact test).

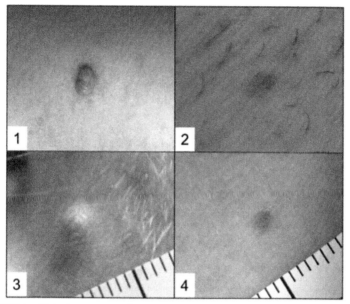

FIGURE 1.—Clinical presentations of MBAITs. MBAITs have variable clinical presentations including pink polypoid papules (1, from shoulder of patient W-F1-IV-9), raised pink papules (2, from groin of L-F1-IV-15), and lightly pigmented papules (3, from cheek of L-F1-IV-4). These lesions were clinically difficult to distinguish from banal dermal nevi, as pictured in (4), which shows a clinically similar lesion also from the chest of the same patient pictured in (2). (Reprinted from Carbone M, Ferris LK, Baumann F, et al. BAP1 cancer syndrome: malignant mesothelioma, uveal and cutaneous melanoma, and MBAITs. *J Transl Med.* 2012;10:179, with permission from Carbone et al.; licensee BioMed Central Ltd.)

Results.—Melanocytic tumors: of the five members of the L family studied, four (80%) carried a germline *BAP1* mutation (p.Gln684*) and also presented one or more atypical melanocytic tumors; of the seven members of W family studied, all carried a germline *BAP1* mutation (p.Pro147fs*48) and four of them (57%) presented one or more atypical melanocytic tumors, that we propose to call "melanocytic *BAP1*-mutated atypical intradermal tumors" (MBAITs). Meta-analysis: 118 individuals from seven unrelated families were selected and divided into a *BAP1*-mutated cohort and a *BAP1*-non-mutated cohort. Malignant mesothelioma, uveal melanoma, cutaneous melanoma, and MBAITs prevalence was significantly higher in the *BAP1*-mutated cohort ($p \leq 0.001$).

Conclusions.—Germline *BAP1* mutations are associated with a novel cancer syndrome characterized by malignant mesothelioma, uveal melanoma, cutaneous melanoma and MBAITs, and possibly by other cancers. MBAITs provide physicians with a marker to identify individuals who may carry germline *BAP1* mutations and thus are at high risk of developing associated cancers (Figs 1 and 2, Table 2).

▶ Although uveal melanoma typically occurs sporadically, a small number of patients demonstrate familial clustering and develop other malignancies, suggestive of a cancer syndrome. Several candidate genes for hereditary uveal melanoma

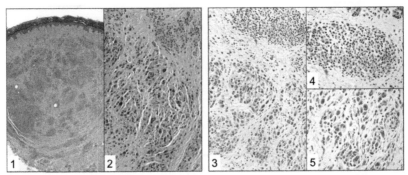

FIGURE 2.—Histology and immunohistochemistry of MBAITs. Representative biopsy from individual W-III-04. The histologic examination (hematoxylin and eosin, H/E, of the nevi at the low power (H&E, 4X Original Magnification) magnification shows an intradermal melanocytic nevus with superficial nests and deeper single melanocytic units. This background melanocytic nevus shows maturation with depth. A second distinct, central, circumscribed population of melanocytes is identified at the mid-reticular dermis (1). This second population of melanocytes on higher power (H&E, 20X Original Magnification) shows variably sized, large epithelioid and spindled melanocytes. There is marked cytologic atypia comprised of pleomorphic, hyperchromatic nuclei (2). The immunohistochemistry for BAP1 demonstrates distinct staining between the background melanocytic nevus and the embedded clusters of atypical epithelioid melanocytes. Identified is strong nuclear positivity in the background melanocytic nevus and negative nuclear staining in the large epithelioid cells (3: BAP-1, 20X Original Magnification). On higher power, the background melanocytes show strong nuclear staining in this superficial nest (4: BAP-1, 40X Original Magnification). Large epithelioid cells with their pleomorphic nuclei demonstrate negative nuclear staining with variable cytoplasmic staining (5: BAP-1, 40X Original Magnification). (Reprinted from Carbone M, Ferris LK, Baumann F, et al. BAP1 cancer syndrome: malignant mesothelioma, uveal and cutaneous melanoma, and MBAITs. *J Transl Med*. 2012;10:179, with permission from Carbone et al.; licensee BioMed Central Ltd.)

have been proposed, including CDKN2A, BRCA2, and p14/ARF. However, germline alterations in any of these genes are extremely rare in uveal melanoma. Recently, BRCA1-associated protein 1 (BAP1) gene on chromosome 3p21 has emerged as another candidate for familial uveal melanoma cancer syndrome. BAP1 encodes a tumor-suppressor protein with varied functions, which are not yet fully understood. Of particular importance in uveal melanoma pathogenesis is BAP1's role as deubiquitinating enzyme. A recent study identified a high frequency (27/57, 47.4%) of somatic mutations in BAP1 in uveal melanoma.[1] Most of the mutations were either truncating or involved the ubiquitin carboxyl terminal hydrolase domain of BAP1 and occurred in tumors with monosomy 3, suggesting that loss of chromosome 3 uncovered a somatic mutation in BAP1. However, a single patient (1.7%) in the study had a germline mutation in BAP1, raising a question of familial uveal melanoma. Several groups have subsequently identified germline mutations in BAP1 in uveal melanoma and demonstrated familial clustering of uveal melanomas and other tumors in these patients. For example, Abdel-Rahman et al identified a pathologic germline truncating BAP1 mutation in 1 of the 53 UM patients studied (1.9%).[2] This mutation segregated in several family members and was identified in other lesions (meningioma and lung adenocarcinoma).

Carbone et al further characterized autosomal dominant BAP1 cancer syndrome through their study of 2 affected families and meta-analysis of all previously published patients (Table 1 in the original article). Of interest, they found that in a patient cohort with germline BAP1 mutation, 18% had uveal melanoma,

TABLE 2.—Comparisons of Gender, Age and Cancer Rates Between *BAP1*-Mutated and Non-Mutated Cohorts

Variable	*BAP1*-Mutated N = 63*	*BAP1*-Nonmutated N = 55	*p*-Value	OR (95%CI)
Gender				
Male	22 (36.7%)	31 (56.4%)		
Female	38 (63.3%)	24 (43.6%)	0.034	-
Age of follow-up				
Number known	46	42		
Mean age (Std. Err.)	53.2 (2.1)	51.0 (2.3)	0.4851	-
At least 1 cancer				
Yes	40 (63.5%)	5 (9.1%)		17.39
No	23 (36.5%)	50 (90.9%)	<0.001	(6.07-49.83)
Malignant mesothelioma				
Yes	13 (21.0%)	0 (0.0%)		
No	49 (79.0%)	55 (100%)	<0.001	-
Uveal melanoma				
Yes	11 (17.7%)	0 (0.0%)		
No	51 (82.3%)	55 (100%)	0.001	-
Cutaneous melanoma				
Yes	8 (12.9%)	0 (0.0%)		
No	54 (87.1%)	55 (100%)	0.007$	-
MBAITs**				
Yes	24 (66.7%)	0 (0.0%)		
No	12 (33.3%)	12 (100%)	<0.001	-
Lung cancer				
Yes	3 (4.8%)	0 (0.0%)		
No	59 (95.2%)	55 (100%)	0.246$	-
Breast cancer***				
Yes	3 (7.9%)	1 (4.1%)		
No	35 (91.9%)	23 (95.9%)	0.621$	-
Renal cancer				
Yes	2 (3.3%)	0 (0.0%)		
No	60 (96.7%)	55 (100%)	0.497$	-

Abbreviations: OR: Odds Ratio, CI: confidence interval.
*62 informative, 1 *BAP1*-mutated patient had cancer of unknown origin.
**Calculated only in individuals belonging to present study, ref. 7 and ref. 10.
***Calculated only in women, -: not calculated; NS: non significant; Std. Err.: standard error.
$Two-tailed Fisher's exact test.

8% had cutaneous melanoma, and 67% had intradermal atypical melanocytic nevoid-like proliferations, which the authors termed MBAITs (melanocytic BAP1-mutated atypical intradermal tumors) (Table 2). These MBAIT lesions clinically present as long-standing, indolent, dermal-based pink to tan nodules and histologically appeared as intradermal lesions composed of large epithelioid and spindled melanocytes, with marked cytologic atypia and pleomorphic, hyperchromatic nuclei, but no appreciable mitotic activity (Figs 1 and 2). Frequent association with a nearby compound or intradermal nevus was also observed. Molecular genetic studies demonstrated germline BAP1 mutations and BRAF (V600E) mutations in all MBAIT lesions.

Although the frequency of germline BAP1 mutations and BAP1 familial cancer syndrome in patients with uveal melanoma appears to be quite small, it is worthy of note for several reasons. Identification of MBAIT lesions, which seem to occur early in BAP1 cancer syndrome, may prompt close oncologic surveillance and enable earlier detection of other tumors, including uveal melanoma. Conversely, in a patient with a known uveal melanoma and new cutaneous dermal-based atypical melanocytic lesion, a misdiagnosis of metastases may be averted through careful histopathologic, immunohistochemical, and molecular genetic investigations.

T. Milman, MD

References

1. Harbour JW, Onken MD, Roberson ED, et al. Frequent mutation of BAP1 in metastasizing uveal melanomas. *Science*. 2010;330:1410-1413.
2. Abdel-Rahman MH, Pilarski R, Cebulla CM, et al. Germline BAP1 mutation predisposes to uveal melanoma, lung adenocarcinoma, meningioma, and other cancers. *J Med Genet*. 2011;48:856-859.

In Vivo Evaluation of Focal Lamina Cribrosa Defects in Glaucoma

Kiumehr S, Park SC, Dorairaj S, et al (New York Eye and Ear Infirmary)

Arch Ophthalmol 130:552-559, 2012

Objectives.—To assess focal lamina cribrosa (LC) defects in glaucoma using enhanced depth imaging optical coherence tomography and to investigate their spatial relationships with neuroretinal rim and visual field loss.

Methods.—Serial horizontal and vertical enhanced depth imaging optical coherence tomographic images of the optic nerve head were obtained from healthy subjects and those with glaucoma. Focal LC defects defined as anterior laminar surface irregularity (diameter, >100 μm; depth, >30 μm) that violates the normal smooth curvilinear contour were investigated regarding their configurations and locations. Spatial consistency was evaluated among focal LC defects, neuroretinal rim thinning/ notching, and visual field defects.

Results.—Forty-six healthy subjects (92 eyes) and 31 subjects with glaucoma (45 eyes) were included. Ninetyeight focal LC defects representing various patterns and severity of laminar tissue loss were found in 34 eyes with glaucoma vs none in the healthy eyes. Seven of 11 eyes with glaucoma with no visible focal LC defect had a deeply excavated optic disc with poor LC visibility. Eleven focal LC defects presented clinically as an acquired pit of the optic nerve, and the others as neuroretinal rim thinning/notching. Focal LC defects preferably occurred in the inferior/inferotemporal far periphery of the LC including its insertion. Eyes with focal LC defects limited to the inferior half of the optic disc had greater sensitivity loss in the superior visual hemifield and vice versa.

Conclusions.—Mechanisms of LC deformation in glaucoma include focal loss of laminar beams, which may cause an acquired pit of the optic nerve in extreme cases. Focal LC defects occur in tandem with neuroretinal rim and visual field loss.

▶ The classic histopathologic characteristics of advanced glaucomatous optic nerve damage include posterior bowing and compression of the lamina cribrosa, associated with axonal atrophy and thickening of the fibrovascular pial septa.

However, not many are aware of the influence of regional variation in normal lamina cribrosa histology on predisposition to glaucomatous axonal damage and of histopathologic changes in the lamina cribrosa in early glaucomatous eyes. In 1981, Quigley and Addicks described the regional differences in the fine structure of the lamina cribrosa in normal cadaveric eyes. They noted that the superior and inferior parts of the lamina at the level of the sclera appear to contain larger pores and thinner connective tissues support for the passage of nerve-fiber bundles than the nasal and temporal parts of the lamina. This observation led the authors to hypothesize that the differences found in laminar structure in these locations may explain the characteristic arcuate scotomatous pattern of early glaucomatous field loss.[1] A decade later, Quigley and colleagues noted the disruption of both collagen and elastin at the laminar insertion sites in human and monkey optic nerve heads with early glaucomatous damage.[2] Recently, Bellezza et al described the histopathologic changes in the lamia cribrosa in an experimental model of early glaucomatous optic neuropathy.[3] The researchers noted significant deformations of the lamina cribrosa with or without an enlargement of the anterior scleral canal opening in the monkey eyes with experimental increased intraocular pressure and early glaucoma.

This study by Kiumehr et al describes the lamina cribrosa defects in glaucomatous eyes using enhanced depth imaging optical coherence tomography (EDI OCT). The authors beautifully correlate the clinical appearance of the optic nerve head and visual field defects with the EDI OCT findings (Figs 1-4 in the original article). The EDI OCT images provide amazing anatomical detail. Although lack of histopathologic correlation is a limitation of the study, this work offers insight into in vivo changes in the lamina cribrosa, which can be potentially affected by postmortem or post-enucleation artifact.

T. Milman, MD

References

1. Quigley HA, Addicks EM. Regional differences in the structure of the lamina cribrosa and their relation to glaucomatous optic nerve damage. *Arch Ophthalmol.* 1981;99:137-143.
2. Quigley HA, Dorman-Pease ME, Brown AE. Quantitative study of collagen and elastin of the optic nerve head and sclera in human and experimental monkey glaucoma. *Curr Eye Res.* 1991;10:877-888.
3. Bellezza AJ, Rintalan CJ, Thompson HW, Downs JC, Hart RT, Burgoyne CF. Deformation of the lamina cribrosa and anterior scleral canal wall in early experimental glaucoma. *Invest Ophthalmol Vis Sci.* 2003;44:623-637.

LOXL1 Deficiency in the Lamina Cribrosa as Candidate Susceptibility Factor for a Pseudoexfoliation-Specific Risk of Glaucoma
Schlötzer-Schrehardt U, Hammer CM, Krysta AW, et al (Univ of Erlangen-Nürnberg, Germany)
Ophthalmology 119:1832-1843, 2012

Purpose.—To test the hypothesis that a primary disturbance in lysyl oxidase-like 1 (LOXL1) and elastin metabolism in the lamina cribrosa of

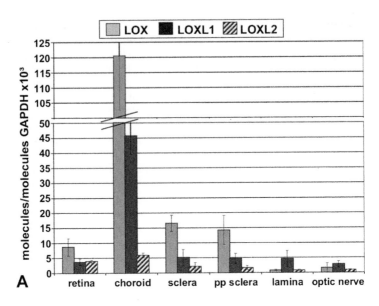

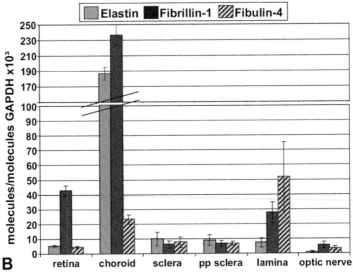

FIGURE 1.—Expression of (**A**) lysyl oxidase isoenzymes LOX, LOXL1, and LOXL2, and (**B**) elastic fiber components in posterior segment tissues from normal human donors (n = 7; mean age, 78.7 ± 7.2 years) using real-time polymerase chain reaction technology. The expression levels were normalized against glyceraldehyde-3-phosphate-dehydrogenase (GAPDH), and the results are expressed as molecules of gene of interest per molecules GAPDH. The values represent mean values ± standard deviation of 6 separate experiments. pp sclera = peripapillary sclera. (Reprinted from Ophthalmology. Schlötzer-Schrehardt U, Hammer CM, Krysta AW, et al. LOXL1 deficiency in the lamina cribrosa as candidate susceptibility factor for a pseudoexfoliation-specific risk of glaucoma. *Ophthalmology.* 2012;119:1832-1843, Copyright 2012, with permission from the American Academy of Ophthalmology.)

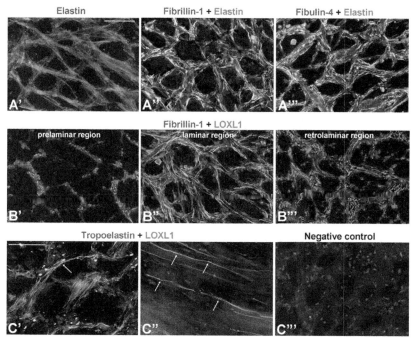

FIGURE 2.—Immunofluorescence labeling of elastic proteins and LOXL1 in cross-sections of the lamina cribrosa of a normal human donor eye (age, 63 years). Positive signals are indicated by green or red fluorescence in contrast to blue fluorescence of nuclei stained with 4,'6-diamidino-2-phenylindole. **A,** Single staining for (**A′**) elastin and double staining for (**A″**) elastin and fibrillin-1 or (**A‴**) elastin and fibulin-4 showing distinct populations of elastic fibers and elastic microfibrils. **B,** Double staining for LOXL1 and fibrillin 1 in the (**B′**) prelaminar, (**B″**) laminar, and (**B‴**) immediate retrolaminar regions showing a predominant location of LOXL1 within astrocytes. **C,** Double staining for LOXL1 and tropoelastin showing colocalization along extracellular elastic fibers (*arrows*) within the (**C′**) laminar beams and the (**C″**) peripapillary sclera. No staining reactions were seen after omission of primary antibodies (**C‴**). Magnification bars = 100 μm in (**A**) and (**B**) and 50 μm in (**C′**) and (**C″**). For interpretation of the references to color in this figure legend, the reader is referred to web version of this article. (Reprinted from Ophthalmology. Schlötzer-Schrehardt U, Hammer CM, Krysta AW, et al. LOXL1 deficiency in the lamina cribrosa as candidate susceptibility factor for a pseudoexfoliation-specific risk of glaucoma. *Ophthalmology*. 2012;119:1832-1843, Copyright 2012, with permission from the American Academy of Ophthalmology.)

eyes with pseudoexfoliation syndrome constitutes an independent risk factor for glaucoma development and progression.

Design.—Observational, consecutive case series.

Participants.—Posterior segment tissues obtained from 37 donors with early and late stages of pseudoexfoliation syndrome without glaucoma, 37 normal age-matched control subjects, 5 eyes with pseudoexfoliation associated open-angle glaucoma, and 5 eyes with primary open-angle glaucoma (POAG).

Methods.—Protein and mRNA expression of major elastic fiber components (elastin, fibrillin-1, fibulin-4), collagens (types I, III, and IV), and lysyl oxidase crosslinking enzymes (LOX, LOXL1, LOXL2) were assessed in situ by quantitative real-time polymerase chain reaction, (immuno)histo-chemistry, and light and electron microscopy. Lysyl oxidase-dependent

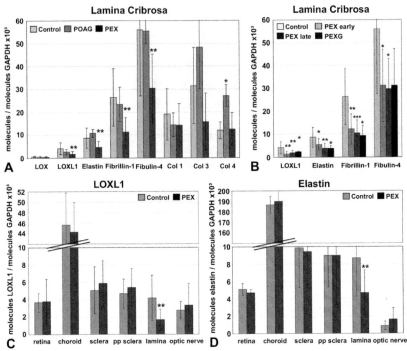

FIGURE 3.—A, Expression of LOX, LOXL1, elastin, fibrillin-1, fibulin-4, collagen type I, collagen type III, and collagen type IV in the lamina cribrosa of normal human donor eyes (control; n = 20), eyes with primary open-angle glaucoma (POAG; n = 5), and eyes with pseudoexfoliation (PEX) syndrome (n = 20) using real-time polymerase chain reaction technology. B, Expression of LOXL1, elastin, fibrillin-1, and fibulin-4 in the lamina cribrosa of normal human donor eyes (control; n = 20), eyes with early stages of pseudoexfoliation (PEX) syndrome (PEX early; n = 10), eyes with late stages of PEX syndrome (PEX late; n = 10), and eyes with PEX-associated open-angle glaucoma (PEXG; n = 5). Expression of (C) LOXL1 and (D) elastin in the retina, choroid, sclera, peripapillary (pp) sclera, lamina cribrosa, and optic nerve of normal human control eyes compared with eyes from patients with PEX syndrome (n = 20 for each patient group). The expression levels were normalized against glyceraldehyde-3-phosphate-dehydrogenase (GAPDH), and the results are expressed as molecules of gene of interest per molecules GAPDH (*P = 0.05, **P = 0.001, ***P = 0.0001). (Reprinted from Ophthalmology. Schlötzer-Schrehardt U, Hammer CM, Krysta AW, et al. LOXL1 deficiency in the lamina cribrosa as candidate susceptibility factor for a pseudoexfoliation-specific risk of glaucoma. Ophthalmology. 2012;119:1832-1843, Copyright 2012, with permission from the American Academy of Ophthalmology.)

elastin fiber assembly was assessed by primary optic nerve head astrocytes in vitro.

Main Outcome Measures.—Expression levels of elastic proteins, collagens, and lysyl oxidases in the lamina cribrosa.

Results.—Lysyl oxidase-like 1 proved to be the major lysyl oxidase isoform in the normal lamina cribrosa in association with a complex elastic fiber network. Compared with normal and POAG specimens, lamina cribrosa tissues obtained from early and late stages of pseudoexfoliation syndrome without and with glaucoma consistently revealed a significant coordinated downregulation of LOXL1 and elastic fiber constituents on mRNA and protein level. In contrast, expression levels of collagens and

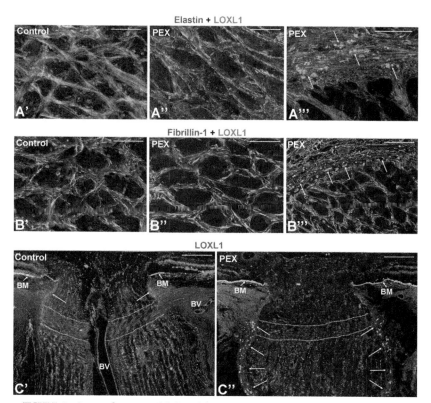

FIGURE 5.—Immunofluorescence labeling of elastic proteins and LOXL1 in optic nerve head tissue of normal human donor eyes and eyes with pseudoexfoliation (PEX) syndrome. Nuclei are stained with 4,′6-diamidino-2-phenylindole (blue fluorescence) in (A) and (B) or with propidium iodide (red fluorescence) in (C). A, Double staining for LOXL1 (red) and elastin (green) showing decreased LOXL1 immunoreactivity and irregular elastin staining in cross-sections of the lamina cribrosa of (A″) PEX syndrome eyes compared with (A′) normal eyes. Pseudoexfoliation material aggregates demonstrating immunopositive labeling for both LOXL1 and elastin (orange, arrows) accumulate in the peripapillary sclera of (A‴) PEX syndrome eyes. B, Double staining for LOXL1 (red) and fibrillin-1 (green) showing decreased LOXL1 immunoreactivity but regular fibrillin staining in the lamina cribrosa of (B″) PEX syndrome eyes as compared with (B′) normal eyes. Pseudoexfoliation material aggregates immunopositive for both LOXL1 and fibrillin-1 (orange, arrows) accumulate in the peripapillary sclera of (B‴) PEX syndrome eyes. C, Sagittal section through the optic nerve head of a (C′) normal eye showing widespread immunostaining for LOXL1 (green) in Bruch's membrane (BM), lamina cribrosa (dotted lines), peripapillary sclera (arrows), and blood vessel (BV) walls. Optic nerve head tissue of a (C″) PEX syndrome eye shows reduced LOXL1 immunostaining within the lamina cribrosa (*dotted lines*), but accumulation of LOXL1-positive PEX material aggregates (arrows) within the peripapillary sclera and optic nerve sheaths. Magnification bars = 100 μm in (A′), (A″), (B′), and (B″); 50 μm in (A‴); 200 μm in (B‴); and 1000 μm in (C′) and (C″). For interpretation of the references to color in this figure legend, the reader is referred to web version of this article. (Reprinted from Ophthalmology. Schlötzer-Schrehardt U, Hammer CM, Krysta AW, et al. LOXL1 deficiency in the lamina cribrosa as candidate susceptibility factor for a pseudoexfoliation-specific risk of glaucoma. *Ophthalmology.* 2012;119:1832-1843, Copyright 2012, with permission from the American Academy of Ophthalmology.)

other lysyl oxidase isoforms were not affected. Dysregulated expression of LOXL1 and elastic proteins was associated with pronounced (ultra)structural alterations of the elastic fiber network in the laminar beams of pseudoexfoliation syndrome eyes. Inhibition of LOXL1 interfered with elastic fiber assembly by optic nerve head astrocytes in vitro.

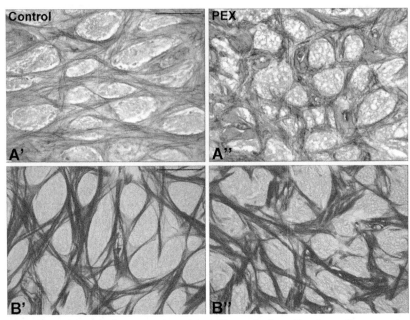

FIGURE 6.—Histomorphometric analysis of elastic fibers and collagen fibers in paraffin cross-sections of the lamina cribrosa of a normal human donor eye (age, 78 years) and an eye with pseudoexfoliation (PEX) syndrome (age, 77 years). A, Light microscopic appearance of representative areas of the lamina cribrosa analyzed for purple-stained elastin fibers using Weigert's resorcin-fuchsin in (**A′**) normal and (**A″**) PEX syndrome tissue specimens. B, Light microscopic appearance of representative areas of the lamina cribrosa analyzed for red-stained collagen fibers using picrosirius red in (**B′**) normal and (**B″**) PEX syndrome tissue specimens. Magnification bars = 100 μm. For interpretation of the references to color in this figure legend, the reader is referred to web version of this article. (Reprinted from Ophthalmology Schlötzer-Schrehardt U, Hammer CM, Krysta AW, et al. LOXL1 deficiency in the lamina cribrosa as candidate susceptibility factor for a pseudoexfoliation-specific risk of glaucoma. *Ophthalmology.* 2012;119:1832-1843, Copyright 2012, with permission from the American Academy of Ophthalmology.)

Conclusions.—The findings provide evidence for a pseudoexfoliation-specific elastinopathy of the lamina cribrosa resulting from a primary disturbance in LOXL1 regulation and elastic fiber homeostasis, possibly rendering pseudoexfoliation syndrome eyes more vulnerable to pressure-induced optic nerve damage and glaucoma development and progression (Figs 1-3 and 5-7).

▶ The pseudoexfoliation process has been shown to be a significant risk factor for glaucomatous optic nerve damage and progression, independent of intraocular pressure. This condition has been characterized as a systemic elastosis, associated with excessive production and abnormal aggregation of elastic proteins, such as elastin and fibrillin-1, into pseudoexfoliation fibrils. Recent genetic studies have demonstrated that polymorphisms in lysyl oxidase-like 1 (LOXL1) gene, a member of the lysyl oxidase family of cross-linking matrix enzymes, play a major role in the development of pseudoexfoliation syndrome and pseudoexfoliation glaucoma. LOXL1 is involved in formation and stabilization of elastic fibers by means of cross-linking tropoelastin monomers into elastin polymers. It has been suggested that abnormalities of elastic components of the

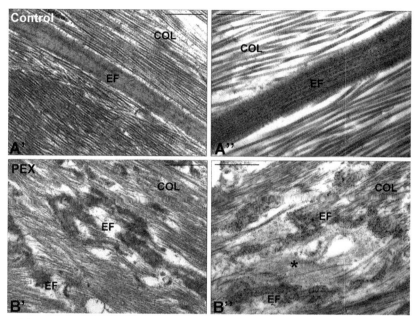

FIGURE 7.—Transmission electron micrographs showing the ultrastructure and anti-elastin immuno-gold staining patterns of elastic fibers in the laminar beams of a normal human donor eye (age, 79 years) and an eye with pseudoexfoliation (PEX) syndrome (age, 83 years). A, Elastic fibers (EFs) with (A′) normal structure and (A″) homogenous anti-elastin immunoreactivity in control tissue. B, Abnormal EFs showing a (B′) moth-eaten structure and consisting of (B″) elastin-positive patches interspersed with amorphous material (asterisks) in PEX syndrome tissue. COL = collagen fibers. Magnification bars = 1 μm. (Reprinted from Ophthalmology. Schlötzer-Schrehardt U, Hammer CM, Krysta AW, et al. LOXL1 deficiency in the lamina cribrosa as candidate susceptibility factor for a pseudoexfoliation-specific risk of glaucoma. *Ophthalmology* 2012;119:1832-1843, Copyright 2012, with permission from the American Academy of Ophthalmology.)

lamina cribrosa are responsible in part for manifestations of glaucoma in patients with pseudoexfoliation syndrome, but whether these abnormalities are primary or secondary to elevated intraocular pressure has been debated.

In this observational, consecutive case series, Schlötzer-Schrehardt et al performed direct sequencing for LOXL1 gene polymorphisms of complementary DNA from 10 donor eyes with early pseudoexfoliation syndrome without glaucoma, 10 donor eyes with late pseudoexfoliation syndrome without glaucoma, and 20 age-matched control eyes. In addition, gene expression studies for lysyl oxidases and elastic fiber proteins were carried out. These molecular genetic studies were also performed on 5 eyes enucleated for end-stage pseudoexfoliation glaucoma and 5 eyes enucleated for end-stage primary open angle glaucoma (POAG). In addition, immunofluorescence analysis for LOXL1, elastin, and fibrillin was performed on 7 donor eyes with pseudoexfoliation syndrome without glaucoma and 7 age-matched controls. Three donor eyes with pseudoexfoliation syndrome and 3 age-matched control eyes were studied with transmission electron microscopy and immunogold labeling with antielastin antibodies. Seven archival eyes with pseudoexfoliation syndrome and age-matched normal control eyes were studied histochemically for elastin and collagen fibers. Lastly, the investigators performed an in vitro elastogenesis assay to assess elastic fiber assembly of normal donor optic nerve head astrocytes cultured with and without LOX inhibitor. The authors found that LOXL1 was the most abundant lysyl oxidase isoform in normal lamina cribrosa, where it is localized primarily to astrocytes in association with complex elastic fiber network, and occasionally colocalized with tropoelastin, supporting the notion of its functional role as a key enzyme in elastic fiber stabilization and maintenance (Figs 1 and 2). This assumption was also supported by in vitro inhibition studies showing that lysyl oxidase cross-linking is required for elastin deposition to the extracellular matrix and for elastic fiber assembly by cultured optic nerve head astrocytes. The investigators observed a statistically significant downregulation of LOXL1 and elastic proteins, both on the messenger RNA and protein levels in the lamina cribrosa of eyes with pseudoexfoliation syndrome and pseudoexfoliation glaucoma, when compared with the age-matched controls and POAG controls (Figs 3 and 5). Furthermore, pseudoexfoliation eyes demonstrated pronounced structural alterations of elastic fibers in the laminar beams when compared with age-matched controls (Fig 6 and 7).

These cumulative data provide evidence that suggests that a primary disturbance in LOXL1 regulation and elastin metabolism negatively affects the structural and biomechanical properties of the lamina cribrosa in the early stages of pseudoexfoliation syndrome, thereby increasing the susceptibility of the optic nerve to intraocular pressure—induced damage.

T. Milman, MD

Differentiation of Malignant Melanoma From Benign Nevus Using a Novel Genomic Microarray With Low Specimen Requirements
Chandler WM, Rowe LR, Florell SR, et al (Dominion Pathology Laboratories, Norfolk, VA; ARUP Inst for Clinical and Experimental Pathology, Salt Lake City, UT; Univ of Utah, Salt Lake City)
Arch Pathol Lab Med 136:947-955, 2012

Context.—Histologic examination of clinically suspicious melanocytic lesions is very sensitive and specific for the detection of malignant melanoma. Yet, the malignant potential of a small percentage of melanocytic lesions remains histologically uncertain. Molecular testing offers the potential to detect the genetic alterations that lead to malignant behavior without overt histologic evidence of malignancy.

Objective.—To differentiate benign melanocytic nevi from malignant melanoma and to predict the clinical course of melanocytic lesions with ambiguous histology using a novel genomic microarray.

Design.—We applied a newly developed single-nucleotide polymorphism genomic microarray to formalin-fixed, paraffin-embedded melanocytic lesions to differentiate benign nevi (n = 23) from malignant melanoma (n = 30) and to predict the clinical course of a set of histologically ambiguous melanocytic lesions (n = 11).

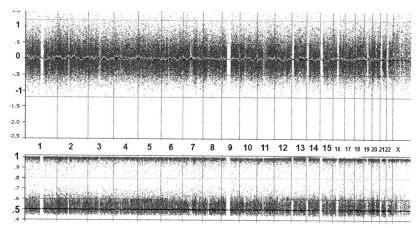

FIGURE 1.—Genome-wide view of probe signal intensity for a benign melanocytic nevus. There are no significant gains or losses of chromosomal material (upper plot) or loss of heterozygosity (lower plot). The y-axis of the upper plot is the number of copies, with normal diploid (2 copies) normalized to 0. The y-axis of the lower plot is dominant allele frequency, with .5 representing a heterozygous state and 1 representing a homozygous state. The x-axis is the chromosome number. (Reproduced with permission of College of American Pathologists. Chandler WM, Rowe LR, Florell SR, et al. Differentiation of malignant melanoma from benign nevus using a novel genomic microarray with low specimen requirements. *Arch Pathol Lab Med.* 2012;136:947-955, permission conveyed through Copyright Clearance Center, Inc.)

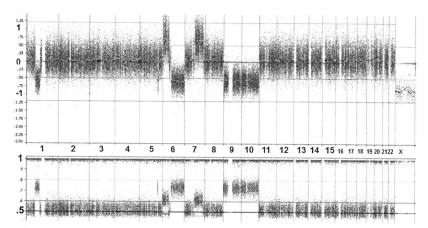

FIGURE 2.—Genome-wide view of probe signal intensity of a malignant melanoma from the arm of a 36-year-old man. The patient died of metastatic melanoma 3 years later. Note the abrupt gains and losses of chromosomal material, characteristic of malignant melanoma (upper plot). The gains and losses correlate well with the dominant allele frequency plot (lower plot), adding further confidence to the copy number calls. The y-axis of the upper plot is the number of copies, with normal diploid (2 copies) normalized to 0. The y-axis of the lower plot is dominant allele frequency, with .5 representing a heterozygous state and 1 representing a homozygous state. The x-axis is the chromosome number. (Reproduced with permission of College of American Pathologists. Chandler WM, Rowe LR, Florell SR, et al. Differentiation of malignant melanoma from benign nevus using a novel genomic microarray with low specimen requirements. *Arch Pathol Lab Med.* 2012;136:947-955, permission conveyed through Copyright Clearance Center, Inc.)

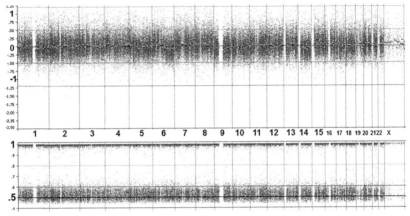

FIGURE 3.—Genome-wide view of probe signal intensity that consensus determined to be equivocal—possibly representing malignant melanoma, possibly representing a benign nevus. Note the subtle copy number decline in 6q and all of chromosome 9. This is a sample of a malignant melanoma from the cheek of a 26-year-old woman who has had no further evidence of disease with 6 years of follow-up. If the subtle copy number changes are real, the low amplitude could have resulted from dilution of the undissected tumor sample with a large quantity of normal-tissue DNA, or alternatively, only a small percentage of tumor cells may have contained the chromosomal copy number aberrations. The y-axis of the upper plot is the number of copies, with normal diploid (2 copies) normalized to 0. The y-axis of the lower plot is dominant allele frequency, with .5 representing a heterozygous state and 1 representing a homozygous state. The x-axis is the chromosome number. (Reproduced with permission of College of American Pathologists Chandler WM, Rowe LR, Florell SR, et al. Differentiation of malignant melanoma from benign nevus using a novel genomic microarray with low specimen requirements. *Arch Pathol Lab Med.* 2012;136:947-955, permission conveyed through Copyright Clearance Center, Inc.)

Results.—For cases with unambiguous histology, there was excellent sensitivity and specificity for identifying malignant melanoma with this genomic microarray (89% sensitivity, 100% specificity). For cases with ambiguous histology, the performance of this genomic microarray was less impressive.

Conclusions.—Without microdissection and with quantities of DNA one-tenth what is required for more commonly used microarrays, this microarray can differentiate between malignant melanoma and benign melanocytic nevi. For histologically ambiguous lesions, longer clinical follow-up is needed to confidently determine the sensitivity and specificity of this microarray. Some of the previous technical hurdles to the clinical application of genomic microarray technology are being overcome, and the advantages over targeted fluorescence in situ hybridization assays currently in clinical use are becoming apparent (Figs 1-6, Table 1).

▶ The accurate diagnosis of cutaneous melanocytic lesions, typically based on clinical characteristics coupled with microscopic examination, can be challenging. As a result, there has been an ongoing search for optimal molecular genetic technique to facilitate differentiation between the benign and malignant cutaneous melanocytic proliferations. Recent studies have described the usefulness of comparative genomic hybridization (CGH, array/microarray CGH) and

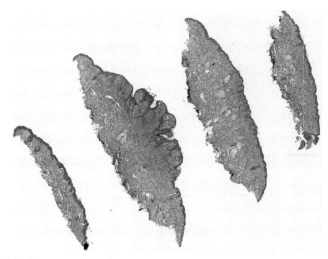

FIGURE 4.—Low-power image of the malignant melanoma from the cheek of a 26-year-old woman shown in Fig 3. Note the large amount of normal tissue (epidermis, dermis, and adnexa). This melanoma is nevoid and may be arising in a preexisting nevus (hematoxylin-eosin, original magnification ×20). (Reproduced with permission of College of American Pathologists. Chandler WM, Rowe LR, Florell SR, et al. Differentiation of malignant melanoma from benign nevus using a novel genomic microarray with low specimen requirements. *Arch Pathol Lab Med.* 2012;136:947-955, permission conveyed through Copyright Clearance Center, Inc.)

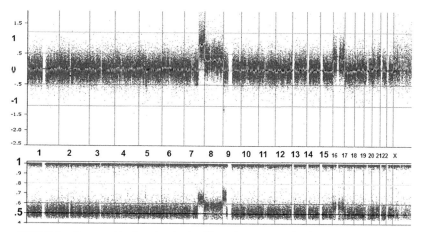

FIGURE 5.—Genome-wide view of probe signal intensity for a case of malignant melanoma from the arm of an 85-year-old woman. The upper plot shows chromosome 9 to be copy number—neutral (diploid). The lower plot reveals a loss of heterozygosity involving the majority of the short arm of chromosome 9. In sum, this is a copy number—neutral loss of heterozygosity. Also of note, the copy number changes detected in this malignant melanoma did not involve regions targeted by the melanoma fluorescent in situ hybridization assay. The y-axis of the upper plot is the number of copies, with normal diploid (2 copies) normalized to 0. The y-axis of the lower plot is dominant allele frequency, with .5 representing a heterozygous state and 1 representing a homozygous state. The x-axis is the chromosome number. (Reproduced with permission of College of American Pathologists. Chandler WM, Rowe LR, Florell SR, et al. Differentiation of malignant melanoma from benign nevus using a novel genomic microarray with low specimen requirements. *Arch Pathol Lab Med.* 2012;136:947-955, permission conveyed through Copyright Clearance Center, Inc.)

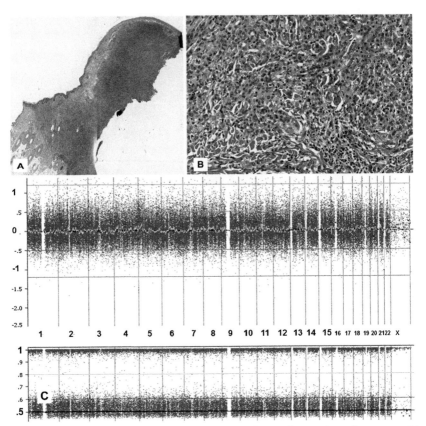

FIGURE 6.—A, Low-power view of the melanocytic lesion of uncertain malignant potential (MLUMP) from a 19-year-old who developed a positive sentinel lymph node (SLN). B, Higher-power view of the MLUMP lesion from a 19-year-old who developed a positive SLN. C, Genome-wide view of probe signal intensity for the primary MLUMP lesion from a 19-year-old who developed a positive SLN. There are no significant gains or losses of chromosomal material or loss of heterozygosity, making it indistinguishable from a benign melanocytic nevus. The y-axis of the upper plot is the number of copies, with normal diploid (2 copies) normalized to 0. The y-axis of the lower plot is dominant allele frequency, with .5 representing a heterozygous state and 1 representing a homozygous state. The x-axis is the chromosome number (hematoxylin-eosin, original magnifications ×20 [A] and ×200 [B]). (Reproduced with permission of College of American Pathologists. Chandler WM, Rowe LR, Florell SR, et al. Differentiation of malignant melanoma from benign nevus using a novel genomic microarray with low specimen requirements. *Arch Pathol Lab Med.* 2012;136:947-955, permission conveyed through Copyright Clearance Center, Inc.)

fluorescence in situ hybridization (FISH) in the diagnosis of cutaneous melanocytic tumors. Some of the limitations of these techniques include lack of widespread availability of molecular diagnostic methods, the expense of molecular diagnostic testing, relatively large tissue sample requirement (array CGH), and the potential for low sensitivity in the diagnosis of malignant melanoma (FISH, 60%-87%).[1,2]

The study by Chandler and colleagues describes the researchers' experience with a novel single nucleotide polymorphism (SNP) genomic microarray

TABLE.—Diagnosis, Clinical Follow-Up, and Genomic Microarray Designation of Melanocytic Lesions of Uncertain Malignant Potential

Diagnosis[a]	Anatomic Location	Age at Biopsy, y/Sex	Length of Follow-up, y	Clinical Outcome	Consensus Array Call
Severely atypical compound melanocytic neoplasm, worrisome for nevoid melanoma	Postauricular	18/F	0.2	SLN+	N
Unusual Spitz nevus	Cheek	33/F	0.1	LTFU	N
Compound Spitz nevus with mild atypia	Thigh	40/F	0	LTFU	N
Favor malignant melanoma in situ developing within a Spitz	Shin	37/F	6.5	NED	N
Somewhat markedly atypical Spitz nevus	Calf	23/M	3	NED	MM
Atypical compound Spitz nevus	Knee	15/T	5.5	NED	N
Compound spitzoid melanocytic lesion of indeterminate biologic potential	Lower abdomen	24/M	3.8	NED	N
Favor malignant melanoma [with Spitz features]	Upper back	35/M	3.2	OPM	MM
Ulcerated, mitotically active Spitz nevus	Midfoot	5/M	0	LTFU	N
Atypical spindle and epithelioid cell nevus (Spitz)	Anterior calf	49/F	16.4	NED	MM
Atypical epithelioid and spindle cell dermal [melanocytic] neoplasm	Lower back	4/M	0	LTFU	MM

Abbreviations: LTFU, lost to follow-up; MM, malignant melanoma; N, benign nevus; NED, no evidence of additional related disease; OPM, other primary melanomas; SLN+, positive sentinel lymph node biopsy.
[b] Designation rendered by participating authors based solely upon the single-nucleotide polymorphism genomic microarray whole-genome view for the sample.
[a] Diagnosis rendered by the dermatopathologist at the time of biopsy. Text in brackets [] was not in the diagnostic line, but was mentioned elsewhere in the report.

(GMA) in confirming the microscopic diagnosis of melanoma and nevus and in refining the diagnosis in melanocytic lesions of uncertain malignant potential (MLUMPs). Genomic microarray hybridization was performed on the formalin-fixed, paraffin-embedded tissue. The authors analyzed 64 melanocytic lesions: 23 benign nevi, 27 primary malignant melanomas, 3 metastatic melanomas (all from different body sites on the same patient), and 11 MLUMPs (Figs 1-5, Table). The microarray employed 330 000 molecular inversion probes targeting SNPs spanning the genome to identify changes in copy number and loss of heterozygosity. The advantages of this molecular genetic diagnostic methodology include the small DNA sample requirement (50 ng of DNA) and the breadth and quantifiable detail of the results.

Although the results of this study are encouraging, they highlight the limitations of the current molecular genetic diagnostic methods. Although SNP-based molecular inversion probe GMA appears to be a sensitive and highly specific method for detecting melanoma in the cohort with a definitive histologic diagnosis (89% sensitivity, 100% specificity), its ability to predict the malignant potential in cases with ambiguous histologic diagnosis is less impressive. Of the 11 MLUMPs analyzed, 4 showed gains and losses consistent with malignant melanoma but had a benign clinical course. Conversely, one MLUMP displayed malignant behavior but had an SNP-GMA pattern consistent with a benign nevus (Fig 6, Table).

Despite the limitations of this assay, the authors predict that the breadth and specificity of information available from an SNP-GMA will make this technology cost-effective, particularly as mutation-specific therapies for malignant melanoma become standard. In addition to enhancing the diagnostic accuracy, this assay can be optimized to screen for clinically relevant SNPs, such as the BRAF V600E, thereby playing a role in directing the potential targeted therapies.

Although there is currently no ideal molecular genetic method to accurately diagnose histologically ambiguous melanocytic lesions, this study and the recent research in the field offer hope that cost-effective, widely available, sensitive, and specific molecular genetic testing for melanocytic lesions will soon become a reality.

T. Milman, MD

References

1. Bauer J, Bastian BC. Distinguishing melanocytic nevi from melanoma by DNA copy number changes: comparative genomic hybridization as a research and diagnostic tool. *Dermatol Ther.* 2006;19:40-49.
2. Gerami P, Li G, Pouryazdanparast P, et al. A highly specific and discriminatory FISH assay for distinguishing between benign and malignant melanocytic neoplasms. *Am J Surg Pathol.* 2012;36:808-817.

Immunocytochemical Diagnosis as Inflammation by Vitrectomy Cell Blocks in Patients with Vitreous Opacity

Matsuo T, Ichimura K (Okayama Univ Med School and Okayama Univ Graduate School of Medicine, Japan)
Ophthalmology 119:827-837, 2012

Purpose.—To describe the clinical and cytopathologic characteristics in patients with vitreous opacity of unknown cause or preceding inflammation, diagnosed cytopathologically as inflammation.

Design.—Retrospective case series.

Participants.—Forty-three consecutive patients (61 eyes) who underwent vitrectomy for vitreous opacity of unknown cause or preceding inflammation and were diagnosed cytopathologically with inflammation at one institution in 6 years from 2005 to 2010. During the same period, 11 consecutive patients with vitreous opacity of unknown cause were diagnosed cytopathologically with lymphoma (large B-cell lymphoma) and were excluded from the study.

Methods.—Cell blocks were made by centrifugation of vitrectomy fluid and embedded in paraffin for immunocytochemistry.

Main Outcome Measures.—Cytopathologic and immunocytochemical diagnosis using vitrectomy cell blocks.

Results.—Histiocytes (macrophages), small lymphocytes, neutrophils, and eosinophils were predominant cells, with no atypical large cells on hematoxylin—eosin staining. Immunocytochemically, most predominant cells were CD68-positive histiocytes (macrophages), followed by CD3-positive

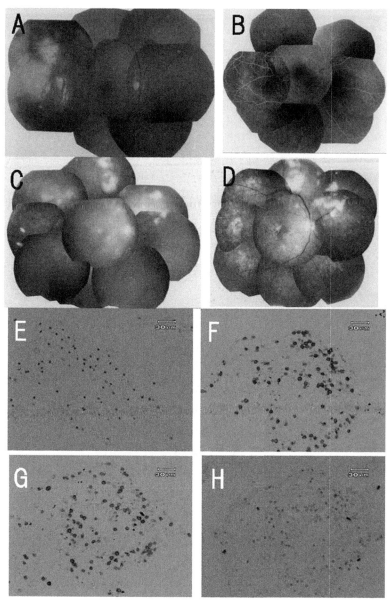

FIGURE 1.—Case 1: a 74-year-old woman. Merged fundus photographs (**A**) and fluorescein angiograms (**B**) of the right eye in December 2002, showing yellowish subretinal lesions with minimal fluorescein leakage in the temporal midperiphery. New yellowish subretinal lesions appear in the upper half midperiphery and in the macular area, whereas the initial lesion in the temporal midperiphery resolved in July 2005 when vitrectomy was performed for concurrent vitreous opacity (**C**, before vitrectomy; **D**, after vitrectomy). A hematoxylin and eosin stain (**E**) of the vitrectomy specimen of the right eye shows predominant small lymphocytes that are positive for CD3 (**F**) and CD5 (**G**), but negative for CD20 (**H**). For interpretation of the references to color in this figure legend, the reader is referred to web version of this article. (Reprinted from Ophthalmology. Matsuo T, Ichimura K. Immunocytochemical diagnosis as inflammation by vitrectomy cell blocks in patients with vitreous opacity. *Ophthalmology*. 2012;119:827-837, Copyright 2012, with permission from the American Academy of Ophthalmology.)

232 / Ophthalmology

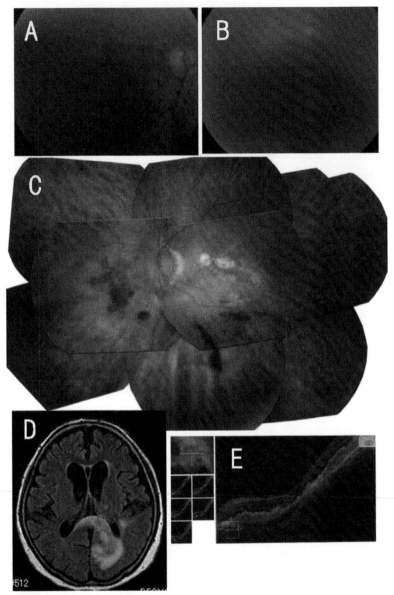

FIGURE 2.—Case 34: a 77-year-old woman with preceding brain diffuse large B-cell lymphoma in November 2008. Vitreous opacity in the right eye (**A**) and opacity with yellowish retinal lesions in the left eye (**B**) in November 2009. Merged fundus photographs in the left eye (**C**) in December 2009 after vitrectomy. Recurrent brain lymphoma (**D**) in February 2010. Optical coherence tomography scan of the left eye (**E**) in December 2009 at the same time of **C**, showing subretinal infiltration. For interpretation of the references to color in this figure legend, the reader is referred to web version of this article. (Reprinted from Ophthalmology. Matsuo T, Ichimura K. Immunocytochemical diagnosis as inflammation by vitrectomy cell blocks in patients with vitreous opacity. *Ophthalmology*. 2012;119:827-837, Copyright 2012, with permission from the American Academy of Ophthalmology.)

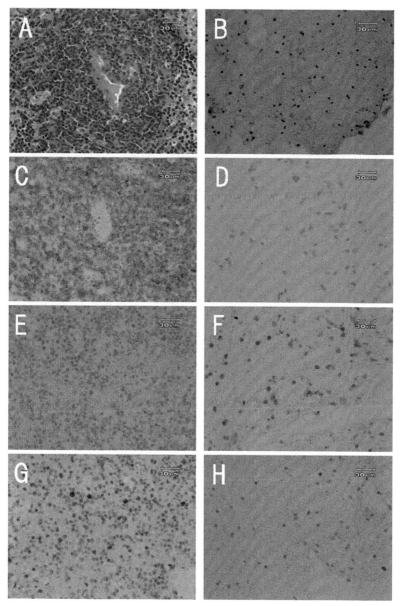

FIGURE 3.—Case 34: a 77-year-old woman. Brain biopsy at the initial presentation in November 2008 (*left column*) shows large cells infiltrating around a blood vessel (hematoxylin and eosin [H&E] stain in **A**) that are positive for CD20 (**C**), negative for CD3 (**E**), and positive for Ki67 (**G**), consistent with the diagnosis of diffuse large B-cell lymphoma. In contrast, vitrectomy specimen in the left eye in November 2009 (*right column*) shows small lymphocytes (H&E stain in **B**) that are negative for CD20 (**D**), positive for CD3 (**F**), and negative for Ki67 (**H**). (Reprinted from Ophthalmology. Matsuo T, Ichimura K. Immunocytochemical diagnosis as inflammation by vitrectomy cell blocks in patients with vitreous opacity. *Ophthalmology*. 2012;119:827-837, Copyright 2012, with permission from the American Academy of Ophthalmology.)

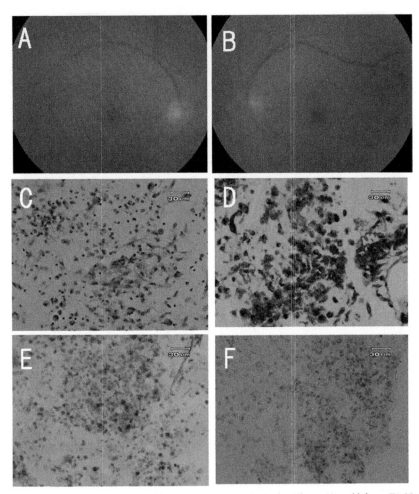

FIGURE 4.—Case 36: a 64-year-old woman. Vitreous opacity in the right eye (A) and left eye (B). No retinal lesions are present in either eye. A hematoxylin and eosin stain (C) of vitrectomy specimen in the right eye shows histiocytes that are positive for CD68 (D). Small lymphocytes are positive for CD3 (E) but negative for CD20 (F). (Reprinted from Ophthalmology. Matsuo T, Ichimura K. Immunocytochemical diagnosis as inflammation by vitrectomy cell blocks in patients with vitreous opacity. *Ophthalmology.* 2012;119:827-837, Copyright 2012, with permission from the American Academy of Ophthalmology.)

T cells, but CD20- or CD79a-positive B cells were rarely present. Epithelioid cells, positive for CD68, were found in 4 patients with or without an established diagnosis of sarcoidosis, and giant multinucleated cells were found in 2 patients with suspected preceding self-limiting Vogt-Koyanagi-Harada disease, based on the presence of depigmented red fundi. Inflammation was diagnosed in 2 patients with vitreous opacity who had a preceding onset of brain lymphoma or systemic lymphoma.

Conclusions.—The presence of macrophages, combined with small T lymphocytes, was a major sign in intravitreal inflammation, manifesting

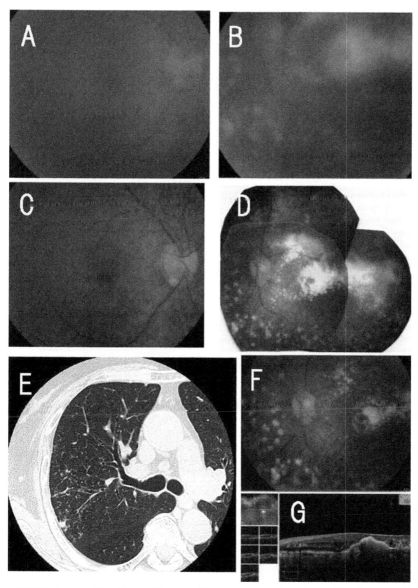

FIGURE 5.—Case 39: a 78-year-old woman. Vitreous opacity in the right eye (**A**) and opacity with yellowish retinal lesions in the left eye (**B**) in May 2010. The right fundus photograph (**C**) and left fundus photograph (**D**) after vitrectomy. Chest computed tomography (**E**) in May 2010 after vitrectomy, showing granular lesions in the bilateral lung fields. The fundus photograph (**F**) and optical coherence tomography (**G**) scan of the left eye in September 2010, showing that yellowish subretinal lesions have resolved spontaneously to some extent. For interpretation of the references to color in this figure legend, the reader is referred to web version of this article. (Reprinted from Ophthalmology. Matsuo T, Ichimura K. Immunocytochemical diagnosis as inflammation by vitrectomy cell blocks in patients with vitreous opacity. *Ophthalmology.* 2012;119:827-837, Copyright 2012, with permission from the American Academy of Ophthalmology.)

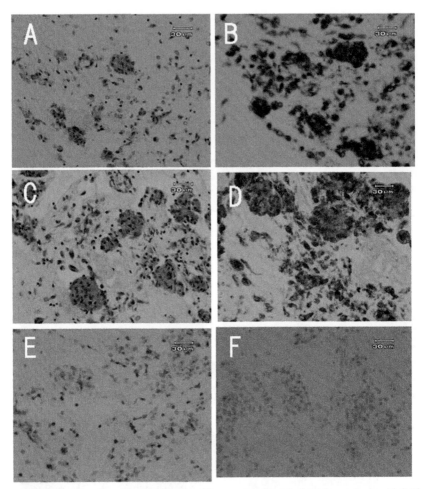

FIGURE 6.—Case 39: a 78-year-old woman. Vitrectomy specimen in the right eye shows epithelioid cells (hematoxylin and eosin [H&E] stain in **A**) that are positive for CD68 (**B**). Vitrectomy specimen in the left eye also shows epithelioid cells (H&E stain in **C**) that are positive for CD68 (**D**), admixed with small lymphocytes that are positive for CD3 (**E**) but negative for CD20 (**F**). (Reprinted from Ophthalmology. Matsuo T, Ichimura K. Immunocytochemical diagnosis as inflammation by vitrectomy cell blocks in patients with vitreous opacity. *Ophthalmology.* 2012;119:827-837, Copyright 2012, with permission from the American Academy of Ophthalmology.)

as vitreous opacity. A simple technique of cytopathology and immunocyto-chemistry, using vitrectomy cell blocks, can be performed in most pathology laboratories (Figs 1-7).

▶ In this retrospective case series of 61 eyes of 43 consecutive patients who underwent vitrectomy for vitreous opacity of unknown etiology or with prior diagnosis of inflammation, Matsuo and Ichimura report their experience with cytology and immunocytochemistry of cell block preparation of vitreous fluid. The authors

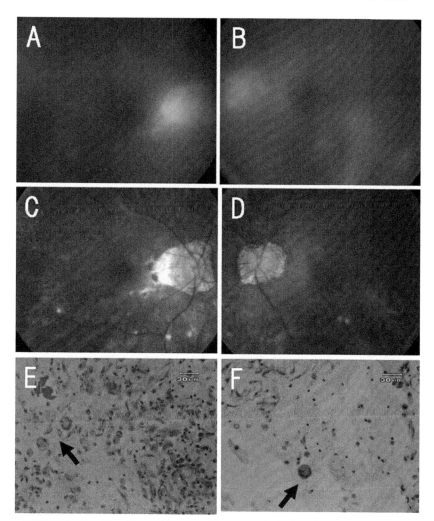

FIGURE 7.—Case 23: a 78-year-old woman. Vitreous opacity in the right eye (**A**) and left eye (**B**). Depigmented red fundus in the right eye (**C**) and left eye (**D**) after vitrectomy. Giant multinucleated cells (*arrows*) are found in vitrectomy specimens of the right eye (**E**) and left eye (**F**); hematoxylin and eosin stain. For interpretation of the references to color in this figure legend, the reader is referred to web version of this article. (Reprinted from Ophthalmology. Matsuo T, Ichimura K. Immunocytochemical diagnosis as inflammation by vitrectomy cell blocks in patients with vitreous opacity. *Ophthalmology.* 2012;119:827-837, Copyright 2012, with permission from the American Academy of Ophthalmology.)

excluded all patients who had vitreoretinal large B-cell lymphoma and exogenous or endogenous endophthalmitis in the same time period (2005–2010; Figs 1-7). Matsuo and Ichimura observed predominantly CD68-immunoreactive macrophages and CD3-immunoreactive T-lymphocytes in all vitrectomy cell blocks. In patients with granulomatous diseases, such as sarcoidosis or Vogt-Koyanagi-Harada disease, granulomatous inflammation predominated. Of note, 2 patients with prior diagnosis of systemic lymphoma and intraocular involvement had non-neoplastic vitritis diagnosed but succumbed to their systemic disease in the follow-up period (Figs 2 and 3). The other 41 patients responded to postoperative anti-inflammatory and immunosuppressive treatments and did not have malignancy on follow-up. The authors conclude that cytopathology and immunohistochemistry are relatively simple and inexpensive techniques that can be effectively used in general pathology practice for diagnosis of intraocular inflammation.

Although this study adds to the body of literature on cytopathologic and immunohistochemical findings in non-neoplastic vitritis, it has several limitations, including the retrospective nonmasked design and exclusion of patients with diagnosis of vitreoretinal lymphoma and infectious vitritis. The observation of predominantly macrophagic (including multinucleated histiocytes) and T-cell inflammatory infiltrate in intraocular fluid is not unique to inflammatory process. The same findings can be observed in evolving intraocular lymphoma, in which the reactive inflammatory infiltrate either obscures the underlying neoplastic process or the neoplastic cells are still primarily in subretinal location. The 2 patients in the study who were diagnosed with vitreous inflammation despite concordant systemic lymphoma, may exemplify this pattern. Conversely, the rare reactive B-lymphocytes can occasionally be observed in vitreous fluid of the eyes with an infectious process, such as herpes-viral retinitis.

Thus, although cytology continues to remain the gold standard in diagnosis of intraocular inflammatory, infectious, and neoplastic vitreous opacity and is greatly aided by immunohistochemistry, the diagnostic accuracy of these methods can be greatly aided by other ancillary techniques, including molecular genetic studies, interleukin levels, and, in some cases, flow cytometric analysis.

T. Milman, MD

Predictive Value of the Seventh Edition American Joint Committee on Cancer Staging System for Conjunctival Melanoma

Yousef YA, Finger PT (New York Univ School of Medicine)
Arch Ophthalmol 130:599-606, 2012

Objective.—To evaluate the predictive value of the seventh edition American Joint Committee on Cancer (AJCC) staging system for conjunctival melanoma.

Methods.—Retrospective, observational case series of 42 eyes of 42 patients with conjunctival melanoma studied by reviewing medical records, pathology reports, and color photographs. The main evaluated outcomes were demographic information, laterality, tumor size, thickness, pathologic diagnosis, seventh edition AJCC stage (clinical and pathologic), recurrence, metastasis, and duration of follow-up.

Results.—There was no sex preference, and the median age was 61 years. Recurrent disease was noted in 33% of patients (n = 14 of 42), with 64% occurring at a median of 2.5 years (range, 1-5 years) after primary treatment. Metastasis was noted in 19% of patients. The significant predictive factors for high risk of tumor recurrence were tumors involving more than 1 quadrant

TABLE 1.—Malignant Melanoma of the Conjunctiva: Seventh Edition AJCC Staging System

	Clinical Primary Tumor		Pathologic Primary Tumor
TX	Primary tumor cannot be assessed	TX	Primary tumor cannot be assessed
T0	No evidence of primary tumor	T0	No evidence of primary tumor
Tis	Melanoma confined to the conjunctival epithelium	Tis	Melanoma confined to the conjunctival epithelium[a]
	Malignant Conjunctival Melanoma of the Bulbar Conjunctiva		
T1		pT1	
T1a	≤1 quadrant[b]	pT1a	Melanoma ≤ 0.5 mm thick, with invasion of the substantia propria
T1b	>1 to 2 quadrants	pT1b	Melanoma > 0.5 mm to 1.5 mm thick, with invasion of the substantia propria
T1c	>2 to 3 quadrants	pT1c	Melanoma > 1.5 mm thick, with invasion of the substantia propria
T1d	>3 quadrants		
	Malignant Conjunctival Melanoma of the Nonbulbar (Palpebral, Fornical, Caruncular)		
T2		pT2	
T2a	Noncaruncular, ≤1 quadrant	pT2a	Melanoma ≤0.5 mm thick, with invasion of the substantia propria
T2b	Noncaruncular, >1 quadrant	pT2b	Melanoma >0.5 to 1.5 mm thick, with invasion of the substantia propria
T2c	Any caruncular, ≤1 quadrant	pT2c	Melanoma >1.5 mm thick, with invasion of the substantia propria
T2d	Any caruncular, >1 quadrant		
	Any Malignant Conjunctival Melanoma With Local Invasion		
T3		pT3	Melanoma invades the eye, eyelid, nasolacrimal system, sinuses, or orbit
T3a	Globe		
T3b	Eyelid		
T3c	Orbit		
T3d	Sinus		
T4	Tumor invades the central nervous system	pT4	Melanoma invades the central nervous system
	Clinical Regional Lymph Nodes		**Clinical Distant Metastasis**
NX	Regional lymph nodes cannot be assessed	M0	No distant metastasis (no pathologic M0; use clinical M to complete stage group)
N0a (biopsy)	No regional lymph node metastasis, biopsy performed		
N0b (no biopsy)	No regional lymph node metastasis, biopsy not performed		
N1	Regional lymph node metastasis	M1	Distant metastasis

Abbreviation: AJCC, American Joint Committee on Cancer.

[a]pT(is) melanoma in situ (includes the term *primary acquired melanosis*) with atypia replacing greater than 75% of the normal epithelial thickness, with cytologic features of epithelioid cells, including abundant cytoplasm, vesicular nuclei or prominent nucleoli, or the presence of intraepithelial nests of atypical cells.

[b]Quadrants are defined by clock hour, starting at the limbus (eg, 6, 9, 12, and 3 o'clock) and extending from the central cornea to and beyond the eyelid margins. This will bisect the caruncle.

$(P = .02)$, tumors thicker than 0.5 mm $(P = .04)$, and tumor multifocality $(P = .04)$. The significant predictive factors for high risk of tumor metastasis were tumors thicker than 0.5 mm $(P = .005)$, tumor invasiveness $(P = .04)$, pathologic diagnosis of conjunctival melanoma rather than melanoma in situ $(P = .04)$, and tumor recurrence $(P < .001)$. Similarly, increasing AJCC T stages (clinical and pathologic) were associated with unfavorable outcomes.

TABLE 2.—AJCC Classification (Clinical and Pathologic) for 42 Patients With Conjunctival Melanoma

Classification	Patients, No. (%)	Recurrence, No. (%)	Metastasis, No. (%)
T stage[a]			
Tis	16 (38)	3 (19)	0
T1	15 (36)	4 (27)	3 (20)
T1a	6 (14)	0	0
T1b	9 (21)	4 (44)	3 (33)
T1c	0	0	0
T1d	0	0	0
T2	3 (7)	1 (33)	0
T2a	0	0	0
T2b	2 (4.8)	1 (50)	0
T2c	0	0	0
T2d	1 (2.4)	0	0
T3	8 (19)	6 (75)	5 (63)
T3a	0	0	0
T3b	2 (5)	1 (50)	0
T3c	5 (12)	4 (80)	4 (80)
T3d	1 (2)	1 (100)	1 (100)
T4	0	0	0
P stage[b]			
pTis	16 (38)	3 (19)	0
pT1	13 (31)	4 (31)	2 (15)
pT1a	7 (17)	0	0
pT1b	4 (10)	3 (75)	1 (25)
pT1c	2 (5)	1 (50)	1 (50)
pT2	5 (12)	1 (20)	1 (20)
pT2a	4 (10)	1 (25)	1 (25)
pT2b	0	0	0
pT2c	1 (2)	0	0
pT3	8 (19)	6 (75)	5 (63)
pT4	0	0	0
N stage			
N0	37 (90)	0	0
N1	4 (10)	0	0
M stage			
M0	35 (83)	0	0
M1	7 (17)	0	0

Abbreviation: AJCC, seventh edition American Joint Committee on Cancer staging system for conjunctival melanoma.
[a]T stage is the initial clinical stage of the tumor.
[b]pT stage is the pathologic stage of the tumor.

For example, clinical stage—related recurrence rates were 19% (Tis), 27% (T1), 33% (T2), and 75% (T3). Clinical stage—related lymphatic and distant metastasis rates were 0% (Tis), 20% (T1), 0% (T2), and 63% (T3).

Conclusions.—Advanced AJCC T-stage (clinical and pathologic) tumors were at higher risk for recurrence and metastasis. In this study, the seventh edition AJCC staging system was predictive of local control and systemic spread of conjunctival melanoma (Tables 1-3).

▶ American Joint Committee on Cancer (AJCC) classification system has been increasingly used in pathologic staging of conjunctival melanoma. The current AJCC classification system is a TNM-based staging system. The T stage is dependent on tumor location (bulbar vs conjunctival nonbulbar vs eyelid), tumor

TABLE 3.—Correlations Among Tumor Features, Recurrence, and Metastatic Rate

Feature	Patients, No. (%)	Recurrence, No. (%)	P Value	Metastasis, No. (%)	P Value
Sex					
Male	21 (50)	7 (33)	>.99	4 (19)	>.99
Female	21 (50)	7 (33)		4 (19)	
Visual acuity					
OD	19 (45)	8 (42)	.54	4 (21)	>.99
OS	23 (55)	6 (26)		4 (17)	
Size, quadrant					
≤ 1	13 (31)	0	.02	0	.09
> 1 to 2	18 (43)	7 (39)		3 (17)	
> 2 to 3	7 (17)	4 (57)		2 (29)	
> 3	4 (9)	3 (75)		3 (75)	
Thickness, mm					
< 0.5	23 (55)	3 (13)	.04	0	.005
> 0.5	19 (45)	11 (58)		8 (42)	
Focality					
Monofocal	29 (69)	5 (17)	.05	3 (10)	.12
Multifocal	13 (31)	9 (69)		5 (38)	
Morphology					
Focal	20 (48)	6 (30)	>.99	4 (20)	>.99
Spreading	22 (52)	8 (36)		4 (18)	
Location(s)					
Bulbar alone	26 (62)	6 (23)	.23	4 (15)	.70
Tarsus or fornix	6 (14)	4 (67)		2 (33)	
Caruncle alone	2 (5)	0		0	
Caruncle + (tarsus/fornix)	7 (17)	4 (57)		2 (29)	
Invasion					
Conjunctival	32 (76)	8 (25)	.19	3 (9)	.04
Globe	0				
Lid	5 (12)	2 (40)		1 (20)	
Orbit	1 (2.4)	1 (100)		1 (100)	
Sinus	1 (2.4)	1 (100)		1 (100)	
Eyelid + orbit	2 (4.8)	1 (50)		1 (50)	
Eyelid + orbit + sinus	1 (2.4)	1 (100)		1 (100)	
AJCC pathologic stage					
PTis	16 (38)	3 (19)	.34	0	.04
pT1	13 (30)	4 (31)		2 (15)	
pT2	5 (12)	1 (20)		1 (20)	
pT3	8 (19)	6 (75)		5 (63)	
AJCC clinical stage					
Tis	16 (38)	3 (19)	.34	0	.04
T1	15 (36)	4 (27)		3 (20)	
T2	3 (7)	1 (33)		0	
T3	8 (19)	6 (75)		5 (63)	
T4	0				
Recurrence					
Yes	14 (33)			8 (50)	<.001
No	28 (77)			0	
NM stage					
N1	4 (10)	4 (100)	.10		
N0	38 (90)	4 (11)			
M1	7 (17)	7 (100)	<.001		
M0	35 (83)	1 (3)			

Abbreviations: AJCC, American Joint Committee on Cancer staging system for conjunctival melanoma (for subgroups, see Table 1); TNM, tumor, node, and metastasis.

invasiveness, and tumor thickness, whereas N and M refer to the presence of nodal and distant metastases. The clinical and pathologic AJCC classification systems for conjunctival melanoma differ slightly: the clinical staging is primarily based on clinically apparent tumor involvement, whereas pathologic staging is focused on tumor thickness and less extensively on tumor location (Table 1).

In this study, Yousef and Finger examined the predictive value of the seventh edition AJCC staging system for conjunctival melanoma (local control and metastasis) by retrospectively reviewing the medical records, pathology reports, and color photographs of 42 patients with conjunctival melanoma (Figs 1-3 in the original article, Table 2). The authors confirmed a trend between recurrence and clinical stage (cTis vs cT1 vs cT2 vs cT3), but this trend was not statistically significant. There was a significant difference in recurrence rate, however, between the tumors involving less than 1 quadrant (T1a) and those involving more than 1 quadrant. In addition, there was a statistical difference in recurrence rate of previously treated and multifocal tumors, the 2 variables currently not included in prognostic AJCC staging. Yousef and Finger also noted a correlation between tumor recurrence and pathologic staging for pTis, pT1, pT2, and pT3 tumors. When evaluating for risk of metastasis, there was an imperfect trend between the clinical AJCC stage and metastatic risk (0% for cTis, 20% for T1, 0% for cT2, and 62% for cT3). There was no significant relationship between the clinical tumor invasiveness (orbit, sinuses, or eyelid) and metastases. The relationship between the higher stage and the risk of metastases was stronger when tumors were staged pathologically (0% for pTis, 15% for pT1, 20% for pT2, and 62% for pT3) (Fig 4 in the original article, Table 3).

Retrospective design and relatively low patient number are important limitations of this study. Thus, its results have to be interpreted with caution. Future large, multicenter, prospective studies are needed for validation and for refinement of the current AJCC staging system.

T. Milman, MD

Congenital Ectropion Uvea and Mechanisms of Glaucoma in Neurofibromatosis Type 1: New Insights

Edward DP, Morales J, Bouhenni RA, et al (Summa Health System, Akron, OH; King Khaled Eye Specialist Hosp, Riyadh, Saudi Arabia; et al)
Ophthalmology 119:1485-1494, 2012

Objective.—To describe the clinicopathologic features of congenital ectropion uvea associated with glaucoma in neurofibromatosis-1 (NF-1).

Design.—Retrospective case series.

Participants and Controls.—Five cases of NF-1 associated with glaucoma, from which enucleated eyes were available, and 2 eye bank eyes used as controls.

Methods.—The clinical features and courses of these patients were reviewed. Formalin-fixed, paraffin-embedded eyes were examined by light and electron microscopy. Immunohistochemistry using antineurofibromin, anti—glial fibrillary acidic protein, and antivimentin was performed in

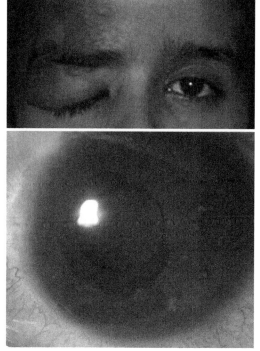

FIGURE 1.—Images from patient 4. **Top,** Photograph showing plexiform neurofibroma on the right side of the face. **Bottom,** Slit-lamp photograph of the iris showing ectropion uvea with Lisch nodules. (Reprinted from Ophthalmology. Edward DP, Morales J, Bouhenni RA, et al. Congenital ectropion uvea and mechanisms of glaucoma in neurofibromatosis type 1: new insights. *Ophthalmology.* 2012;119:1485-1494, Copyright 2012, with permission from the American Academy of Ophthalmology.)

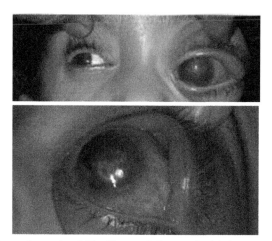

FIGURE 2.—Images from patient 5. **Top,** Photograph showing a buphthalmic eye and corneal scarring with periocular neurofibromatosis. **Bottom,** Photograph showing the large cornea with scarring. Ectropion uvea is not easily visible clinically because of corneal scarring, but was evident on histopathologic examination of the enucleated specimen. (Reprinted from Ophthalmology. Edward DP, Morales J, Bouhenni RA, et al. Congenital ectropion uvea and mechanisms of glaucoma in neurofibromatosis type 1: new insights. *Ophthalmology.* 2012;119:1485-1494, Copyright 2012, with permission from the American Academy of Ophthalmology.)

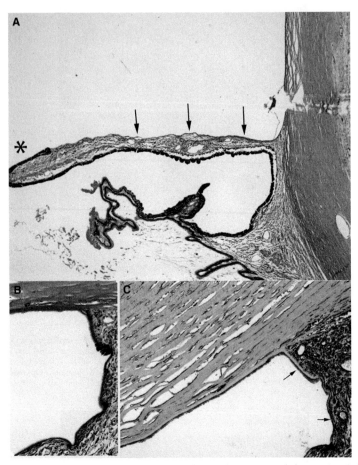

FIGURE 3.—Photomicrographs from patients 1 and 5. **A**, Photomicrograph from patient 1 showing endothelialization of the iris surface (arrows) with ectropion uvea (stain, hematoxylin—eosin; original magnification, ×4). **B**, Photomicrograph from patient 1 showing descemetization of the anterior chamber angle (*; stain, periodic acid—Schiff; original magnification, ×16). **C**, Photomicrograph from patient 5 showing immunostaining with antivimentin antibody. There was no positive labeling of proliferating corneal endothelial cells that cover the anterior chamber angle (arrow; stain, 3—3′-diaminobenzidine hydrochloride chromogen; original magnification, ×20). * = ectropion uvea. (Reprinted from Ophthalmology. Edward DP, Morales J, Bouhenni RA, et al. Congenital ectropion uvea and mechanisms of glaucoma in neurofibromatosis type 1: new insights. *Ophthalmology*. 2012;119:1485-1494, Copyright 2012, with permission from the American Academy of Ophthalmology.)

3 patients. Gene expression of the mitogen-activated protein kinase (MAPK) signaling pathway was examined in corneal endothelial cells in 1 patient.

Main Outcome Measures.—Cause of glaucoma in patients with ectropion uvea and NF-1.

Results.—The age of patients at the time of glaucoma diagnosis ranged from birth to 13 years. Four of the 5 patients had megalocornea and buphthalmos at presentation. Ectropion uvea was noted clinically in 2 patients,

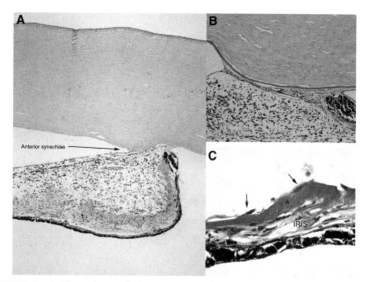

FIGURE 4.—A, Photomicrograph from patient 5 showing anterior synechiae formation with membrane over iris surface (stain, hematoxylin—eosin; original magnification, ×4). B, Photomicrograph from patient 4 showing iridocorneal adhesion at higher magnification with proliferating endothelial cells and basement membrane formation over the anterior iris surface (original magnification, ×4). C, Photomicrograph showing the iris surface with a thick peripheral anterior synechiae-positive basement membrane covering the atrophic iris surface (arrows; stain, periodic acid—Schiff; original magnification, ×20). (Reprinted from Ophthalmology. Edward DP, Morales J, Bouhenni RA, et al. Congenital ectropion uvea and mechanisms of glaucoma in neurofibromatosis type 1: new insights. *Ophthalmology.* 2012;119:1485-1494, Copyright 2012, with permission from the American Academy of Ophthalmology.)

but was demonstrated histopathologically in all 5 patients. On histopathologic examination, all patients had varying degrees of angle closure secondary to endothelialization of the anterior chamber angle. Uveal neurofibromas were noted in all patients; anteriorly displaced ciliary processes were noted in 4 of 5 patients who demonstrated ciliary body involvement with neurofibromas. Absence of Schlemm's canal was observed. The endothelial cells lining the closed angle demonstrated positive stain results with the vimentin antibody. Positive antineurofibromin immunolabeling was detected in normal control corneal endothelium, but was absent in corneal endothelium in patients with endothelialization of the angle. Upregulation of genes from the MAPK signaling pathway was demonstrated in the corneal endothelial cells isolated from the NF-1 eyes.

Conclusions.—Ectropion uvea in NF-1 glaucoma is secondary to endothelialization of the anterior chamber angle and is associated commonly with severe pediatric glaucoma in NF-1 patients. The endothelial cell proliferation may be related to overexpression of the Ras (Rat sarcoma)-MAPK genes in these eyes (Figs 1-7, Tables 1 and 2).

▶ In this beautifully illustrated retrospective case series of 5 patients with severe pediatric neurofibromatosis-1 (NF-1) glaucoma with unique features of endothelialization of the iridocorneal angle and ectropion uveae, the authors describe the

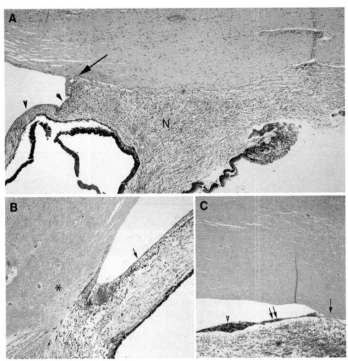

FIGURE 5.—Photomicrographs from patients 4 and 5. A, Diffuse neurofibroma (N) infiltrating the ciliary body with formation of the pseudoangle and endothelialization of the anterior chamber angle (arrow) and iris surface (arrowheads). Note absence of trabecular meshwork and Schlemm's canal (stain, hematoxylin–eosin; original magnification, ×10). B, Closure of the anterior chamber angle with endothelial cells and basement membrane-like structure mixed with pigmented melanocytic cells covering the trabecular meshwork. The membrane also covers the anterior iris surface (arrow). A Lisch nodule is noted in the angle. Note absence of Schlemm's canal (*; stain, hematoxylin–eosin; original magnification, ×10). C, Iridocorneal adhesion with pigmented membrane (double arrows) and Lisch nodule (arrowhead) covering the anterior surface (stain, hematoxylin–eosin; original magnification, ×20). (Reprinted from Ophthalmology. Edward DP, Morales J, Bouhenni RA, et al. Congenital ectropion uvea and mechanisms of glaucoma in neurofibromatosis type 1: new insights. Ophthalmology. 2012;119:1485-1494, Copyright 2012, with permission from the American Academy of Ophthalmology.)

phenotype and propose the possible mechanisms of glaucoma in this specific entity (Figs 1 and 2, Table 1). The main recognized mechanisms of NF-1 associated glaucoma include: (1) direct infiltration of the anterior chamber angle by neurofibromas, (2) developmental angle abnormalities (analogous to primary congenital glaucoma), (3) secondary angle closure resulting from neurofibromatous thickening of the ciliary body and choroid, and (4) fibrovascular synechial angle closure and neovascular glaucoma.

Edward et al noted variable degree of descemetization and endothelial cell proliferation in the anterior chamber angle and on the surface of the iris, associated with ectropion uvea (Table 2, Figs 3-5). Immunofluorescence studies demonstrated absence of NF1 in the endothelial cells (Fig 6). Electron microscopy showed multilayered proliferation of corneal endothelial cells and basement

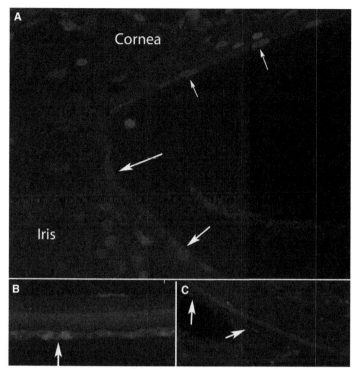

FIGURE 6.—Results of immunostaining of the cornea and anterior chamber angle with anti—neurofibromatosis 1 (NF1) antibody in patients 4 and 5. A, Note the faint to absent staining in the endothelial cells lining the iris surface and cornea (arrows) in patient 4 (stain, Alexa Fluor 488; original magnification, ×40). B, Normal corneal endothelial cells showing intense staining in the cytoplasm (arrows) in patient 4. C, Lack of anti NF-1 immunoreactivity seen in corneal endothelium (arrows) in patient 5 (stain, Alexafluor 488; original magnification, ×100). (Reprinted from Ophthalmology. Edward DP, Morales J, Bouhenni RA, et al. Congenital ectropion uvea and mechanisms of glaucoma in neurofibromatosis type 1: new insights. *Ophthalmology.* 2012;119:1485-1494, Copyright 2012, with permission from the American Academy of Ophthalmology.)

membrane material over the anterior chamber angle and iris (Fig 7). The authors did not comment on whether cytokeratin filaments or desmosomes were observed. Gene expression profiling studies on the corneal endothelium of 1 NF1 patient and 2 controls were performed and showed upregulation of RAS-MAP-ERK-MAPK signaling pathway.

The authors propose that endothelialization and descemetization of the anterior chamber angle, possibly related to loss of NF1 expression and upregulation of MAPK signaling pathway, may contribute to development of severe pediatric glaucoma in a subset of NF1 patients. They point out, though, that other mechanisms likely play a role in NF1-related glaucoma, based on their observation of neurofibromatous anterior chamber angle and ciliary body infiltration, absence of Schlemm canal, and anteriorly rotated ciliary body processes in the eyes of patients in this case series. Regardless of relative contributions of these factors to developmental glaucoma, observation of ectropion uveae clinically in NF1

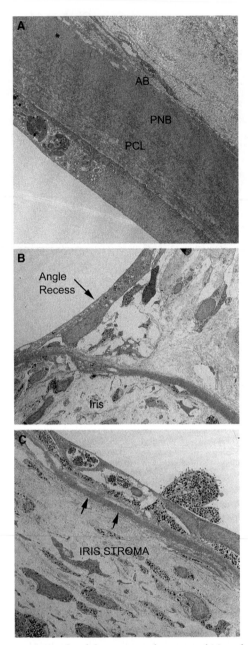

FIGURE 7.—Electron micrographs of the cornea, angle recess, and iris surface from patient 4. A, Descemet's membrane showing normal anterior branded zone (AB), thickened posterior nonbanded zone (PNB), and posterior collagenous layer (PCL). The corneal endothelial cells show prominent rough endoplasmic reticulum (original magnification, ×11 000). B, Amorphous basement membrane covering the anterior chamber angle recess (original magnification, ×2500). C, Multilayered endothelial cell proliferation mixed with melanocytic cells along with amorphous basement membrane (arrows) cover the iris surface (original magnification, ×4000). (Reprinted from Ophthalmology. Edward DP, Morales J, Bouhenni RA, et al. Congenital ectropion uvea and mechanisms of glaucoma in neurofibromatosis type 1: new insights. *Ophthalmology*. 2012;119:1485-1494, Copyright 2012, with permission from the American Academy of Ophthalmology.)

TABLE 1.—Summary of the Clinical Features of Neurofibromatosis-1 Patients

Patient No.	1	2	3	4	5
Gender	Male	Female	Female	Female	Male
Age at glaucoma diagnosis (enucleation), yrs	Birth (8)	Birth (12)	Birth (5)	13 (27)	Birth (3)
Ipsilateral orbitofacial involvement	Present (LPNF)	Absent	Present	Present (LPNF)	Present (LPNF)
IOP at presentation (mmHg)	Not available	24	Not available	25	23
Megalocornea/ buphthalmos	Present	Present	Present	Absent	Present
Ectropion uvea	Absent	Absent	Absent (iris not visible)	Present	Present
Lisch nodules	Present	Absent	Not recorded	Present	Present
Gonioscopy	No view	Not done	No view	PAS noted at time of presentation	PAS noted at time of presentation
Previous glaucoma surgery	None	Trabeculotomy; MMC trabeculectomy, GDD	None	MMC trabeculectomy	MMC trabeculectomy, diode CPC ×2
Clinical course	NLP at time of diagnosis	Presented at birth with buphthalmos; several glaucoma procedures; RD repair; 4-yr clinical course before enucleation	NLP at diagnosis	Failed trabeculectomy; RD noted at last visit with low IOP 14-yr clinical course before enucleation	IOP progressively increased to 30s; ectropion noted after first surgery more prominent with time; painful eye developed with NLP over 3 yrs before enucleation

CPC = cyclophotocoagulation; GDD = glaucoma drainage device; IOP = intraocular pressure; LPNF = lid plexiform neurofibroma; MMC = mitomycin C; NLP = no light perception; PAS = peripheral anterior synechiae; RD = retinal detachment.

TABLE 2.—Summary of the Histopathologic Findings in Neurofibromatosis-1 Patients

Patient No.	1	2	3	4	5
Eye size (mm)	35	22	37	25	33
Cornea	Corneal scarring plus endothelial degeneration	Pannus, stromal scar and new vessels, band keratopathy	Edema+, stromal scar, endothelial degeneration	Prominent corneal nerves	Endothelial degeneration
Angle/iris/ciliary body	Complete angle closure, descemetization of iris surface, anterior displaced ciliary processes	Focal ectropion uvea, complete angle closure, descemetization of the anterior iris, peripheral anterior synechiae	Iris descemetization, complete angle closure, anterior displaced ciliary processes	Normally placed ciliary processes, anterior synechiae	Anteriorly displaced ciliary processes, absent Schlemm's canal
Ectropion uvea	Present	Present	Present	Present	Present
Retina	Retinal ganglion cell loss	Retinal detachment with proliferative vitreoretinopathy, retinal ganglion cell loss	Atrophic retina with retinal ganglion cell loss and gliosis	Subretinal hemorrhage, retinal detachment, retinal ganglion cell loss	Retinal ganglion cell loss
Ocular neurofibromatosis	+Ciliary body, +choroidplexiform	+Ciliary body, +choroids	+Choroid	+Ciliary body, +choroids	+Ciliary body, +choroids
Immunohistochemistry S100 (IHC)	Not performed	Not performed	+In choroid NF	+In choroid and CB NF	+In choroid and CB NF
GFAP (IHC)	Not performed	Not performed	+In choroid NF	+In choroid and CB NF	+In choroid and CB NF
Vimentin	Not performed	Not performed	+Along iris and angle membrane	+Along iris and angle membrane	+Along iris and angle membrane

CB = ciliary body; GFAP = glial fibrillary acidic protein; IHC = immunohistochemistry; NF = neurofibromatosis.

patients will now enable us to better understand the pathology of the anterior chamber angle. Future studies are needed to determine if this NF-1—related glaucoma phenotype has a distinct biologic behavior.

T. Milman, MD

Article Index

Chapter 1: Cataract Surgery

Chapter 2: Refractive Surgery

Chapter 3: Glaucoma

Chapter 4: Cornea

Chapter 5: Retina

Chapter 6: Oculoplastic Surgery

Chapter 7: Pediatric Ophthalmology

Chapter 8: Neuro-ophthalmology

Chapter 9: Imaging

Chapter 10: Ocular Oncology

Chapter 11: Pathology

Author Index

A

Agar A, 61
Agoumi Y, 60
Ahlskog JE, 174
Al-Qahtani AS, 136
Alagöz N, 42
Aldave AJ, 203
Alió JL, 47
Almer Z, 154
Alniemi ST, 143
Anshu A, 71
Arevalo JF, 108
Arsava EM, 182
Artornsombudh P, 103
Artürk N, 120
Asp S, 28
Auffarth GU, 32
Aung T, 12
Avisar I, 135

B

Baba T, 109
Baiocchi S, 78
Bangsgaard R, 149
Bansal AS, 98, 164
Baratz KH, 194
Barnett MH, 177
Barreau G, 2
Barsam A, 1
Baumann F, 212
Bauza A, 145
Bell CM, 63
Belzunce A, 52
Bilyk JR, 138, 208, 210
Blair MP, 168
Blaydon S, 121
Bouhenni RA, 242
Boyce AM, 173
Brauner SC, 66
Brenner LF, 47
Brøndsted AE, 8
Brown DM, 102
Brown DP Jr, 178
Brown GC, 101
Brucks M, 53
Brugnoli de Pagano OM, 150
Buckley EG, 175
Buttanrı IB, 119

C

Campbell RJ, 63
Caporossi A, 78
Carbone M, 212
Celik HU, 42
Chandler WM, 224
Chappell MC, 200
Char DH, 200
Chee S-P, 14
Chen J, 96
Chen S, 45
Cheng J, 81
Chin KJ, 196
Chong KK, 128
Chow CC, 168
Clark WL, 102
Colby KA, 90
Cole TB, 200
Colin J, 19
Comer GM, 106
Corcòstegui B, 165
Costello F, 167
Craven ER, 68
Cursiefen C, 85

D

Davagnanam I, 163
Dawson E, 144
Dexl AK, 30
Diehl N, 143
Diehl NN, 155
Dietrich-Ntoukas T, 85
Dorairaj S, 216
Drack AV, 203
Duan Y, 178
Dugel PU, 113

E

Eagle RC Jr, 208
Edward DP, 242
Elmann S, 121
Espana EM, 36
Eustis HS, 146

F

Fayet B, 131
Fazıl K, 119

Fechtner RD, 57
Feit H, 157
Feng Y, 45
Ferris FL III, 112
Ferris LK, 212
Fethke NB, 194
Filkorn T, 5
Finger PT, 185, 196, 238
Fitting A, 32
Fledelius HC, 149
Florell SR, 224
Fong CS-u, 4
Fraser CL, 163
Friedman DS, 156
Fuertes I, 165
Fujizuka N, 161

G

Gagné S, 60
Gangnon RE, 110
Garcia-Martin E, 165
Garg SJ, 98, 164
Garrick R, 177
Gazzard G, 12
Gevorgyan O, 103
Ghanem EA, 39
Ghanem RC, 39
Ghanem VC, 39
Gibson CR, 40
Gilbert ME, 210
Gilhooley MJ, 83
Gill HS, 169
Gill SS, 63
Glover M, 173
Gobin YP, 188
Goldstein JN, 182
Gomes BAF, 36
Gonzalez E, 24
Gregory-Roberts EM, 165
Grentzelos MA, 37, 76
Griepentrog GJ, 143
Guillon M, 140

H

Hagiwara A, 109
Hammer CM, 217
Hammersmith KM, 86
Hatch BB, 41

Printed and bound by CPI Group (UK) Ltd, Croydon, CR0 4YY

08/05/2025

01864755-0004